dancing the flame of life

of the

of life

the vital
principles
of yoga

Dona Holleman started studying Oriental philosophy at the age of 12 while living on the island of Java. Her main focus was Buddhism and Taoism, but since a very early age her real interest has been the body, the mystery of the body. Thus, when she came in contact with yoga in the 50s, it became immediatly her main path. In the mid 60s she met and studied with BKS Iyengar, but has since then spent the last 40 years exploring the various aspects of yoga in her own practice and teaching, learning only from her own body. Her belief is that the final answer lies within the body, and that each human being has to find this for him or herself alone, guided only by the inner light, the inner teacher which is in each of us.

dancing the flame of life

the vital principles of yoga

DONA HOLLEMAN

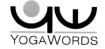

YOGAWORDS

Dancing the Flame of Life:
the vital principles of yoga

First published by YogaWords Ltd 2009

Copyright © Dona Holleman 2009

Part two: The Asanas first appeared in Dancing the Body of Light
by Dona Holleman and Orit Sen-Gupta, published 1999 by Pandion Enterprises

Dona Holleman has asserted her moral right to be identified
as the author of this work in accordance with the
Copyright, Designs and Patents Act of 1988

ISBN 978-1-906756-00-0

British Library Cataloguing-in-Publication Data
A catalogue record for this book is available from the British Library

Set in MetaPlus

Printed and bound in Great Britain by
Athenaeum Press Ltd, Gateshead, Tyne & Wear

This book has been printed on paper that is sourced and
harvested from sustainable forests and is FSC accredited

YogaWords Ltd
32 Clarendon Road
London N8 0DJ

www.yogawords.com

contents

acknowledgments

During the seventies and eighties I started to work on the 'perfect' description of all the asanas that I had learned in the sixties in India from B.K.S.Iyengar for the 'final' book, not realizing that there is no perfect description, only an approximation, and that there can never be a final book. I adhered to the syllabus as we used to practice in those early days with BKS Iyengar, and I also began to outline the rudiments of the vital principles of practice. By the late 1990s the description of the asana had taken much more form, as well as the principles, and thus I started shopping around in the States and Europe to find a publisher who would take on the project of a book. Nobody seemed interested: too big, too sophisticated, too technical, too this, too that.

One evening in 1997 I vented my frustration on my good friend Johanna van der Schaft, who, after not even two seconds, exclaimed: 'Never mind, I will do it, I will be your publisher.'

It was an audacious thing to say, seeing that neither of us had much experience (I had none) in publishing, but in our enthusiasm we decided to form a two-woman publishing company. This was in 2000.

We decided to call our company Pegasus. This magical animal has been in all cultures the symbol of freedom, transporting on its powerful wings poets and heroes to the heavens to bathe in the waters of freedom and immortality.

Alas, we had a disappointment: the name was already in use by another publishing company. So we chose Pandion Enterprises. Pandion, the Latin name for Osprey, is another powerful symbol for freedom and independence, making its nest high up in the trees and diving deep into lakes and oceans to catch its prey. And so it was.

Pandion Enterprises has been pretty busy since that moment: Dancing the Bbody of Light, Centering Down (a reprint of the original one), Harmonic Passages, The Fish in Search of Water, Eyes of Innocence. In all these projects Johanna has stood at my side with her enthusiasm and energy. Each one of us has spent weeks, months, of seven, eight hours a day at the computer, working away at the various projects. Together we have gone through difficult times and good times, navigating our way through obstructions and disappointments, never losing our optimism. Johanna has been the managing director of our brave little company, while I have been the editor.

I thank Johanna from the bottom of my heart for all the tears and laughter we shared, and I hope that Pandion Enterprises will flourish still for a long time to come, even though both of us are very busy.

A generous thanks for Andrea Gennari who, together with his girlfriend Silvia, spent, in the mid 80s, weeks of his time taking photographs of me performing the asanas in my yoga studio in Florence, three thousand in total. These photographs were originally taken for my articles in the Jyotim journals, and later on they formed the fourth chapter of Dancing the body of light.

In order to fit those photographs to the text, Judith Wolters sorted through all three thousand of them, together with Walter Goyen, a professional lay-out man. It was up to her to choose the right photograph for the right text, travelling up and down to Walter's home to work together. Judith has worked close with Johanna and me all these years, sharing her expertise in computers and photography, and has been a wonderful shoulder to lean on when disappointments hit. A heartfelt thanks to her.

An enormous heartfelt thanks to our business partner and friend Sylvia Strike of Los Angeles, who has believed in us from the beginning and has supported us in everything we did. She has often given us invaluable advice, and with her down-to-earth optimism and common sense has helped us through many perplexities and queries; she has also been our main distributor in the States and Canada. She has been a real pal all throughout.

A big hug from both Johanna and me to Toni Montez, who has been for more than twenty years my friend and sister, and who also has helped, supported and encouraged us throughout everything. In her relationship with me she has fulfilled many roles throughout the years: dress chooser, accountant, organizer, tea-maker on cold days when we were working out in the fields for The fish in search of water, trip organizer, willing ear to complain to, to mention only a few.

A heartfelt thanks to Paul Walker of YogaWords, who believed from the start in this book and wanted to bring it to the yoga community at large and the teacher community in particular, as a classical text to be used in schools and training courses.

Last but not least, I want to thank all my students who loyally supported me all these years, and patiently functioned as 'guinea-pigs' for me to 'dissect' each asana and find the right description. To give an idea, some postures took four, five days of repeating, till I had it 'right', with those students generously and enthusiastically participating in this tedious job. The German group, the American one, thanks to all of you for your patience and support.

At the end of all I want to thank my animals, my horses, donkeys and other animals. Whenever I get sick of being indoors, working at the computer, burning my brain, I go and romp around with them, after which my brain is 'brain-washed' and I am ready for more work.

preface

Yoga in daily life

Cisco is standing between the trees, the sun through the leaves making mottled patterns on his skin. When I approach, he looks up, and then comes towards me with a soft nicker. Standing before me he lowers his head, so I can caress him on his forehead, and I reflect for the umpteenth time with wonder how far we have traveled together. Cisco is a rescue horse, and without my forty-five years of yoga, I do not know if we could have arrived where we are now, standing next to each other, content to be in each other's company.

Yoga is an age-old philosophy, but like all philosophies, it remains sterile unless applied in daily life, and not confined merely to memorizing words and concepts. As everyone knows, the word yoga means: union. There are as many interpretations of this word union as there are yoga practitioners. At this moment, reflecting on the struggle of the last three years, and of the peace at the end, my heart overflowing with love for this massive, gentle creature, who taught me that yoga has to be applied in a 360° circle, including everything, even old, abused horses, I am in union with all of life, with all living beings, with the matrix of life.

Often human beings inflict suffering on their relatives, the animals, in a very un-yogic way. Meeting Cisco was for me a highlight in my life, and the chance of my life to apply all that I learned from the yoga philosophy. Physical control and discipline combined with suppleness and letting go at the right moment, and above all, facing one's fears, doubts, and 'un-skillfulness', just the same as in our daily yoga practice. But there is a difference in making one's own body a perfect instrument of skillfulness, and one's own mind clear and confident, or having to do the same thing with a five-hundred kilo flight-animal that has been abused and wants nothing more in life than to run as far away as possible from anything human. Here compassion has to bloom to the full, or the struggle to win is in vain. To move with control and gentleness, and at the same time with determination, to not allow confusion to enter into the game, to make all movement a tai chi dance, a meditation, a perfect asana in order to not set off the flight response, was an extremely rewarding yogic exercise.

One thing I have learned in my dealings with Cisco and my other rescue animals – that without love and compassion any practice, yogic or otherwise, is a practice in vain isolation.

'Whatever is done by force can never be beautiful'
Xenophon in *The Art of Horsemanship*, written 400 BC

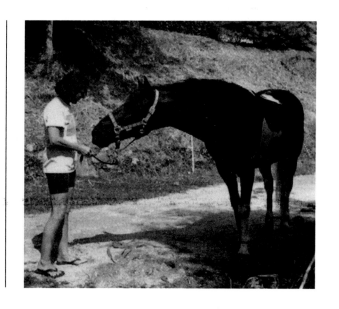

introduction

The story

The Catholic nun carefully steps over the stones on the beach, leading the thin little pony by the bridle. The three-year-old girl in the saddle is beaming with delight as she tells everyone that 'riding a horse is very, very nice'. It is 1946, and the Japanese war is raging in Asia.

My parents were caught in Bangkok when the Japanese troops invaded Thailand, and ended up in a prisoner-of-war camp. Luckily, the camp guards consented to the request of my parents that the children, my brother and me, be allowed to leave the camp and sent to the nuns in Huahin, a small village on the coast. It was there that the nuns, trying to keep us busy and away from the ravages of war, rented the pony on a daily basis, so we could ride on the beach.

There is a famous quote saying: 'Today is the first day of the rest of my life'. Now, sixty-four years later, as I think of that little girl on the pony on the beach in South-East Asia, I reflect that, as age sets in, it is important to look for that child within, to look for that place where the world is always new and 'riding a horse is very, very nice'.

Since those days I have traveled through many countries, cities, situations, meeting people and losing them again, learning new things and forgetting old things, changing, growing, evolving, but always coming back to that secret place where 'riding a horse is very, very nice', where the outer body is only the fragile shell of the inner being – eternal, unchanging, riding the little pony while the years ravage the body. Places where joy is uncontaminated and the spirit is transparent like the waves lapping on the beach beneath the pony's hooves in that timeless moment sixty-four years ago.

If today is the first day of the rest of my life, what do I want to do with the rest of my life?

After having considered several options for a career, I decided on yoga. That was in the late fifties. There was not much going on then – Paul Brunton, Indira Devi, Yesudian, to name a few names.

When I met BKS Iyengar in 1964 during a summer camp of Jiddu Krishnamurti in Saanen, a charming little village in Berner Oberland, I decided to travel to India to study with this teacher. Nine months later I traveled back to Europe, carrying in my baggage all the asanas and breathing techniques that I was able to learn in those months. Back to Poona in 1969, to deepen and develop the practice, going at the same time deeper into Hindu and Buddhist philosophy. Again back to Europe – England, Holland, Italy, practicing and teaching what I had learned.

I owe much to the people who have inspired and helped me along the way, especially Jiddu Krishnamurti, Vanda Scaravelli, BKS Iyengar, Mabel Todd, and Carlos

Castaneda. I first met Krishnamurti in 1960, and spent the next twenty years attending his talks and conducting private interviews with him. Through him I met both BKS Iyengar and Vanda Scaravelli (who became my closest friend and mentor). While these teachers provided encouragement, insight and instruction in the asanas, it was my task to find a balance between the physical practice of Iyengar, the more feminine aspect that Vanda emphasized, and the meditative state of mind that Krishnamurti espoused and embodied. At about this same time in the mid-1960s, I also began a close examination of the works of Carlos Castaneda. From him I learned about 'intent' and (as he calls it) 'the assemblage point' or 'reality tunnel' in which each of us lives. Castaneda underscored the notion that we are free to change this reality tunnel at any time we wish, and that it is sufficient merely to intend such a change.

Then, in 1980, a new element came in – the work of Mabel Todd. This remarkable woman worked in the 1930s with dancers. From her work I learned about alignment, breathing, rooting, the hara (or center), and elongating, which later on developed into the eight principles of practice.

As a result of this I wrote in the same year Centering Down, where I applied the ideas of Mabel Todd to yoga, showing a way to practice yoga with the minimum of wear and tear on the body.

Centering Down became thus a mixture of Krishnamurti, Iyengar, Mabel Todd and Castaneda, and became straight away a classic.

In 1991 I met Renato Turla, ex karate champion of Italy, who became a good friend. Together we started an association called Jyotim, and published a monthly journal, also called Jyotim. In this journal I started to elaborate on the material from Centering Down – the asanas, the eight principles of practice and the philosophy. Slowly the description of the asanas began to grow, as well as the eight principles of practice, which I conceived of initially as eight, then they became five, then seven, and then again eight. Apart from the articles written by Renato and myself we invited several other people to contribute, amongst others Alice Plato, who wrote comprehending articles on scoliosis, herself suffering from this disease, and Orit Sen-Gupta, a student of Hindu philosophy. Orit later on contributed to the book Dancing the Body of Light, which was for a large part a collection of the articles that I had previously published in the Jyotim journal. Then came the publication of Harmonic Passages, which I wrote together with Renato, as well as the video A fish in search of water, brought out by Diana Eichner and Kate Rabinowitch. This video is partly biographical, partly an expounding of a philosophy, in which yoga is taken out of its Hindu wrappings and shown as a universal way of life.

All that was long ago, and as the years roll by, perspectives change, new things are being discovered, old things are discarded, understanding growing, changing, maturing.

In 2003 the circle came back to its beginning sixty-four years ago, the horses came back into my life, and riding a horse is still 'very, very nice', only now maturity has set in, and the capacity and willingness to learn, from anything, anywhere, letting life be the guide and teacher, expanding yoga in new directions, letting peripheral vision be the tool, growing old in body, but younger every day in spirit, as joy is nurtured and carefully kept innocent in the midst of daily life.

Dona Holleman, Soiano del Lago, 2009

part one
centering down

What does centering down mean?

The word centering down comes from the Quaker tradition, and signifies an inner attitude whereby a human being opens her/himself to the life force which is the matrix of all existence, which is the force that holds everything together and is constantly creating and inventing new ways of expressing itself. All things of nature, including the human being – the last arrived child of nature – are nothing else but containers, big or small, for this life force. The birds, the trees, the grass underneath the feet, the lion stalking the deer, the waves of the sea crashing on the sand – all express the life force in its own way and contains it. But if the life force is inside the human being, why do we have to open ourselves up to it? The thing is that we don't; all we need to do is to realise it. This realisation comes when we learn to listen, to pay attention.

Human beings are all too prone to want to change things, to alter their surroundings. This changing or altering is done by the way we classify everything, by our descriptions of reality, in other words, by attaching language, or the human word, to life. The thirst for dominion is so strong, that we even want to classify and change the life force itself by our descriptions, our religions and philosophies. We never realize that life, the life force itself, is beyond human description.

Thus our capacity to listen, to pay attention, that we have in childhood, when everything is new, is diminished, and we lose our sense of belonging to a greater family, the family of life. This alienation drives us further into an ever-increasing search for meaning – in the words of Henry Thoreau: 'Most people live lives of quiet desperation' (Walden).

In the past yoga was practiced in the wilderness. The practice of yoga is meant to soften the hardness of the human body and mind, to make both permeable for life. The human body and mind are made hard by our way of living, of being, of thinking, by the alienation that we ourselves create each day. Through softening our bodies and minds we can again learn to listen to the pulsations of life.

The front of our bodies correspond to our intellectual, human brain, which can compute and think, and which creates language, philosophies, theories, etc. Its original function was – and still is – to allow the defenseless ape-human to survive in a world where eat or be eaten is the rule. In this function the human brain has done only too well, and from a defense tool has turned into an aggressor's tool – the human prey animal developed through evolution, for survival's sake, the mind of the predator.

The back of our bodies correspond to the old or reptilian brain, the one which was there long before the human intellectual brain was developed. It does not know human language, but only the instinctual responses of the body. As such it has infinite capacity for listening. This listening is done not with the ears, not with the eyes, not with any of the senses that we usually use. It is a listening that comes out of the heart, a direct knowledge of the life force, something that the young, frontal, brain does not have.

Centering down consists in the capacity to withdraw at will, on certain occasions, the energy from the frontal brain, the face and the frontal body and move it into the back of the body to access this old knowledge. Frowning, pouting and other hard expressions of our self-centered personalities disappear from the face in the smile and slanting eyes of the Buddha statues, in the almond eyes of old Egyptians paintings. As all our knowledge is put aside we become again in-nocent like children. Innocent means 'harmless' – as we no longer 'harm' life by classifying it and boxing it in.

Thus the new brain has its usefulness for classifying, for thinking, for planning, but its major by-product is alienation through its self-centered activity; one could say that this brain functions in a state of en-stasy as it draws all energy into itself for its self-centered activities.

The old brain is the brain of the heart. The heart knows the life force directly, and thus knows ec-stasy. The words ec-stasy means 'to stand outside oneself'. Ec-stasy is the energy generated by the realisation that the life force is in us – and in all of nature. It is the realisation that we are nature, at a par with everything else, a member of a vast family. In ec-stasy there is no division between 'us and them', no alienation, as we realize the one-ness of all life.

Centering down, or yoga in its purest and simplest form, consists in knowing when to use the intellectual brain, and when to use the old brain. To make the body and mind so flexible that we can easily move back and forth between the two states of our being, the en-stasy of the frontal brain, and the ec-stasy of the old brain or heart. It is the highest form of flexibility in which we have transcended all theories, descriptions and obstructions and flow easily, effortlessly and joyously with the ceaseless flow of life. For the eternal child within, 'riding the horse of life will always be very, very nice'.

Centered yoga

The story

I casually opened the horse-riding magazine that I had bought that morning, and it opened on an article called Centered riding, written by a woman called Sally Swift. A bell vaguely clang in the back of my head as I began to read the article, and then it hit me: I had written that article. No, not really, but it could have been. There they were, all the eight principles of practice: the center, breathing, peripheral vision, alignment, intent. Excitedly I read through the whole article, and then rushed into Amazon.com to order the book. As it turned out, Sally Swift had actually studied with Mabel Todd in the thirties, and had integrated her work in horse riding.

This is where I decided to call my interpretation of yoga: Centered yoga. As simple as that.

What is *Centered yoga*?

Centered yoga is the search for balance between the two polarities of the human being, the en-stasy of the frontal brain, and the ec-stasy of the old brain or heart through the application of the eight principles of practice. It is the understanding and application of the old yin-yang symbol, where the two polarities form one circle. With most of us we manifest one predominant personality. For instance, one person may rely more on the intellectual, human, brain, while another one is quieter, living more from observation. Of course this is not always 100%, and not at all times, hence the dots within the yin-yang circle.

The human, thinking, yang side of us is the one that acts positively upon the world. It tries to change the outer world according to a personal inner idea. This includes judging, classifying and labeling the outer world according to one's personal conditioning. The song of a bird is 'nice'; the sound of an airplane is 'not-nice'. Thus the two sounds are changed by being labeled and classified, put into two different categories. In this we forget that a sound is only a sound, a vibration of air, and that any adjective we apply to it is a purely human and, in addition a purely personal one. For another bird the bird song may not be nice at all, but may mean an aggressive assertion of this-is-my-tree-stay-away, and for an airplane lover the sound of the plane may be music-to-the-ears. The yang side corresponds to our thinking, judging, acting side. *We* are not changed, transformed, but spend our energy on trying to transform the outer world.

The listening, yin side is the one that receives, that allows the world to act upon us, instead of us acting upon the world and trying to change it. It allows the world to act upon up us and – in doing so – to change *us* in ways that more often than not are not subject to verbalization. Thus, instead of labelling the birdsong as 'nice', if we take time to just listen to it without throwing anything back in the form of judgement or labelling, we may find that something happens inside us as a result, something that cannot be defined, but nevertheless takes place. In this *listening* something is touched inside us, and *we* are changed, transformed, and will never be the same again.

This listening corresponds to the capacity – present in each human being, but with most people not as developed as the thinking side – to pay total attention. Total attention is opening the channel from the outer world toward the inner world, allowing the outer world to 'come in' and 'do' to us whatever it has to do.

Our daily life is for the majority spent in the thinking, acting, 'changing the world' mode. This can make us aggressive and domineering. In total attention the person who pays total attention is not there, as the two are mutually exclusive. To think, there has to be a person who thinks, that is at the center of the thoughts. To pay attention, there cannot be a person behind it; there is no center that collects the attention. There is only the act of observation, of attention.

This is the meaning of Centered yoga: the capacity to be in either mode at will, depending on the circumstances; to be able to dance between the two modes of our being. Spending too much time in one mode or the other will bring us out of balance, and will turn us either into hard, self-centered, judgmental people, victims of our own thinking processes, or into helpless dreamers. Therefore it is of vital health for the mind and the heart to be able to revert to either mode at will, whenever and wherever needed.

In my early days, following the guidelines of my various teachers, I began to develop a series of principles that can help us bring our yoga practice into this balance, the balance between acting and listening, in which total attention precedes and sustains the acting. I am also greatly indebted to my superb masters, my horses, who taught me, and continue to teach me, their masterful skill in being attentive to everything around them. Being the prey animals they are, that is their only survival tool. For yoga teachers total attention is a sine-qua-non. Without it we are preying on our students and do not allow them to find their own development and path, thus obstructing them to become confident and harmonious practitioners.

In 1981 I wrote Centering Down. It was my first attempt to describe – not the practice of yoga itself – but the way *how* to practice. Centering Down became straight away a classic and is still in demand. For many schools and practitioners it has become the basic book for practice. In it I describe the beginning and the evolution of what became the eight principles of practice.

Many people are now applying the eight principles of practice, and thus I thought it opportune to give a short history of each one and to explain them in more detail. Further explanation you can find in Centering Down, Dancing the Body of Light, Harmonic Passages, and the Centered yoga Manual.

The eight principles of practice

It takes a lifetime to become simple, and the process seemingly never ends. Traveling through Centering down (1981), Tree of Life (1982), Syllabus for Teacher and Student and Asana in Photo (1984), the Yoga Darsana volumes I and II (1987), the Jyotim journals (1992–), Dancing the Body of Light (2000), A Fish in search of water and Eyes of Innocence (2002), Harmonic Passages (2003), and the Centered Yoga Manual (2005), understanding deepening, shedding notions and words that are more in the way than helpful, I can only try to show that there is a way of practicing yoga, or riding horses, or anything else, that is at once integral and joyous.

In Part II will give a description of the eight principles of practice. For clarity sake I have divided them sequentially, but in reality they form one whole, taking place simultaneously. Each principle contains within it all the others – the first one contains already the last one, and they all come back to centering body and mind in such a way that there is a natural physically and mentally meditative state at all times and everywhere, not at certain times and in certain places or postures. This meditative state guides all actions, making them fluid, graceful and harmonious.

In the application of these eight principles to yoga it is important to understand the physical body, how it is put together and how it functions, before adding the asanas to it. At the same time it is also important to understand the workings of the mind. The application of the eight principles of practice is meant to give the body the maximum inner space and ease by following its natural lines and its relationship with gravity, the air pressure and other stresses imposed on it by the environment that it is subject to. This is only possible if we listen to the body from a meditative state of mind or total attention. In this state of mind we can initiate each movement from the energy body, which then in turn pulls and guides the physical body through the movements.

In the practice of yoga this process is applied to our own physical body. When I ride my horses, I apply exactly the same eight principles on them, with amazing results in fluidity, ease and joy in their movements. The eight principles are universal, as is yoga itself.

In the description of each principle I will also give the source, showing that learning comes from a 360° direction, not just from one narrow band of information.

'If one is *not* a yogi, one *practices* yoga.
If one *is* a yogi, everything that one does *is* yoga.'

The eight principles of practice

1	The meditative state of mind or the not-doing of meditation
2	Relaxation or the not-doing of the body
3	Intent or the not-doing of visualization
4	Rooting or the intelligent use of gravity
5	Centering or the knowledge of hara
6	Bodyscape or the anatomical understanding of the body
7	Breathing or the total use of inner breathing space
8	Elongating or using the total breathing to open the body

1 The meditative state of mind or the not-doing of meditation

It was when I attended the Krishnamurti talks in the sixties and seventies that I first came across the term *meditative state of mind*. Later on, when I was studying the writings of Carlos Castaneda, I came across the term *stopping the internal dialogue*. Both these terms dealt with a state of mind in which thought has stepped aside for a moment so that the listening, ec-static state of mind can take over.

The meditative state of mind or inner silence, that ec-static state of mind, is the matrix, the base on which everything else rests, as well as the glue that holds everything else together. It is not a state of mind that comes at the end of all the other practices as a reward, but it is the departure point for whatever comes afterwards. Without the meditative state of mind the other principles lose their deeper meaning.

The meditative state of mind is not the same as meditation. Meditation is something that you 'do' and involves being in a certain place for a certain amount of time and usually in a certain posture. It is an 'activity'. The meditative state of mind is not bound to location, activity, posture or time. It is not something that you 'do' but something that you 'are'. It is a state of mind in which there is total attention, not to anything in particular, like in concentration, but to the life force itself.

Usually, we pay attention to things to the exclusion of everything else. This is called concentration. The word concentration means to 'move towards the center'. In this there is still an inner tension, which is often expressed in the body, and especially in the face. In this state there is the object of concentration and the subject who concentrates. There is a center.

In the meditative state of mind there is no object of attention and no subject that pays attention, but only the state of attention itself, without object and subject. This is total attention. Total attention is a state of mind in which we pay attention; not to something in particular, but all around, to everything. In this there is complete silence; there is no center as the 'me' who is aware or attentive.

How do we move from our usual thinking to the state of total attention? There is no way. To arrive at total attention you have to pay total attention. There is no road, no technique.

There are some physical techniques that can be helpful, though.

The front of the body corresponds to the new brain. It is the side of the body that we can see, that we are most familiar with. It is the side of the body that is 'hot', where we play out our emotions and thoughts. It resonates with the thinking, calculating brain, and its sense of knowledge is the eyes. Our emotions and thoughts are engraved on the front of the face, in the grooves and wrinkles, in the worry lines or in the laughing 'crow's feet' wrinkles next to the eyes.

The back of the body corresponds to the old brain, sometimes called the reptilian brain. It is 'cold', cannot think in human terms, and does not have the typical human emotions. Its sense is the ears. It does have the 'old' emotions, though, that is, the emotions that belong to the physical body.

It is important to first of all become aware of how much we over-use the frontal side of our body and brain, and secondly to see if we can bring the awareness back into the back of the body and the back of the brain, so that we balance the new and the old part of us, the conscious and the unconscious. In order to do this we can use the eyes.

It is interesting to note how seldom we use the eyes in a conscious way, and how little we know about the different uses one can make of them.

Let us for a moment look at the animal world. The human 'animal' belongs to a category called the mammals. This category is divided in two large groups: the vegetarians and the meat eaters. It is wonderful to reflect how ecological nature is. The vegetarians eat the grasses and other plants, and provide the food for the meat eaters. Thus there is no wastage of material, and everything is in balance.

If we look at the eyes and their use in both the grass eaters and the meat eaters, we see a marked difference. The meat eaters have their eyes on the front of the face. These are the concentric eyes that pick and choose out of a herd of grass eaters the one that is going to be dinner.

These eyes are not concerned with the surroundings; they are only concerned with the one particular object of choice.

On the other hand, the vegetarians, who are the dinner, need to know from which direction the danger is coming. In other words, they need to have a type of vision that can see practically in an arc of 360°. Thus, when we look at horses, or donkeys, or giraffes, all grass eaters, we notice that their eyes are set on the side of their faces, thus providing a peripheral view of their surroundings.

Normally the 'I' of human beings that looks out through the eyes is standing, so to speak, right behind the eyeballs, peeking out through the holes of the eyes. The physical result of this is that the eyes have a certain hardness to them, are dry, round, and their focusing attention is driven through the inner corners of the eyes, giving the eyes an impression of narrowness. This is concentric vision.

Drawing the awareness into the back of the head has the immediate effect of widening the eyes, of making them soft and liquid, and of diffusing their focusing attention through the outer corners, giving them an almost Egyptian slant. This is peripheral vision.

The story

I am sitting next to Cisco while he is eating, enjoying his enjoyment of his food. Suddenly, he jerks up his head to look sharply around. I have not noticed anything unusual, but looking more closely in the direction of his gaze, I pick out a cat strolling in a distant field. With my human eyes I did not notice anything, but for the prey animal anything moving, in whichever direction, is a potential threat and noticed thanks to its peripheral vision.

I began to experiment with these two modes of vision: the concentric vision and the peripheral vision, and found out that the two are profoundly different, and have far reaching effects.

In concentric vision the energy of looking goes through the inner corners of the eyes. This makes the eyes narrow, hard and dry. The vision is focused on one particular object, which stands out sharp and clear and three-dimensionally. The visual field is a sharp, narrow band in front of the eyes: everything else is unfocused, un-important.

In peripheral vision the energy of looking goes through the outer corners of the eyes. This makes the eyes wide, soft and liquid. There is no object of focusing, and therefore everything has the same flatness. Things are slightly unfocused, and nothing stands out, but the field of vision is 180° from left to right. In this broad field anything unusual, a cat walking far away in the field, a bird flying overhead, will immediately sharply draw the attention: the prey animal's survival tool.

Concentric vision is connected to the thinking brain; peripheral vision is connected to the feeling or attentive brain. For the prey animal to detect the predator before it is too late, it cannot go through the slow process of thinking and concentration. Its brain needs to be lightning fast to detect the danger, and thus survive.

The story

I am riding the big stallion Gerrita. It is New Year's Eve. We are pedaling along quite nicely when suddenly, out of the blue, there is this huge BANG. Gerrita immediately swells up to twice his size and takes off in fifth gear, but at the same moment that he does so my body clamps itself onto him like a tic onto a dog and within two seconds he is under my control again. I did not think, plan or feel fear – there is no time for that. My body and 'old brain' knew exactly what to do, and did it, completely bypassing my young, thinking brain.

Thinking, though technically extremely useful, is bound to the slow, time-consuming process of formulating words and concepts. It is accumulative, as it can accumulate words, descriptions, concepts. On the other hand, total attention, which is the survival tool for the prey animal, falls outside the boundaries of verbal memory, and therefore outside the boundaries of time. It cannot accumulate anything verbally. Its memory is linked to surviving, and therefore to 'pictures' of dangerous situations of the past.

Concentric vision is linked to the thinking brain; peripheral vision is linked to the feeling, pre-linguistic brain.

Here are some exercises to experiment with these two modes:

Exercise 1
With the eyes open look ahead of you in the concentric mode, with the energy of your looking going through the inner corners of the eyes, and isolate some object to look at it more closely. You will see that this object becomes sharp, and that everything around it is vague. I like to compare this to the Hubble telescope, where the lens isolates a tiny part of the universe, making it very sharp, while the rest is screened out.
Then, still looking straight ahead, widen the eyes. Imagine that you have your eyes on the sides of your face and that you are looking sideways, the right eye to the right and the left eye to the left, simultaneously. This is called peripheral vision. You will see in this mode that between the two eyes you cover half a circle, in which everything is unclear, but your field of vision is very wide. In this mode it is as if your feeling sense is activated – you feel your surroundings through your eyes.

Exercise 2
In concentric vision, with the energy of your looking going through the inner corners of the eyes, say something to yourself internally, like 'two and two is four'. You will see that this is very easy, as this is what we do all day long. Now try to do the same thing in the peripheral vision mode, that is, say to yourself internally: 'two and two is four'. You will discover that it is impossible. This is precisely because peripheral vision is linked to the old, pre-linguistic brain; it simply cannot formulate words.

Exercise 3
In concentric vision, with the energy of your looking going through the inner corners of the eyes, look internally, with eyes closed, at your body, and isolate, let us say, the right shoulder. This is easy – that is the job of concentric vision. Then go into peripheral vision and try to do the same thing. You will see that you cannot isolate a particular part of your body, but that you are in touch with your body through a listening/feeling sense, in which you feel the whole body, but cannot isolate parts of it.

The same applies to the ears. Here too the 'I,' that habitually stands, as it were, right behind the ear holes, has to move backwards into the back of the head, leaving the ears soft and open and more vulnerable, not only to sounds, but especially to the empty spaces in between the sounds, the silence which is the matrix of sound. This is called peripheral hearing, and is as important as peripheral vision to 'feel' your way through life.

2 Relaxation or the not-doing of the body

The second principle aims at releasing unnecessary tensions in the body. The body needs a certain tone to function at its optimum. However, most of us are either below the healthy level of tone, or way over it – we are stressed.

Over the years the body accumulates emotional and physical stress and stores this in various parts of the body, such as the shoulders, the neck, the lumbar region, and the hip joints, until this becomes an actual problem.

Thus, before imprinting the asanas on the body, we need to learn to release these old patters. This can be done in any given position, or while walking, or riding.

This releasing is not the same as going limp. If, for a moment, we split the body in the skeletal structure and the muscular system, we can say that the body should be upheld by the skeletal structure and the muscles closest to it, while the peripheral muscles, the ones used for dynamic movement, should release their superfluous tension when not called into action. These superfluous tensions are usually unconscious, and are released through the practice of awareness with peripheral vision, which can bring the chi energy into the tense muscle.

This awareness comes from the *inside*. Many people say: 'Oh yes, I have stiff shoulders, but there is nothing I can do about it.' This means that they look at the problem from *outside*, as an external observer. This, in general, has the opposite effect from relaxation, as it fixes the tension or blockage even more in the mind and body, till it becomes 'my stiff shoulders, my stiff hips.' Each repetition of the affirmation further aggravates the situation. This is called *doing*.

In relaxation or the *not-doing* of the body the tension is not confirmed by external observation and affirmation. On the contrary, the awareness crawls, as it were, inside the muscle or joint, without naming the problem, without even calling this tension a problem. The awareness, from inside the muscle or joint, merely observes the tension, the blockage, quietly and with a great deal of clarity and affection. In this quiet observation the body will, by itself, unfold and unwind, gradually allowing air and space to come back into the tense parts. This is called *undoing*, when the muscles and joints unfurl like a tightly closed leaf, to let in the sunlight and the air.

The skin is also included in this process. In the course of the years, the skin tends to become a defensive barrier, protecting the body from the onslaughts of the world, like cold or heat, or from the energies of other people. It becomes like a sharp dividing line between the inner and outer energies, keeping the outer energies out, and the inner energy in.

In deep relaxation the skin becomes again transparent, translucent, like in early childhood, so that the body becomes vulnerable again to the outside energies, and no longer constricts the inner energy. This is one of the most important aspects of relaxation: re-connecting to the surrounding space by, as it were, 'taking the skin away,' making it so transparent that it does not obstruct the free flow of energy from the inside towards the outside, and vice versa.

Part of the reason why we tend so easily to accumulate tensions is due to the structure of the human body. The human body differs from the other animals in that it stands permanently upright on two feet. This has its advantages and disadvantages.

The advantage is that the spinal column is not locked between two pair of weight bearing points, the shoulder joints and the hip joints, like with the animals. Looking at the horse you can see that his spine is horizontal, hanging between the weight bearing shoulder joints and the weight bearing hip joints. Thus the spine is not free and can only move in a limited fashion. A bucking horse can bend his spine like in bakasana, or can twist it if he wants to park his rider somewhere else (like on the ground). Otherwise there is not much movement.

The human spine is, on the contrary, only locked at the base between the weight bearing hip joints, but at the top part it is swinging free between the free-swinging shoulder joints.

Where with the animals the spine is horizontal in relationship to gravity, in the human spine gravity runs vertically through the spine. This makes the balance a little difficult. In fact, if you come to think of it, the human body spends all its life trying *not* to fall. It has to arrange all the time its various parts in such a way that the weight is distributed at all times evenly on the front and the back of the body, as well as on the sides. Any deviation will immediately bring the muscles into the state of alarm, doing their best to maintain the balance. If this situation is chronic – as it is with almost everyone, since we do not learn in childhood how to stand straight, most muscles are in a chronic state of tension.

In order to relax the body, we need to learn to stack the various parts of the body one on top of each other in such a way, that the force of gravity runs straight and smooth through the entire length of the body and the spine, and all the parts hang easy and free from this line. Otherwise we need to use unnecessary muscle power to keep them up.

These parts are the feet, pelvis, chest and head. Ideally, the four main points of the vertical alignment are the ankles, the hip joints, the shoulder joints and the ear holes. By balancing these various parts of the body one above the other, you will reduce the amount of muscle tension and strain used to keep the body upright.

There are some areas in the body where tension builds up very easy. One of them is the neck and shoulder girdle.

The shoulder girdle is the ring that covers the upper ribs and fits like a yoke on top of the rib cage. It consists of the collarbones at the front and the shoulder blades at the back. The arms hang loosely from the shoulder girdle, and thanks to the shoulder blades they have an incredible range of movement. The shoulder blades should be able to slide freely across the rib cage, but more often than not become rigid and are held glued to the ribs, thus preventing the shoulders to move to their maximum. Through the movements in yoga we can learn to loosen again the shoulder blades so that they can function optimally.

The shoulder joint is a ball and socket joint, with the head of the upper arm fitting loosely in a rather shallow socket. Because of the shallowness of the joint (compared with the ball and socket joint of the hip which is very deep and therefore has a major stability), the arm has a wide range of movement.

There is a healthy way to hold the shoulder joint, and a less healthy way. Due to psychological and emotional inhibitions the shoulders are often pulled simultaneously up, forward and inwards towards the sternum, rendering the upper chest narrow on the front and bent on the back. This in turn influences the state of the mind, as the circulation of blood and chi energy is blocked.

The position in which the shoulder joints are at maximum repose is in the position where the upper arms rotate outward. This is the rotation you assume in savasana; therefore I have called it the *savasana rotation*. This rotation is used in most postures, and helps to open the upper chest, releasing the muscles.

Exercise in awareness of tensions

Stand in tadasana with the feet at hip width. Close your eyes. With concentric vision search your body mentally from the feet up to the top of the head for places that are tense in an effort to keep you upright. Check your feet, toes, ankles, calves, knees, thighs and buttocks for any spots of tension. Go up through the hip joints, the pelvis, the abdomen, the chest, shoulders, neck and throat. You will probably find many tight places. Much of this tightness is an unconscious and unnecessary effort to cope with gravity. Gravity is always trying to pull us down. You can learn to cope with the problem of gravity without tension through an understanding of the body and correct balance.

Then use peripheral vision. In this mode feel your body and *un-do* the tensions from inside. This is done through *intent*.

Once you have learned to do this in tadasana you can apply the same technique in all the postures or asanas, as each asana is a different way of balancing the body on the gravitational force, and therefore, if the alignment is correct, you need to spend much less energy than if the alignment is incorrect and you thus have to rely on a lot of muscle tension to keep your body from falling.

3 Intent or the not-doing of visualization

The story

I have just bought Cisco and he is frightened to death, running as fast as he can away from me when I approach him. He does not like human beings. There is nothing I can do but to stand still, and focus my *intent* on him. I *will* him to come to me. I tell him internally that I will not harm him. I *will* him to trust me. Then I slowly move towards him. His legs are shaking and his eyes are wide open, but then – he slowly turns towards me. Carefully I stretch my hand out to him, and he stretches his neck as far as he can in order to sniff my hand. It is the beginning of a deep friendship.

Intent is the most fascinating of the eight principles of practice, and has been extensively discussed in the books of Carlos Castaneda.

Regarding the practice of yoga, most people will apply their personal effort to the performance of the postures. This effort more often than not exceeds the amount of energy needed to actually perform the pose. If we learn to apply intent to the practice of the poses, we can do them with a lot less effort, and what we get back is a more abundant flow of energy throughout the body as well as a sense of freedom, lightness and beauty.

We apply personal effort because we think we have to 'learn' the asana. Thinking that we have to 'learn' postures is a mistake. The body knows how to do them. In reality, there is nothing that the body can learn which is not already there, from birth onward. Inviting the body to do what is knows to do is intent. Intent is the projection of a clear picture of the movement that we want to perform, while keeping the body in a state of relaxation and the mind in the meditative state, inviting the body to 'produce' the movement.

To understand how to feel what the energy of intent feels like, we can do the following exercise:

Exercise borrowed from tai chi: The unbendable arm

In the *unbendable arm*, two people stand facing each other. One student extends her arm sideways and the other student tries to bend her arm, with the first one resisting with all her strength. This is a muscular act, in which the stronger person wins. The other way is to visualize that you do not have muscles and bones, but chi energy. This energy comes from the hara, and the hara gets its energy from the ground, so you have to root the feet and 'sit' in the lower belly. The energy from the feet goes to the hara and from there to the arm. Let that energy run through the arm and out through the fingers. To let the energy flow feely, the eyes should relax, looking with peripheral vision. Relax the arm and keep elongating the chi energy; the more you relax the eyes and the arm, the freer and stronger the energy can flow out through the fingers and the more unbendable the arm becomes. Now the other person cannot bend the arm. This is your intent, which you can use in all the postures. The intent is when you project your chi energy to do a certain pose; then the body has to follow, it cannot not follow.

How do we apply intent to a posture? In order to experience the working of intent we can do a couple of exercises.

Paschimottanasana

One way of doing paschimottanasana is to bend forward, hold the feet with the hands and pull the trunk forward with muscular force. The other way is to quietly sit down on your mat, take a moment to relax your body, scanning with the inner eye the places where you know you habitually carry tensions, and undo those tensions with your awareness, with your peripheral vision. Whenever we put our attention or our intent on a particular part of the body, we bring chi energy into that part; the very awareness will undo the tension through the application of chi energy.
At the same time go into peripheral vision with soft and meditative eyes. Then, in your mind, in your inner 'video', you 'do' paschimottanasana, without actually moving your physical body. If your body and mind are

relaxed and still, and this inner video is clear and quiet, it will, at a certain moment, pull the physical body into paschimottanasana. The body *cannot refuse*. It *has* to follow the intent, thus is the power of intent. This would be another way of describing intent; as a mental force that has the power of self-fulfillment. It is the carrot that you dangle in front of the energy body, at which the energy body *has* to initiate the posture, pulling the physical body with it. Thus intent consists of a conscious image of the execution of a movement or posture before actually doing it, visualized by the inner eye: the inner video.

Twist in Siddhasana
Sit in siddhasana, with the right foot on the left thigh. Extend the right arm sideways and, bringing it around the back, hold the right foot. The left hand rests on the right knee. Imagine that you do not have eyes on your face, but rather on your upper chest, halfway between the sternum and the shoulder heads. Let those be the eyes that look, not the ones on the face. In that way you feel that automatically the whole upper chest opens, because those eyes want to look out. If we use the image of horses, then we can say that sometimes horses have blinkers, so they can look only forward. The shoulder heads are like those blinkers: if the shoulders come forward, they form the' blinkers' for the eyes on the upper chest, so that they cannot look. You have to move those blinkers out of the way, so that those eyes can look. If you then turn to the right side, it is not your head that wants to turn, but those eyes want to turn and see what is behind you. If you imagine those eyes on the upper chest wanting to turn and look, the body turns by itself, because images are strong, they are an integral part of intent. Having a strong image like that is already the intent, because the body follows the image; the body *has* to follow. The intent is the carrot for the energy body, and the energy body pulls the physical body. The physical body is the slowest part: the physical body is pulled by the energy body and the energy body is pulled by intent.

The story
The big stallion Gerrita is a little sleepy, and I wonder why. Then I realize that I am also a little sleepy. We both toddle along listlessly. Shaking myself out of it I *will* myself forward, pulling him along. He immediately picks up my energy and starts to trot faster and faster. Since I came back to horse riding, I apply intent regularly while on the horse, with remarkable success. Horses cannot compute, but they have an enormously large and well functioning motoric brain, and are extremely sensitive to human body language. This can have its positive and negative results. The negative ones are of course that the horse feels if its rider is nervous, and thus it also gets nervous. The horse can feel human energy. When

I ride, the moment I project my energy forwards, to go a little faster, the horse immediately picks this up and goes faster. If, on the other hand, he wants to have a little fun on his own, without my consent, I intend calmness and control. In this way, I have an immediate feed-back on the quality of my intent.

4 Rooting

Gravity and the rebound force: rooting

In order to understand the art of rooting we need to understand the third law of Newton. Gravity pulls everything to the center of the ground, but because the ground itself is compact, when gravity draws a body down to the ground, the compact ground resists. That resistance is a bounce, a force upward, opposite to and equal to the downward pull of gravity. When we understand that the rebounding force is *always equal* to the downward pull, we can manipulate this by increasing the downward pressure in certain areas in order to lighten it in others.

In yoga our problem is that too often we try to provide all the upward activity ourselves, instead of allowing our bodies to use the bounce provided by the ground. In order to do this we have to learn the art of rooting in whatever we do, as well as the art and knowledge of the *Russian bar*.

Rooting is the act of using that part of the body, which is in direct contact with the ground, to let it ride downward on the gravitational pull, but *more so than usual*. In other words, it is an elongation downward of that small part of the body that is on the ground. If that part is an arch, the counterthrust of the ground back up is caught in the arch and then channeled through the alignment of other arches or bandhas, joints and muscles to run throughout the entire body, bringing opening and chi energy to the entire body. Thus the quality of the asana as well as our daily life can improve by not abandoning ourselves to the downward pull of gravity, but by knowing how to bounce up like a cork.

When you talk about rooting you are talking in the first place about feet.

Tadasana
(For the action of the bandhas see page 34). Stand with the feet parallel to each other at hip width. Bend forward and with your hands spread each toe separately on the floor, straightening them onto the floor. The big toes follow the line of the inner arch, and the little toes the line of the outer arch. Then let a helper try to pull the toes up from the floor: they should not come up. This is leading you into rooting and pada bandha. A bandha is a circle with a suction cup action, like the octopus. It is a hollowness that 'sucks' the energy out of the ground. A common mistake is to start the suction of the feet in the tips of the toes, which means that the toes curl up. The toes form the rooting rim of the cup, not the cup; the suction is only between the metatarsals and the heels, by pulling the metatarsals back to the heels. Thus the knuckles of the toes should stay down and the toes remain straight; they do not curl up. The toes do slide slightly back towards the

heels, but not becomes you are pulling them up, but because you are pulling the metatarsals back to the heels. This is the action of the stirrup in the *spring joints* (see page 35). Glue and lengthen the bottom of the toes on the floor. When the feet root In this way, the 'echo' takes place in the pelvic joints: the pelvis will automatically lift up from the femur heads (mula bandha).

The Russian bar

The concept of the Russian bar is extremely useful and interesting. This is a circus program where two men hold a flexible rod on which they balance a young and agile girl. Their job is to toss the girl up in the air and catch her again on the rod, and her job is to do various exercises while being tossed up, like landing on the rod in hanumanasana or in full arm balance. Since the men carry the girl they are called the 'porteur' (circus language is traditionally French), while the girl is called the 'agile'.

This concept of the porteur and the agile fits exactly our perception of rooting: the part of the body which roots is always on the ground, and therefore stable, deriving its stability from the ground, while the rebounding force that is guided through the joints above the rooting part opens those joints, as they are free from the stabilizing effect of the ground. This lifts the aligning parts up from the underlying one, thus rendering them unstable but agile. Thus in all postures we have a stable basis (the porteur) and a mobile and light part (the agile) on top of the stable basis. To give this lightness and also a certain security or stability to the agile part of the body, the basis has to be well grounded and stable. To understand this concept we can do the following exercises as examples:

Full arm balance
Through the action of hasta bandha rooting results in an elongation of the arms and a lifting up of the chest from the shoulder heads.

Vasisthasana I
Applying pada bandha and hasta bandha in this pose rooting results in a lifting of the pelvis off the femur heads and the chest off the shoulder heads.

5 Centering

The skeletal structure of the pelvis
The pelvis divides the vertical body into two equal halves, and forms the bridge between the legs and the spine. It consists of the two iliac wings, the pubic bone, and the ischias or sitting bones. The pelvis can rotate forward, backward or stay in a neutral position in the middle.

In the middle position of the pelvis the spinal processes have just disappeared into the back, but the back muscles are still relaxed. It is important to understand that a natural 'hollow' back is normal. If the pelvis is rolled too far forward, this hollowness becomes too deep, and the back muscles become hard, narrow and tense, with the result that the spine locks and free movement is no longer possible in the lumbar vertebrae. If, on the other hand, the pelvis is rotated so far back that the lumbar spine is totally straight or even bent backwards, we violate the natural curve and render the spine vulnerable to shocks and sudden movements.

A good reminder for the neutral position of the pelvis is that in all postures the sacrum should move in a straight line away from the lumbar spine, which means in many positions, towards the heels. A coccyx that is tipped up into the lumbar spine results into an extreme lordosis in the lumbar; on the other hand, tucking the coccyx under results in a flattening of the lumbar.

The pelvis as center of gravity, power and movement: the hara
In the human body the center of gravity is in the lower abdomen, as well as the center of control and motion. This center of control is called in Japanese the hara. It is the main recipient and container for the force called chi.

Being the center of the body, ideally all movements should flow into the hara and flow out of it again; the rebounding power of the ground flows up from the feet through the action of pada bandha into the hara and from the hara into the rest of the body. In the section on breathing we show that the breathing too should flow into and out of the hara. This power is called chi energy.

This chi energy is subtler than muscular force. It is the extra energy derived from awareness that allows you to do more than muscles alone could possibly do. Your chi is in action when you move with a minimum of effort, resulting in lightness, vigor, correctness and beauty.

Though breathing is the main source of chi intake, it needs a vehicle for distribution. That vehicle is attention or awareness. By placing the attention on certain parts of the body, chi is directed there. This attention is part of intent.

The story
The horse, with its horizontal spine, has two centers of power. The first one is in the pelvis, where his motoric center is, as well the sexual one. An average horse weighs 500 kilo. To drive this mass forward, the horse has to use his buttock muscles and thigh muscles. The buttock muscles are the motor of the body. The center of gravity in the horse is right behind the shoulder blades – this is where we put the saddle if we want to ride him, so that we sit right on his center of gravity, and thus our weight is carried in the most economic way by him. When the human ape assumed the permanent upright position, though, these centers, the motoric one, the sexual one and the gravitational one, all ended up in the same spot: the middle of the pelvis. You can find it in the following way: Divide the body three times in two: from the hip joints up and down (this is the same length), left and right of the spinal column (same width), and front and back of the body. Where these three lines cross is the center: right in the middle of the pelvis. The Japanese call this center the hara.

6 Bodyscape

The physical body consists of hundreds of muscles, bones, organs, ligaments and nervous connections. There is general information circulating amongst all of these parts, guided and computed by the brain. When I raise my hand, the movement has first been conceived by the brain, after which the brain gives the communication to the muscles to execute the movement.

These movements, which we also find in the yoga postures, follow certain pathways that most often are determined by habits, by copying other people, like one's parents, or by sheer laziness. On a daily basis this may be good enough. However, we can change the quality of the movement by changing these unconscious and habitual pathways of information. This is done by guiding the movements consciously along certain lines that I have called *bodyscape*. A river, flowing in a hilly landscape, will not force its way through the hills, but will flow easily around them, always looking for the path of least resistance.

In rooting, the part of the body that rests on the ground becomes a conduit through which our energy flows down into the earth's energy field, and the earth's energy in turn flows back up into us. This is part of the gravitational pull that the earth exerts on the body. The ground, feeling the weight of the object (our body), offers resistance. That resistance is the rebounding force. The joint closest to the point of contact between body and ground is where the energy flows in both directions, where it splits.

This rebounding energy does not stop at the first joint, but will attempt to flow through a series of joints and muscles to reach all of the body. To facilitate this, the bodyscape must be such that it will enable the energy to flow easily through natural pathways.

If we look at the physical body as looking at a landscape, we can see that certain bones, joints and muscles have a closer communicating network than others. One could compare it to electrical wires: when the raw points of two electrical wires are at a distance from each other, the spark (electrical information) cannot make the jump. Two wires that are close together, though, and have their raw points pointing at each other, can easily shoot the energy through.

This is how the bodyscape functions. By consciously guiding the movement and the breath through certain muscle chains and joints, the information or communication travels faster and more efficient. If we then combine this with the principles of rooting and breathing, we get a powerful, and at the same time almost effortless, expansion from inside, called *elongation*.

In general terms, the energy travels through all the major joints: the ankles, knees, hips, spinal column, shoulder joints, elbows and wrists. These joints should not only be in contact with each other through our awareness, but they should also be physically aligned with one another. This enables them to receive the energy and, in turn, send it on to the next joint.

For this to function best, these joints should be open and aligned on smooth straight or round lines, never on angular lines. This will allow the energy to travel on in an even flow, without being held up or even cut off by sharp angles; therefore, all movements in yoga are done on round, generous lines.

The muscles form another, no less important energy pathway, as they connect certain places in the body where energy is gathered. These gathering places are called *bandhas*. Energy is collected in these bandhas and sent on to the next bandha or gathering point through specific muscle chains. Finding the entrance door to those muscle chains results in *non-local* action.

Local action versus non-local action

An action is local when it is confined only to the area where it takes place. We can compare this to a leaf that falls in a pond. The pond does not have an entrance or an exit, and so all the leaf can do is turn around and around in that little space, without going anywhere.

A non-local action is comparable to a leaf falling in at the spring of a river: it will traverse the full length of the river and touch many areas on its way.

One can do thousands of local actions in the body, but that is laborious and time consuming, and does not take you much further in understanding the unity of the body. Moreover, these local actions may have a benefit in a certain area, but go contrary to other areas. It is therefore more fun and healthier for the body in the long run to look for non-local actions.

These non-local actions run through certain connecting lines. These lines can go either through certain joints, or through certain muscle chains, or through the bandhas, which are energy arches or containers.

To initiate a non-local action, we need to find the entrance to the connecting line. Once you find the entrance, all you need to do is set the movement in motion, and the connecting line will carry it *automatically* and harmoniously through the entire body, without you having to go through the, what I call, start-stop process, which means that every movement comes immediately to a halt and then the next one is started *by an act of will*. If the action runs through the connecting line, there is no start-stop process, and the action is carried forward without the employment of will.

A beautiful movement is a movement in which there is no stop/start situation, not even a hint of it, but the energy flows fluently and uninterrupted.

The story

I am watching the dressage Olympics in Aachen. Those horses move like snakes; as the energy starts in the buttocks and hind legs, it is carried forward in a smooth, beautiful, undulating movement throughout their whole body, making these horses look as if they do not have any blockage of energy anywhere in their bodies, in spite of their size and power. They move like waves incarnate.

The ulnar wrist point

Non-local actions are almost always initiated in a bandha, though there is one addition. This addition is a point on the inside of the wrist on the side of the little finger. In acupuncture this point is called the *gate to paradise*, and is a powerful entrance point. I call this point the *ulnar wrist point*, as it is located on the ulnar or little finger side of the wrist.

This point is used extensively in martial arts, like brick breaking in karate, in sword fighting, in horse riding and even in such mundane activities as hammering a nail into the wall.

> *Exercise*
> Two students stand facing each other. One student stretches her arm forward with the palm facing down. The other student places her hand palm facing up on top of that hand, and tries to push it down, with the first student resisting. Then the second student tries again, this time with the palm facing down. Then a third time, this time making a loose fist, placing the ulnar wrist point on the hand of the other student and pushing down. She can now clearly feel how both the pectoralis and the latissimus dorsi muscles jump into action, and how the other student has very little chance to hold up against the pressure.

Bandhas

All other non-local actions are initiated in a bandha. In general one can say that these non-local actions are the result of rooting and the rebounding force of gravity, and travel through the entire body. As such the bandhas are indispensable as they serve as conduits for the rebounding energy and the breathing wave.

In the classical yoga texts the bandhas are described as forceful (concentric) contractions done on the exhalation. What we describe here as a bandha is a lifting upwards, on the inhalation, of an arch that serves as a conduit for the rebounding force. It is not a concentric contraction, but rather an 'eccentric' lifting of the arch of the bandha, a widening, in particular of the muscular and ligamental part of it.

Perhaps the easiest way to understand a bandha is to compare it to a cyclone or a whirlwind, in which all the action takes place on the rim, on the periphery: the rim twirls around a center, called the eye of the cyclone. We can see this clearly on meteorological charts: the energy is trapped and compressed towards the center.

In the cyclone, when the energy is compressed towards the center, the center is pushed upwards; one can see leaves (in a small whirlwind) or clouds (in a cyclone) being sucked up towards the sky, into the center or eye of the cyclone, which is the highest point.

In the body a bandha functions in the same way. It is a particular place where energy is trapped and then sent on to the next bandha. This is the meaning of non-local action.

One of the main characteristics of energy is, however, that it can only be trapped in a round container, or an arch. Therefore all the bandhas are found in those parts of the body where there is an arch-construction of bones, usually with a ligamental floor. The sole of the foot, with its arch structure and the ligamental 'stirrup,' the arch of the pelvis with the pelvic diaphragm, the arch of the lower ribs with the lower thoracic diaphragm, even the arch of the jaw bones with the floor of the tongue, the palm of the hand with the ligamental plate of the palm: these are the places where we find the bandhas.

To trap the energy inside the arch, the peripheral rim of muscles and joints is slightly constricted inwards towards the center. If the arch is in contact with the ground, this rim is also rooted into the ground, creating the rebounding force or the *Normal Force* of Newton. The combination of rooting and constricting the energy towards the center creates the eye of the storm, in other words, the center is lifted and the energy is pushed upwards.

We can distinguish five major arch formations in the body useable as bandhas for the rebounding force:

    a. Pada bandha or the arch in the foot
    b. Mula bandha or the pelvic arch
    c. Uddhyana bandha or the arch formed by the lower thoracic diaphragm
    d. Jalandhara bandha or the arch formed by the upper thoracic diaphragm
    e. Hasta bandha or the arch in the hand

a Pada bandha or the arch in the foot
For the purpose of creating lightness and bounciness in the body we have to first look at those joints in the foot which serve the act of walking, or the so-called *spring joints*: the *upper and lower spring joints.*

The upper spring joint is the joint between the ankle and the foot. The ankles fit over the foot like a horse rider on the back of the horse, with the legs hanging down. This joint can only move forwards and backwards, which is necessary for walking (it is especially evident in skiing), but it is not an arch joint. Therefore it is not usable for collecting the rebounding force.

The lower spring joint is the joint between the heel bone, the talus bone and the navicular bone. Nava means boat in Latin, and the virtue of this bone and this joint is that it is very mobile in all directions: it can 'rock' like a boat. This is of vital importance for us human beings, who have to walk on two feet, which is a controlled 'falling': the lower spring joint is constantly engaged in correcting the balance, together with the toes. You can find this joint underneath the highest point of the foot arch.

Pada bandha is the easiest to understand and activate in tadasana:

Tadasana
The foot has three major arches: the inner arch, the outer arch and the transverse arch. Pada bandha consists in magnetizing or *rooting* the outer rim of the entire foot on the floor and 'sucking' the center of the sole of the foot up. You can compare this to the suction cups on the tentacles of an octopus. The foot becomes like a suction cup, where the metatarsals are pulled slightly back towards the heel, while leaving the toes long

and straight on the floor, serving as the magnetizing or rooting part. A common mistake is to start the suction in the tips of the toes, which means that the toes curl up. The toes form the rooting rim of the cup, not the cup; the suction is only between the metatarsals and the heels, by pulling the metatarsals back to the heels. Thus the knuckles of the toes should stay down and the toes remain straight; they do not curl up. The toes do slide slightly back towards the heels, but not because you are pulling them up, but because you are pulling the metatarsals back to the heels. This is the action of the stirrup in the lower spring joints. Glue and lengthen the bottom of the toes on the floor.

As the metatarsals are pulled back towards the heel, the lower spring joint is pushed upwards, the arch of the foot becomes higher and the energy of the ground is collected. Supporting the lower spring joint are several muscles, in particular two muscles called together the 'stirrup': the tibialis posterior and the peroneus longus muscles. These muscles form the beginning of the muscle chains that cover the inner and outer legs to end up in the front and back of the trunk, where the trunk muscles carry on the movement. The energy generated in the arch of the foot through the action of pada bandha travels upwards through the tibialis posterior on the inner leg to run through the adductors on the thighs into the ilio-psoas muscle, which attaches on the anterior rim of the iliac crest and the anterior surface of the lumbar vertebrae, while on the outer leg it travels through the peroneus longus into the tensor fascia lata and then into the back of the trunk where it connects with the latissimus dorsi, which attaches on the posterior rim of the iliac crest and the posterior surface of the lumbar vertebrae. Thus the rebounding force, collected in the center of the sole of the foot, is carried up into the lower abdomen (the hara or central point of gravity and power), which then results in the lifting of the pelvic floor in the so-called mula bandha.

b Mula bandha or the pelvic arch

The pelvis consists of the two iliac wings, the pubic bone, and the sitting bones. As the word says, we sit on the sitting bones, while the pubic bone and the coccyx (which forms part of the spinal column, not of the pelvis) are usually suspended, unless one rotates the pelvis strongly forward (so that we 'sit' on the pubis), or backward (so we 'sit' on the coccyx). Roughly speaking these bones are connected by a ligamental plate called the pelvic floor or the pelvic diaphragm. When rooting the sitting bones into the floor (in sitting), or when movement is carried up from pada bandha through the legs, this pelvic floor is lifted and widened. This is called mula bandha.

Mula bandha is used in all postures, but in particular in breathing. The very act of keeping the awareness always in the hara in all movements gives stability to the body and centers it in a natural way, and keeping the hara always supported by the mula bandha in all movements brings coordination and grace to those very movements.

c Uddhyana bandha or the arch formed by the lower thoracic diaphragm

At the base of the rib cage we find the thoracic diaphragm. This is a muscle in the shape of an umbrella that divides the rib cage from the abdominal cave. At the center of the diaphragm is a ligament. Anatomically this center goes down on the inhalation into the abdominal cave, thus colliding with the intestines. The lungs are like a sponge, you can compress them and open them, in the same way as you can squeeze a sponge and let go. This is necessary for breathing. On the other hand, the intestines are tightly bundled up together and non-compressible. When the center of the diaphragm goes down on the inhalation it collides with the non-compressible intestines and therefore the stomach goes forwards. This is generally called abdominal breathing.

In the classical yoga texts uddiyana bandha is described as a contraction of the diaphragm after the exhalation, pulling it up into the rib cage. Here we use it differently. As the center of the diaphragm goes down on the inhalation and collides with the intestines, the abdominal muscles refuse to yield forward. Hence the movement cannot go anywhere, but is forced to return back up again along the inner spinal column and ends up in the lower ribs that widen as a result. Thus, even though the center of the diaphragm goes down, the diaphragm as a whole widens and moves slightly up into the rib cage. This moving in and widening of the diaphragm is of special importance in backbends, as in this way the lumbar spine is lengthened and widened in the backward curve, and therefore protected from getting squashed in the middle between the pelvis and the rib cage.

d Jalandhara bandha or the arch formed by the upper thoracic diaphragm
Jalandhara bandha is the act of bringing down the jawbone to the sternum. This has to be done during the breathing and in a specific way.

The rib cage is divided in the upper part and the lower part. In the lower part the ribs are attached to each other by cartilage, and thus they are very mobile and widen to the sides on the inhalation. The ribs in the upper part of the chest are attached on the frontal side of the body to the sternum and on the back to the upper thoracic vertebrae. Therefore they cannot widen laterally, but are lifted during the inhalation. This lifting forms the lower level in jalandhara bandha. The upper level of jalandhara bandha is formed at the front by the jawbones and at the back by the base of the skull, which is joined to the atlas vertebra. This is a sliding joint (actually an old ball and socket joint).

As this bandha forms part of the mula bandha breathing, we start with that.

In mula bandha breathing the inhalation starts at the bottom of the spinal column, in the region of the sacrum, and then moves upwards through the kidney area to the top of the spine along the interior part of the spine. Thus, the upper chest lifts and the shoulder blades widen and are lowered. In this way, not only is there no strain in the trapezius muscle, but there is actually a release as the shoulder blades widen and descend. This is the vertical lifting action of the lower level of jalandhara bandha on the inhalation.

The second phase is the lowering of the chin towards the sternum at the height of the inhalation. This is made possible due to the fact that the joint between the first vertebra and the head is a sliding joint (the old ball and socket joint, which has the shape of a bean). The joint surfaces between the atlas or first cervical vertebra and the skull permit a horizontal sliding movement forwards and backwards. Thus the head can slide horizontally forward before coming down, maintaining the concavity of the neck. These joints are similar to the joints between the sacrum and the ileum, the sacro-iliac joints. Both these pairs of joints have roughly the shape of a bean, and permit a slight sliding action. It is interesting to note that these two sliding joints are at the extreme ends of the spinal column, and are actually the first and last joints that connect the spine to the rest of the body.

As the jaw moves forward and down you have to get close to the sternum, but not touch it. The sternum and the jaw remain parallel to each other, elongating the corners of the jaws (right underneath the ears) forwards. Keep that length in the jaws and the freedom and openness in the fleshy part underneath them as the chin comes down to the upcoming sternum. Thus chin and sternum meet halfway and there is no strain anywhere.

The trapezius muscle covers the cervical vertebrae and part of the thoracic vertebrae. When the thoracic spine is elongated due to mula bandha breathing, the upper ribs are lifted and spread, together with the sternum and the collarbones. In order for that to happen, the trapezius muscle has to be kept fairly relaxed, which is not possible if the chin is brought down at a sharp angle.

If the chin would be brought sharply down to the sternum, that movement would start from a backward position of the joint. As a result of that the upper cervical vertebrae are pushed out backwards (you can feel this very clearly with your fingers) and there is a strong tension in the trapezius muscle.

If, on the other hand, one *first* slides the head forward horizontally in the joint, in between the atlas and the skull (the so-called 'swan neck movement') and *then* bends the head down, the bending starts from a more forward position of the skull on the atlas vertebra. The result is that there is much less strain on the muscles and ligaments of the neck and in the trapezius muscle, and the upper cervical vertebrae are not pushed out backwards, but remain in, concave, the way they should be according to their natural curve (again you can feel this easily with your fingers).

Even though in anatomy this would be considered nonsense, you move in your imagination the jaw forward and down, and the back rim of the head back and up. This is one of those anatomical contradictions, that is, that even though the jaw extends forwards, the back of the head moves backwards and lifts up. Anatomically speaking this is impossible, but energically it is quite possible and a very obvious feeling. It gives you actually a feeling of great width across the upper neck. Again to use images, the symbol of yoga is traditionally the cobra, *kundalini*. The cobra has its tail curled up in a spiral, which is the spiral of the crossed legs. Then the spine (the body of the snake) lifts upwards out of the spiral of the legs in a powerful and graceful curve and ends up in the neck, which is broad, with the head pointing forward and down (jalandhara bandha).

In the breathing, these three bandhas, mula bandha, uddiyana bandha and jalandhara bandha, do not take place in a time sequence. The moment the lower abdomen moves backward, as a result of the pelvis moving forward with the mula bandha movement, the kidneys move *back* and the jaw extends *forward*. It cannot stay in place. The movement of the breathing is therefore a zigzag movement: the pelvis moves forward, the kidneys move backward, and the jaw moves forward.

e Hasta bandha or the arch in the hand

This bandha is used in all the poses where the palms of the hands are on the ground (as in the hand balancings) and the body needs to get its rebounding energy from this contact. This energy then travels through the arms and shoulder joints to lift the body up from those shoulder joints.

The hand has the same structure as the foot, so we have to apply the same movements as in pada bandha. That is, as the weight of the body in pada bandha has to be shifted from the heels (the upper spring joints) to the central bones of the feet (the lower spring joints), so also in hasta bandha the weight of the body has to be shifted from the wrists (which correspond to the upper spring joints of the feet) to the central bones of the palms (which correspond to the lower spring joints of the feet). Then the center of the palms is sucked upward in the same way as for the pada bandha, trapping the energy in the typical arch construction and sending it upward through the arms and shoulder joints. The fingers are kept long and flat on the earth and they root together with the wrists, forming the rim of the bandha. This corresponds to the action in the pada bandha, where the toes are elongated on the earth and root together with the heel bones.

7 Breathing

I use mainly two types of breathing: one I call the *soft awareness breathing*, and the other one the *accentuated awareness breathing*.

Generally speaking, the soft awareness breathing is associated with concentric vision, while the accentuated awareness breathing is associated with peripheral vision.

The soft awareness breathing is the one that is maintained during the day, while the accentuated awareness breathing is the one used for performing the yoga postures or to give more energy to whatever movement one wants to make. This last one is also called the mula bandha breathing, as its trajectory is through the bandhas, while the soft awareness breathing does not follow a particular trajectory.

Both types of breathing require awareness in order to bring the best out of them. Normally we are not aware of our breathing, as it is supposed to be an automatic process of the body. Awareness, however, is always associated with chi energy, and so breathing with awareness, in addition to bringing a greater amount of oxygen to the body, also brings a greater amount of chi energy. Moreover, with the awareness one can direct the breathing to go wherever oxygen or chi energy is lacking, thus filling in the gaps in energy.

Both these types of breathing are described in part three on breathing.

8 Elongating

In our use of language we have to be aware that there is a profound difference between the words *stretching* and *elongating*. Stretching is a mechanical lengthening of a certain muscle, produced by shortening another one, and takes place on a purely physical level. Therefore, there is a limit to stretching, beyond which the muscle will rip. This ripping happens when the power of the shortening muscle exceeds the capacity of the other muscle for being stretched.

Muscles can either be contracted or stretched, but there is a third possibility in which the muscle *elongates*.

Deep within the fibers of the muscles there is a hidden door, which is opened by awareness and breathing and, once opened, allows the muscle to *undo* itself, that is, to elongate without the aid of another muscle shortening itself. For example, whereas in order to stretch the biceps muscle of the arm we contract the triceps, and vice versa, in elongating we experience both muscles *undoing* themselves simultaneously and elongating. As always, the conscious awareness of the movement of elongating enhances its power.

Whereas in stretching there is the danger of ripping, in elongating there seems to be no limit at all. Rather, both muscles seem to simultaneously ride on the flow of energy. Thus, not only is there no danger involved, but there is also no fatigue or residue, as in the case of stretching, where the shortening muscle is left with the residue of lactic acid.

Thus we see that elongation is done by visualization or intent, and is a movement that travels in two opposing directions as the result of awareness and breath flowing through the alignment.

part two
the asanas

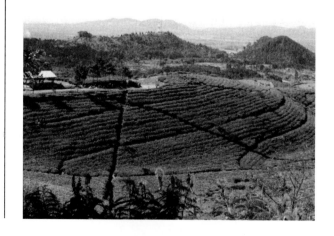

Introduction

This chapter gives the technique of the asanas. If you cannot study with a competent teacher, it will give you a fairly good understanding of how to practice the poses on your own, using the text within the blocks at the beginning of each chapter as your sequence of practice. By taking a different sequence each day, you will cover all the poses in a balanced way.

All the asanas are done on a yoga mat. For some positions, though, like head balance and shoulder balance, it is advisable to use a padding for the head, like a folded blanket. Otherwise, no aids and props are mentioned in this book. External tools, aids and props tend to distract the attention from the real pose, and give a false sense of accomplishment. It is better to do the poses slowly and to your capacity, even if that capacity is limited, rather than force the body with the aid of props to do what its own innate intelligence is not yet capable of handling.

The second issue not tackled in this book is that of physical problems and diseases. If treated well, the body is a self-healing organism. As such, yoga in itself is the greatest aid there is. Without going into specific details, just practicing the whole of yoga, including the breathing, creates the ideal condition for the body to take care of most normal physical problems. For major diseases, one should refer to a qualified doctor and eventually practice yoga under his or her guidance.

The third issue is that of dealing with physical and mental fatigue due to stressful living. The body is not only a self-healing organism, but it thrives on a finely tuned balance between exercise and rest. This balance is provided by the method of practicing yoga as described in this book. The feeling of resting is provided by the relaxation, the breathing and the elongation described in the *Eight Principles*. Practicing all the following asanas, guided by the Eight Principles, gives the body the balance which it needs to feel in optimum health and vitality.

The last issue is that of aging. In the "Hatha Yoga Pradipika", it is written that anybody can practice yoga, old, young, healthy and ill. There is no need to fear the effect of aging; the body can be as young as you want it to be. Disease and age are held at bay by cultivating the habit of happiness and joy, and above all, by a real love for this marvelous instrument, the body, and for this greatest gift of all, yoga.

Before going into the various groups of asanas, it is interesting to have a closer look at the basic posture, tadasana or straight standing pose, which contains all the postures in the same way as white light contains all the colors of the rainbow.

Part 1 Tadasana/Standing Straight

tada=mountain

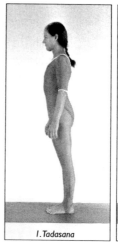
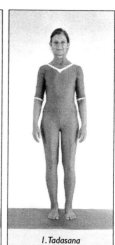

1. Tadasana   *1. Tadasana*

Technique

The feet

Stand with the feet at hip width, parallel to each other. Keep the feet even, and the toes straight forward; do not turn them in or out. On the back of the body, the fibers of the latissimus dorsi and those of the gluteus maximus cross over the lumbar vertebrae with a strong ligamental plate, the fascia thoraco-lumbaris. If the feet are turned outward, these fibers slacken and the lumbar spine sags inward, exaggerating the natural curve. To protect the lumbar spine from sagging, the feet must be parallel to each other, or even slightly turned inward for those who have a weak or excessively curved lumbar spine. This tightens the fibers of the gluteus maximus and consequently tightens the fascia thoraco-lumbaris. The weight of the body is evenly distributed between the two feet; the soles of the feet should be conscious of their contact with the earth, as if the feet had roots going deep into the earth with the force of gravity (rooting, the fourth of the Eight Principles).

The foot has three arches: the inner (long) arch, the outer (short) arch and the frontal or transverse arch. The inner arch is supported by the abductor hallucis, which runs from the heel to the big toe and abducts it. The outer arch is supported by the abductor digitis minimus, which runs from the heel to the little toe and abducts it. The transverse arch is supported mainly by two muscles, the peroneus longus and the tibialis posterior. The longus runs underneath the sole of the foot and up on the outer side of the lower leg to the head of the fibula. The tibialis posterior runs from the navicular bone in the foot over the heel up to the back of the lower leg. These two muscles together form a kind of stirrup which supports the transverse arch. These three arches must be raised to rebounce the weight of the body back upwards against the downward pull of gravity. The arches of the feet form the ultimate point where the weight of the body is received. As the upper body weight falls onto the pelvis, it divides into two, flowing through the hip joints into the thigh bones. The weight divides again in the knee joints and flows downwards through the fibula and tibia into the ankles and arches, where it is divided over the many bones of the feet. As the feet are small compared to the rest of the body, they need a special structure in order not to collapse under the weight of the body. This structure is the arch.

Arches are also used in architecture to hold great weights. For instance, the dome of a cathedral is copied from the arch of the feet; only thus can the weight of the roof of the cathedral be supported. In the body we find many domes. Two of them are key points in bearing the weight of the body: the feet and the pelvis. It is interesting to note that the central point of gravity is in the dome of the pelvis, while the dome of the feet is the place where the body roots into the earth. Thus the first rebounce action takes place in the arches and ankles, the second in the pelvis and the third in the spinal vertebrae.

To lift the three arches, the distance between the big and little toes has to increase by abduction of these toes: the big toe continues the curve of the inner arch and the little toe the curve of the outer arch, so that the triangle of the foot (heel-big toe-small toe) occupies the maximum floor space and the toes are fully spread. In the beginning, the hands can be used to spread the toes. Bend forward; with the fingers spread the toes and elongate them away from the metatarsals, so that the toes are straight, not curled (the result of wearing shoes). Animals have four points to stand on, but we have only two, which makes for a difficult balance while standing and walking. Therefore the toes serve to maintain the equilibrium of the body. We have to learn to use our feet like hands in all the postures, so the toes are like fingers on the earth, especially the big toes and the little ones. To check how the toes serve for balance, sway to right and left, and feel how each time the toes correct the balance of the body. Then try the same thing while walking. Walking is a form of controlled 'falling'; when you walk, you 'fall' from the ball of one foot onto the heel of the other one. Here too, you can feel how the toes serve to keep the balance in this unstable movement. The bottom of the toes, the distal heads of the metatarsals (especially those of the big and little toes) and the heels should be rooted in the earth. Without disturbing the toes, pull the cushions underneath the heels backwards with your fingers, so that the heels are extended on the earth. Then lift the central metatarsals up to form the transverse arch.

Learn to use both the outer and inner arches evenly. With weak inner arches, the outer ankles are caved in, so that the inner ankles are pushed out, towards each other. To lift the inner arches, you have to root the base of the big toes into the earth and elongate the other toes. Then bring the body weight diagonally towards the outer heels, so that the inner ankles move in and the outer ankles move out. Keeping that action, bring the body weight onto the center bones of the feet, in particular the talus bone (between the metatarsals and the ankles), and raise the outer arches up. To check the arches, you can experiment with a pen. Most people are aware of the long inner arch, but few people are aware of the short outer arch. Lifting the arches, see if you can pass the pen underneath them from the outer edge of the foot towards the inner edge, through the outer and the inner arches. Lift the inner and outer ankles of both feet evenly. As the weight of the body is transmitted through the legs to the ankles, the ankles have to rebounce that weight back upwards together with the arches; they should not be passive. The inner and outer ankles should have the same height.

The legs
Elongate the back of the knees. The knee caps are embedded within the knees, but do not overstretch the back of the knees; the legs should not be bowed backwards. The knees face straight forward, with the inner knees in line with the inner ankles and the outer knees in line with the outer ankles. Create space in the knee joints, they continue rebouncing the weight of the body back upwards.

The pelvis
Anatomically the shoulder joints, hip joints and ankle joints should be aligned vertically, so that the lower legs are at right angles to the soles of the feet. Thus the weight of the body is transmitted to the feet in a straight line. As described later in this chapter, for the purpose of making the body light we will change this angle. For the moment, however,

we will base the rest of the description on this classical anatomical alignment.

Keeping these three joints in line and keeping the knees straight, the next step is to assess the position of the pelvis. The pelvis is a bowl-like construction at the lower end of the spinal column. It is attached to the spinal column in the sacro-iliac joints, which connect the ileum part of the pelvis to the sacral part of the spine, and to the legs in the hip joints, which connect the ilea with the femurs.

These are the two pair of joints where the pelvis moves in relation to the spine and legs. However, these joints are also heavily protected, the sacro-iliac joints by the irregularity of their joint surfaces, and the hip joints by their strong ligaments and muscles. As a result, the pelvis usually moves in relation to the rest of the trunk in the lumbo-sacral joint, where there is very little protection. This joint connects the sacrum with the lumbar spine and is already a stress point for most people. Eventually this joint and the rest of the lumbar spine weaken, which can lead to damage of its vertebrae and discs.

The pelvis can assume three positions. The correct one is the neutral position, in which the pelvis is vertical and the buttock bones point straight down. When the hip joints, knees and ankles are in line, the hip joints are thus fully extended (a hundred and eighty degrees). This position is quite rare. Sometimes the pelvis is rotated too far backward, causing the lumbar spine to come too far back, and sometimes it is rotated too far forward, causing the lumbar spine to curve too far inward as the sacrum and coccyx are tilted up, in which case the abdominal muscles become slack as the angle between pelvis and femur is less than a hundred and eighty degrees.

In both cases the pelvis has to be brought to a vertical position. The most common incorrect posture is the one in which the pelvis is rotated forward around the femur heads. This can easily be checked in the following way: choose an outer corner where two walls meet and stand with the back against it. Keep the heels two inches away from the corner, but rest the sacrum and the back of the head against it. Then put the hands in the small of the back. If there is a wide gap between the lumbar area and the corner, the pelvis is rotated forward, thus pulling the lumbar spine into the body. To correct this, practice as follows: move the feet forward until they are about a foot away from the corner, but keep the sacrum and the back of the head on the corner. Bend the knees a little and rotate the pelvis back around the femur heads, until the lumbar spine is in touch with the corner. Then straighten the knees again. Repeat this movement for a couple of weeks, gradually moving the heels closer to the corner as the mobility in the hip joints increases, until the heels are two inches away from the corner. It is not the intention to eliminate the natural curve of the lumbar spine, but only to reduce it. Thus a gap can remain of about two inches between the lumbar spine and the corner.

This is a see-saw action. Rotating the pelvis backward around the femur heads means that the two frontal hip bones move *up* towards the ribs, while the coccyx moves *down* and forwards towards the pubic bone. Many people cannot do this without bending the knees. This shows that the hip joints are unable to extend fully and therefore the knees have to give in to allow the pelvis to rotate backward. This is the see-saw action of pelvis and knees at the periphery around the central axis of the hip joints. Thus, when the knees are fully extended and the hip joints are in line with the ankle joints, the pelvis is stuck in that forward rotated position.

There are two points in the pelvis where the body often resorts to see-saw action:

I. See-saw action around the hip joints

This is the action described above. To open the hip joints, the following movements are necessary:

a. Rotate the pelvis backwards until it is vertical and the buttock bones point straight down to the earth.

b. At the same time, straighten the knees fully.

c. Constrict the following muscles around the pelvis slightly inwards towards each other: the tensor fascia lata muscles, which run from the frontal hip bones through the ileo-tibial tract of the fascia latas to the outer sides of the knees, the adductors on the inside of the thighs, the iliopsoas muscles and the rectus abdominus. When these muscles are toned, they stabilize the pelvis and lift it up from the femur heads. Do not tighten the gluteus maximus.

Steps a. and b. are simultaneous peripheral dynamic movements in opposite directions around the static axis of the hip joints. As a result, these joints open fully and the groins and sides of the hips are extended. Thus, in the correct movement the two frontal hip bones move up and the knees resist backwards simultaneously. Just resisting the knees backwards tends to cause the pelvis to rotate forwards, while just lifting the two frontal hip bones up towards the ribs without resisting the knees tends to cause the pelvis to rotate backwards (see-saw action I).

II. See-saw action around the sacro-iliac joints

To open the sacro-iliac joints the following movements are necessary:

a. Keeping the pelvis (the compound bone of ileum, ischias and pubis) vertical, move the two frontal hip bones forward and up towards the ribs, and the knees back (see-saw action I).

b. At the same time, the compound bone of sacrum and coccyx has to make a movement which is called counter-nutation, that is, it has to rotate backwards in relation to the pelvis. This means that the coccyx moves forward towards the pubic bone and the sacrum becomes vertical.

c. Constrict the tensor fascia lata muscles and the adductors of the inner thighs slightly inwards towards each other and tighten the iliopsoas and rectus abdominus.

Steps a. and b. are simultaneous peripheral dynamic movements in opposite directions around the static axis of the sacro-iliac joints. As a result, these joints open and the – now vertical – sacrum moves forwards into the space between the two ilea, wedging them slightly apart. The entire pelvis widens laterally and lifts vertically up from the femur heads.

Moving the two frontal hip bones forwards without anchoring the coccyx would cause the entire pelvic bowl to rotate forwards and the coccyx to be tipped back and up. On the other hand, moving the coccyx forward towards the pubic bone without also moving the two frontal hip bones forward would cause the entire pelvic bowl to rotate backwards. Thus, in the correct movement the pelvis (ilium+ischias+pubis) and the sacrum (+coccyx) move separately, rotating in opposite directions: the pelvis rotates forward and the sacrum rotates backward around the axis of the sacro-iliac joints. Thus these joints are opened.

The result of movements I and II together is that the pelvis becomes vertical, is widened laterally, moved vertically forward against the femur heads and lifted up from those femur heads.

The spine and chest

The upper rim of the sacrum is connected to the lumbar spine in the lumbo-sacral joint. When the pelvis and sacrum become vertical through the dual action in the hip and sacro-iliac joints, the lumbo-sacral joint is pulled slightly backward and down. This causes the rest of the lumbar vertebrae to come back too and thus the whole lumbar spine is elongated.

Thus, the first action of rebouncing the weight of the body back up takes place in the arches of the feet and the ankles. Lifting the pelvis up from the femur heads is the second rebounce action. The elongation of the spinal column, which starts in the lumbar vertebrae and continues through the thoracic and cervical vertebrae, is the third.

When the lumbar spine moves back, the shoulders move neither forward nor backward, but the shoulder joints remain in line with the hip and ankle joints. Do not bend the spine in the lumbar or thoracic area and do not collapse the chest or abdominal area between the navel and the lower ribs.

The weight of the body is brought onto the back and the pelvis and back are widened laterally. At the same time the distance between the two frontal hip bones widens, so that the lower abdomen moves in and up towards the navel. This tones the muscles of the lower abdomen and strengthens the internal organs.

As the pelvis and back widen laterally, the spine 'grows' out of the pelvis by itself. If the spine is pulled up by the rib cage, the shoulders and the shoulder blades, the body is not centered in the pelvis and the pelvis has not widened. It is important to learn this movement first, as all the other asanas depend on it.

As the lumbar spine 'grows' out of the pelvis, the thoracic spine continues that movement. Move only the spine, elongating it upward; do not push the lower ribs forward in the mistaken idea that you are lifting the spine. The spine elongates up through its own internal liberating force and the rib cage is merely suspended from it, without any strain or tension on the solar plexus: as the spine elongates, the rib cage is also lifted, but vertically and passively. The result is the same as in the pelvis: the rib cage widens laterally.

Summarizing

Keep the ears, shoulder joints and hip joints in a line with the ankle joints, and the knees straight. Then move the top of the sternum (corresponding to the first two thoracic vertebrae) and the pubic bone (corresponding to the coccyx) forward. At the same time move the lower ribs (corresponding to the lower thoracic vertebrae) and the navel (corresponding to the lumbar vertebrae) backward. Do not bend any part of the spine. As a result, the whole back is widened laterally and the spine is elongated vertically. When you practice this on the corner between two walls, the sacrum and the back of the head are in touch with the corner, but not the thoracic vertebrae or the heels.

To open the upper part of the chest do as follows
a. Keep the ears in line with the shoulder joints, the hip joints and the ankles.
b. Keep the lower ribs down and in as described above.
c. Elongate the neck upward as if you were balancing a book on the head. Keep the face vertical, do not tilt the chin up.

Steps *a.* and *c.* are the two simultaneous peripheral actions around the axis of the upper chest. As a result, the upper chest opens.

A healthy and harmoniously developed spine shows an even groove from the sacrum to the first thoracic vertebra. Many people have a deep groove in the lumbar area and none on the sacrum or between the shoulder blades. This shows an unhealthy and uneven development of the spine. To get an even groove, center the body in the pelvis and draw the groove down to the sacrum, at the same time drawing it up through the area between the shoulder blades to the first thoracic vertebra with the movements described above.

The shoulders, shoulder blades and arms hang passively; do not pull the shoulders back forcefully, and do not pull the shoulders and arms up. The arms and hands are suspended passively from the shoulder joints, held to the body by their ligaments, not by the muscles above the shoulders (the trapezius muscles). As the back and rib cage widen, the shoulders and shoulder blades widen too and go down automatically if the arms are dropped, in other words, if one gives the full weight of the arms to the force of gravity.

The neck and head

Elongate the neck up, keeping the face vertical. Do not tilt the chin up and do not push the head forward. The ears remain in line with the shoulder joints. The neck can only elongate if you are aware of the tensions which shorten the muscles at the back of the neck. Gently *undo* these tensions from inside and ease the neck upwards. The correct position of head, neck and shoulders is that adopted by women in more primitive cultures when carrying water basins on their heads.

Tadasana is the basic position for all the other ones, and, if understood fully, will greatly facilitate the understanding of the other positions. The above description is the purely anatomical explanation. This has to be understood first, before one can, as it were, explode the physical frame, so that the Body of Light can take over. This goes for all the other techniques given in this book. Note that the words 'earth' and 'sky' have been used, instead of the usual 'floor' and 'ceiling'. This is to maintain a certain awareness of the human body as a link between the energy of the earth and the energy of the sky. After all, the physical body is made of the substance of the earth, but the Body of Light, the Energy Body, is made of the light of the sun, the light of the stars, lighting up the earth body from within.

The anatomical posture is, taken literally, a limiting posture. How can we make the transition from this purely physical description of the pose into the liberation of the Energy Body, loosening the grip of gravity on the body. What is the key, if there is a key?

A key there is, and a very interesting one too. At this point we need to take a closer look at the bones of the feet, and especially the joints. The bones of the lower legs, the tibia and the fibula, end in what is commonly known as the ankles, the inner and the outer ankles. The inner and outer ankles form a kind of vice into which is wedged a particular bone, called the talus. You can compare the talus to a wooden horse in a gym, with somebody (the lower leg bones) sitting astride on it. This joint is called the talocruralis joint, and is more commonly known as the *upper spring joint*. It is vital in the movements of walking, running and jumping, as it permits the lower legs to bend forward in relation to the foot. The entire weight of the body is transmitted from the tibia and the fibula through the talocruralis joint to the talus. Underneath and on the front of the talus are two other joints. The one underneath is called the subtalar or talocalcanean joint. It connects the talus to the heel bone (the calcaneus). The one on the front of the talus is connected both to the frontal part of the heel bone as well as to the first bone in the arch of the foot, the navicular bone. Therefore it is called the talocalcaneonavicular joint. It is also called the *lower spring joint* and is situated slightly forward from the ankles, on top of the arch. It permits the sideways rocking movement of the bones of the foot necessary in walking, running and jumping, to maintain the balance (the word 'navicular' comes from *nava*, which means 'boat').

The job of the talus is to divide the weight of the body over the heel and the bones of the arch, respectively through the subtalar joint and through the talocalcaneonavicular joint. Not only are these joints used for dividing the weight of the body, but they are also used for walking, running and jumping, hence their name *spring joints*.

Of the two, the talocalcaneonavicular joint is the more complex. As described previously, it is supported by the peroneus longus and the tibialis posterior. The tibialis posterior has the function of shortening the distance between the navicular bone and the heel bone, in which process the navicular bone slips partially under the talus, thus raising the arch. The fibers of the two muscles are intertwined, and the force of the action of the tibialis posterior is thus transmitted to the peroneus longus.

These two muscles form a kind of stirrup underneath the medial arch of the foot, supporting and lifting the lower spring joints. This action of lifting is called *pada bandha* (*pada* is 'foot' in Sanskrit and *bandha* means 'bound'). Pada bandha is the first of the major bandhas in the body and at once supports and motivates the other bandhas. Seen from this point of view, the rest is easy to deduce.

The key to lightness is to not keep the pelvis aligned with the upper spring joints or talocruralis joints, but to keep it aligned with the lower spring joints or talocalcaneonavicular joints. One can compare this to the stance of Olympic ski jumpers. The angle of the ski jumper to his skis is never ninety degrees, but less. In the case of tadasana, the entire body is kept at an angle of about eighty degrees forward. This brings the lower abdomen vertically above the lower spring joints.

As described earlier, most people follow the anatomical description and stand completely vertical, with the shoulder and hip joints aligned with the ankles or upper spring joints. Thus the weight of the body falls on the talocruralis joints and through the subtalar joints onto the heels. In this way it is very difficult to rebounce the weight of the body back upwards. Leaning the physical body slightly forward, so that more of the body weight is transmitted by gravity to the talocalcaneonavicular joints permits those joints to take responsibility for the rebounce action by using the tibialis posterior and the peroneus longus, pulling the arches up and continuing that action up to the knees. In this action these two muscles are supported by the abductors of the big toes and the little toes, and the result is not only that the body is extremely 'bouncy', but also stable at the same time.

Thus the real rebounce action is not in the ankles or lower legs, but in the lower spring joints, the talocalcaneonavicular joints.

As mentioned before, this is the result of leaning the *physical body* slightly forward over the arches of the feet. However, the *inner energy*, the weight of the inner awareness, has to move backward, towards the back of the body (see also the description of padmasana, sitting and savasana). This double action of moving physically forwards and energy-wise backwards, coupled with the action of the spring joints, liberates the energy from the rooting feet towards the lower abdomen and from there up along the spine towards the top of the head. This is what is called, in the Eight Principles, *connecting*.

Part 2 Surya Namaskar/Sun Salutation

Surya namaskar or the *sun salutation* is a classical way to connect the various asanas into one continuous, flowing event. Combined with the breathing, it helps the body to perform all the asanas without interruption and therefore without a break in the flow of energy. We have suggested in this book that most groups of asanas can be done in this way, as an alternative to the start-stop-start method, in which each pose is performed separately from the other, with a break in between. This last method is fruitful in order to learn the precision of the asanas but, as indicated above, it also involves an inevitable break in the rhythm of the body and the breathing, as well as in the flow of energy.

Even though the practice of yoga in general is not conditioned by physical states such as disease or aging, or by mental states, such as depression, surya namaskar in particular has a beneficial effect on the minds and bodies of people who tend to have minor physical diseases, or who struggle with the physical and mental effects of aging, due to its influence on the blood circulation and the flow of the breath and the energy. Specially in the case of aging, the start-stop-start method not only tends to cool the body off in between the asanas, but also makes it hard to start up the energy, the motor, each time again. Combining the various asanas with a mild form of surya namaskar, without straining, can help the body – and the mind – to retain its heat, the flow of the breath and of the energy, as well as the physical and mental concentration necessary to perform the asanas. This is the purificatory effect of the flow, after which the body and mind feel refreshed and optimistic, having, as Patanjali states, burned the impurities of the body and the nervous system in the fire (tapas) of the practice.

In the sequence of surya namaskar it is important to concentrate on the synchronization of the breathing and the movement, so that the two form one, uninterrupted unit. I have coined surya namaskar in combination with the asanas mala. A *mala*, in Sanskrit, is a necklace, a rosary, a circle of beads or pearls (the asanas) strung together on a string (surya namaskar).

The sequence

1. Stand in **tadasana** (*tada=mountain*) on a mat with the feet together. Keep the body slightly slanted forward so that the weight of the body falls directly onto the lower spring joints. On a mula bandha inhalation, raise the arms over the head, using the rebounce action in the lower spring joints (pada bandha) to trigger off the mula bandha (photo 1b).

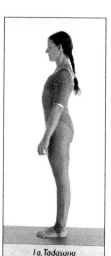 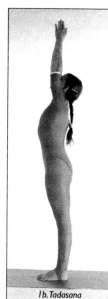

1a. Tadasana   1b. Tadasana

2. On the exhalation bend forward, keeping the legs perpendicular, and place the hands on the mat next to the feet. Bring the trunk and head to the thighs and shins. This position is called **uttanasana** (*uttana=intense stretch*).

3. On the inhalation, raise the head and curve the whole spine up, from the sacro-iliac joints to the first cervical vertebra.

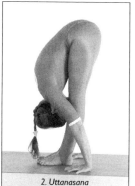 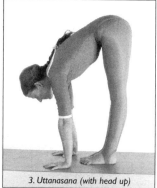

2. Uttanasana   3. Uttanasana (with head up)

4. On the exhalation, lean the body weight on the hands and jump with the feet backwards. At the same time bend the arms and lower the chest, till the shoulder joints are above the hands with the elbows pointing backwards and the upper arms parallel to the earth. The head, trunk and legs are parallel to the earth and the weight of the body is supported only on

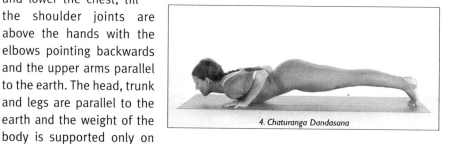

4. Chaturanga Dandasana

the hands and the balls and toes of the feet. This position is called **chaturanga dandasana** or *crocodile pose* (*chatur=four; anga=limb; danda=staff*).

5. On the inhalation, raise the head and chest till the arms are straight and perpendicular, rooting the hands and performing hasta bandha. Keep the legs parallel to the earth. Pull the pubic bone slightly forward, so that the trunk can curve upwards and backwards. Elongate the neck as in jalandhara bandha, so that the sternum is raised high, and then curve the head backwards. This position is called **urdhvamukha**

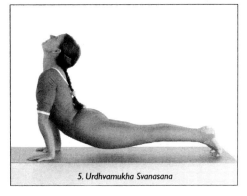

5. Urdhvamukha Svanasana

svanasana or *upward facing dog pose* (urdhva=upwards; mukha=face; svana=dog).

6. On the exhalation, raise the pelvis and thighs and bring them backwards, keeping the arms straight and the hands and feet *rooted,* till the chest, the head and the spinal column form one line with the arms. Thus the whole body forms a triangle, with the coccyx as the highest point. This position is called

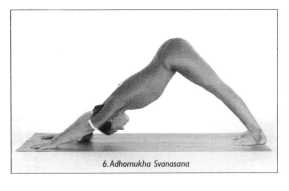

6. Adhomukha Svanasana

adhomukha svanasana or *downward facing dog pose* (adho=downwards; mukha=face; svana=dog).

7. On the exhalation, bend the knees and jump forward into **uttanasana**, rooting the hands as in adhomukha vrksasana (see page 178) and shifting the weight of the body to the hands as you jump. Lift the head and keep the bending of the knees minimal, so that when the feet land in between the hands the hips are high and the knees can straighten immediately. Bring the trunk and head to the thighs and shins in **uttanasana**.

8. On the inhalation, stand up again straight in **tadasana** (see 1a).

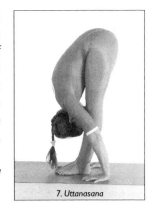

7. Uttanasana

Part 3 Standing Poses

These positions can be done in three different modes:

a. Performing each position separately and holding it for one minute.

b. Vinyasa

Connecting two or more positions by flowing from one into the other, using the breathing. For example:

- Utthita trikonasana » parsvottanasana » parivrtta trikonasana
- Utthita trikonasana » ardha chandrasana » virabhadrasana III
- Virabhadrasana II » virabhadrasana I » virabhadrasana III
- Utthita hasta padangusthasana » urdhva prasarita ekapadasana » virabhadrasana III

Use your imagination to make your own combinations and keep each position for three breaths.

c. Mala

Connecting all the positions, through surya namaskar, in the following way, using the breathing, and holding each of the standing poses for the duration of three breaths:

- Tadasana » inhale extend the arms upwards » exhale uttanasana, inhale raise the head » exhale chaturanga dandasana » inhale urdhvamukha svanasana » exhale adhomukha svanasana, inhale » exhale utthita trikonasana on the right side, stay for three breaths, inhale » exhale adhomukha svanasana, inhale » exhale utthita trikonasana on the left side, stay for three breaths, inhale » exhale adhomukha svanasana, inhale » exhale uttanasana » inhale tadasana, exhale » inhale extend the arms upwards etc.

Standing poses	
1. Tadasana	c. Holding the foot with the opposite hand
2. Garudasana	
3. Vrksasana I	d. Holding the foot with the opposite hand and turning the trunk and head to the side of the raised leg
4. Vrksasana II	
5. Ardha Baddha Padmottanasana	
6. Vatayanasana	e. Holding the foot with both hands and bringing the head to the shin
7. Utkatasana I	
8. Utthita Trikonasana	19. Urdhva Prasarita Ekapadasana
9. Ardha Chandrasana	20. Prasarita Padottanasana
10. Parsvottanasana	a. Hands on earth, head up
11. Parivrtta Trikonasana	b. Hands and head on earth in between feet
12. Parivrtta Ardha Chandrasana	
13. Virabhadrasana II	c. Holding ankles, head on earth in between feet
14. Utthita Parsvakonasana	
15. Virabhadrasana I	d. Namasté II, head on earth in between feet
16. Virabhadrasana III	
17. Parivrtta Parsvakonasana	21. Padangusthasana
18. Utthita Hasta Padangusthasana	22. Padahastasana
a. Holding the foot with the same side hand	23. Uttanasana
b. Holding the foot with the same side hand and bringing it to the side	

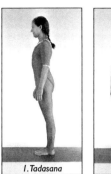 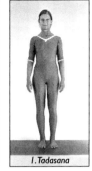

I. Tadasana   I. Tadasana

1.Tadasana
tada=mountain

- See page 43.

2. Garudasana
garuda=eagle
- Stand in tadasana.
- Bend the left knee slightly and wrap the right leg around it.
- Cross the right elbow over the left and join the palms of the hands. The fingers point upwards to the sky, and the right palm will be slightly higher than the left.
- Hold for one minute and then repeat on the other side, changing the crossing of the legs and arms.

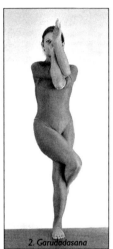 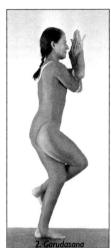

2. Garudasana   2. Garudasana

3. Vrksasana I
vrksa=tree
- Stand in tadasana.
- Lift the right foot and place it as high as possible against the inner left thigh. Extend the right (bent) knee out of the hip joint, down and back, by pressing the heel firmly against the inner left thigh.
- Do not turn the right side of the pelvis backwards. The pelvis should remain straight, facing forward.
- On a mula bandha inhalation lift the arms up over the head. This movement starts with rooting the left foot and performing pada bandha. This movement, traveling upwards through the left leg and the hip joints will elongate them and will activate the mula bandha. Thus the pelvis and trunk are lifted up from the femur heads. The coccyx should remain pointed down to the earth as the lower abdomen moves in and up on the mula bandha inhalation.
- Join the palms of the hands. On each inhalation elongate the left leg further and extend the right thigh further sideways and down out of the right hip joint. Lift the pelvis and lower abdomen so that the hands and arms also go further up. On each exhalation maintain that length of the body.
- Hold for one minute and then repeat on the other side.

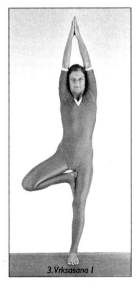

3. Vrksasana I

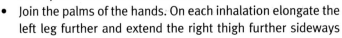

4. Vrksasana II

vrksa=tree

- Stand in tadasana.
- Lift the right foot and place it in the groin of the left leg as for padmasana (see page 71). Extend the right (bent) knee out of the hip joint, down and back, without turning the right side of the pelvis backwards. The pelvis stays straight, facing forward.
- Rotate the right arm around the back and hold the right foot. Do not tilt the pelvis forward, but keep it in a vertical position, and keep the left leg straight.
- On a mula bandha inhalation, lift the left arm up over the head. This movement starts with rooting the left foot and performing pada bandha in the lower spring joint. This movement, traveling upwards through the left leg and the hip joints will elongate them and will activate the mula bandha. Thus the pelvis and trunk are lifted up from the femur heads. The coccyx and the right knee should remain pointed down to the earth as the lower abdomen moves in and up on the mula bandha inhalation.

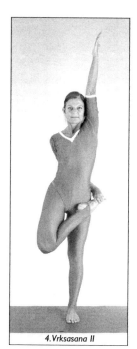

4. Vrksasana II

- On each inhalation elongate the left leg further and extend the right thigh further down out of the right hip joint. Lift the pelvis and lower abdomen so that the left hand also goes further up. On each exhalation maintain that length of the body.
- Hold for one minute and then proceed to 5.

5. Ardha Baddha Padmottanasana

ardha=half; baddha=bound; padma=lotus; uttana=intense stretch

- On an exhalation bend forward, hold the left ankle with the left hand and bring the head to the shin. If the balance is a problem you can keep the left hand on the earth.
- On each mula bandha inhalation lift the pelvis up from the left femur head so that the spine elongates further towards the head.
- On each exhalation slide the head further down on the left shin.

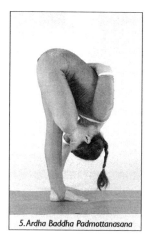

5. Ardha Baddha Padmottanasana

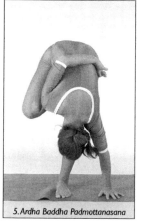

5. Ardha Baddha Padmottanasana

- Hold for one minute, raise the head and trunk on an inhalation and then repeat 4 and 5 on the other side.

6. Vatayanasana

vatayana=horse

- Stand in tadasana.
- Lift the right foot and place it in the groin of the left leg as for padmasana (see page 71). Extend the right (bent) knee out of the hip joint, down and back, without turning the right side of the pelvis backwards. The pelvis stays straight, facing forward.
- On an exhalation bend the trunk forward and place the hands on the earth.

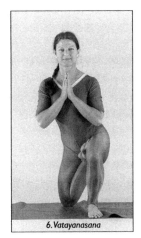
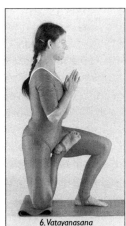

6. Vatayanasana
6. Vatayanasana

- Bend the left knee and place the right knee on the earth behind you in such a way that there is an angle of ninety degrees in the left knee.
- Lift the hands and stand up, balancing on the left foot and the frontal inner edge of the right knee.
- Bring the pelvis and back to a vertical position and rotate the right hip joint forward to come in line with the left one.
- Join the palms of the hands in front of the sternum in namasté I and look straight forward.
- Hold for one minute and then change legs.

7. Utkatasana I

utkata=powerful, fierce

- Stand in tadasana.
- Spread the feet at hip width and, using a mula bandha inhalation, lift the arms up over the head. This movement should start with rooting the feet and performing the pada bandha in the lower spring joints. This movement, traveling upwards through the legs and the hip joints will elongate them and will activate the mula bandha. Thus the pelvis and trunk are lifted up from the femur heads. The coccyx should remain pointed down to the earth as the lower abdomen moves in and up on the mula bandha inhalation.
- Join the palms of the hands. On an inhalation elongate the legs further and lift the pelvis and lower abdomen so that the hands and arms also go further up.
- On the exhalation rotate the pelvis and trunk forward to an inclination of about thirty degrees from the vertical line and bend the knees slowly to an angle of ninety degrees, without changing the inclination of the trunk. The arms stay in line with the trunk.
- Hold for ten seconds and then stand up again.

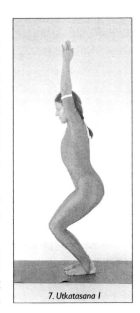

7. Utkatasana I

8. Utthita Trikonasana

utthita=extended; tri=three; kona=angle; trikona=triangle

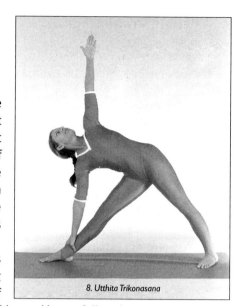

8. Utthita Trikonasana

- Stand in tadasana and spread the legs.
- The distance between the feet is the same as the length of one leg. Turn the left foot forty-five degrees in and the right foot ninety degrees out to the right. The heel of the right foot should be in line with the center of the inner arch of the left foot. Turn the right shin, knee and thigh to face the same direction as the right foot. The pelvis also turns slightly to the right.
- Turn the left shin, knee and thigh out. This lifts the inner knee and ankle of the left leg and brings the weight on the outer edge of the left foot. For the action in the arches, ankles and knees follow the instructions given in tadasana. Root the feet and perform pada bandha on both feet to activate the mula bandha.
- On a mula bandha inhalation elongate both legs and lift the pelvis and trunk up from the femur heads. Lift the arms sideways, in line with the shoulders and parallel to the earth. The palms of the hands face the earth.
- On the exhalation, roll the right side of the pelvis over the right femur head, at the same time extending the right buttock bone towards the left heel. To do this the biceps muscle of the right thigh has to elongate from the knee to the buttock bone. Thus the coccyx points towards the left heel and the right side of the lumbar spine is elongated. Do not turn the left hip bone forward, but keep rolling it out and back.
- As the right buttock bone moves towards the left heel, you have to elongate the whole right side of the body from the groin to the tips of the fingers. Then place the right hand on the right ankle. The right hip bone, waist and lower side ribs should go down faster than the right hand. Do not put any weight on the hand but keep the weight of the body on the pelvis and upper thighs. Keep the outer edge of the heel and the little toe of the left foot firmly on the earth and the left hip bone, thigh, knee and shin rotating outwards.
- The spine should be in line with the line between the feet, and should divide the back in two equal parts. The left and right side of the waist and rib cage should be equally long and parallel to each other.
- Point the left hand straight up towards the sky with the palm facing forward. Keep the head and neck in line with the spine and look up at the left hand.
- On each mula bandha inhalation elongate the body in two opposite directions, splitting in the hip joints. The lower abdomen and spine elongate towards the back of the head, while the right buttock bone, coccyx and left leg extend towards the left heel.
- On each exhalation rotate the left side of the trunk backwards and the left hip bone, thigh, knee and shin outwards. Do not swing the left hand backwards, but keep it pointing straight up towards the sky, and keep the outward rotation of the right thigh and knee.
- Hold for one minute and then proceed to 9.

9. Ardha Chandrasana

ardha=half; chandra=moon

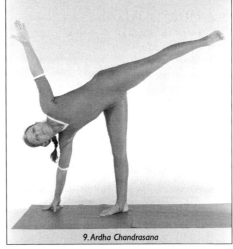
9. Ardha Chandrasana

- On an exhalation bend the right leg and place the right hand on the earth, in line with the feet and about half a meter from the right foot.
- Place the left hand on the left hip, bring the weight of the body forward over the right foot and then straighten the right leg, lifting the left leg up till it is in line with the trunk. The toes point forwards.
- Extend the left arm up and point it straight up to the sky with the palm facing forward. The right arm is parallel to the right leg, so that both the arms are in one line. Keep the head in line with the spine and look up at the left hand. Root the right foot and perform pada bandha to activate the mula bandha.
- On each mula bandha inhalation lift the pelvis up from the right femur head and elongate the body in two opposite directions, splitting in the hip joints. The lower abdomen and spine elongate towards the back of the head, while the coccyx and left leg extend towards the left heel.
- On each exhalation rotate the left side of the trunk backwards and the left hip bone, thigh, knee and shin upwards.
- Do not swing the left hand backwards, but keep it pointing straight up towards the sky, and keep the outward rotation of the right thigh and knee.
- Hold for one minute and then bend the right leg on an exhalation to return to utthita trikonasana (8). Repeat 8 and 9 on the other side.

10. Parsvottanasana

parsva=side, flank;
uttana=intense stretch

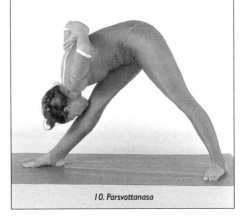
10. Parsvottanasa

- Stand in tadasana and spread the legs.
- The distance between the feet is the same as the length of one leg. Turn the left foot forty-five degrees in and the right foot ninety degrees out to the right. The heel of the right foot should be in line with the heel of the left foot. Turn the right shin, knee and thigh to face the same direction as the right foot. The pelvis also turns slightly to the right.
- Turn the left shin, knee and thigh out. This lifts the inner knee and ankle of the left leg and brings the weight on the outer edge of the left foot. For the action in the arches, ankles and knees follow the instructions given in tadasana. Root the feet and perform pada bandha on both the feet to activate the mula bandha.

- Join the palms on the back in namasté II and press the knuckles of the index fingers together by taking the elbows back.
- On a mula bandha inhalation elongate both legs and lift the pelvis and trunk up from the femur heads. On the exhalation rotate the pelvis and trunk towards the right, rolling over the right femur head, till they face the right foot. The line from hip bone to hip bone across the lower abdomen should be almost perpendicular to the right thigh so that the trunk from the navel upwards faces the same direction as the right foot.
- On a new inhalation lift the pelvis still further up from the femur heads and elongate the biceps muscle of the right thigh from the knee to the buttock bone, extending that bone towards the left heel. On the exhalation bend the trunk forward till the head rests on the right shin.
- On each mula bandha inhalation lift the pelvis up from the right femur head and elongate the body in two opposite directions, splitting in the hip joints. The lower abdomen and spine elongate towards the back of the head, while the right buttock bone, coccyx and left leg extend towards the left heel. On each exhalation slide the head further down on the right shin.
- Keep the elbows raised high and the palms of the hands pressed firmly together.
- Hold for one minute, raise the head and trunk on an inhalation and then repeat on the other side.

11. Parivrtta Trikonasana

parivrtta=turned around; trikona=triangle

- Stand in tadasana and spread the legs.
- The distance between the feet is the same as the length of one leg. Turn the left foot forty-five degrees in and the right foot ninety degrees out to the right. The heel of the right foot should be in line with the heel of the left foot. Turn the right shin, knee and thigh to face the same direction as the right foot. The pelvis also turns slightly to the right.
- Turn the left shin, knee and thigh out. This lifts the inner knee and ankle of the left leg and brings the weight on the

11. Parivrtta Trikonasana

outer edge of the left foot. For the action in the arches, ankles and knees follow the instructions given in tadasana. Root the feet and perform pada bandha on both the feet to activate the mula bandha.
- On a mula bandha inhalation elongate both legs and lift the pelvis and trunk up from the femur heads. Lift the arms sideways, in line with the shoulders and parallel to the earth. The palms of the hands face the earth.
- On the exhalation rotate the pelvis and trunk towards the right, rolling over the right femur head, till they face the right foot. The line from hip bone to hip bone across the lower abdomen should be almost perpendicular to the right thigh, so that the trunk from the navel upwards faces the same direction as the right foot.

- On a new inhalation lift the pelvis and trunk still further up from the femur heads and elongate the biceps muscle of the right thigh from the knee to the buttock bone, extending that bone towards the left heel. Thus the coccyx points towards the left heel and the right side of the lumbar spine is elongated.
- On the exhalation elongate the whole left side of the body from the groin to the tips of the fingers and, rotating the stomach and chest still further towards the right, place the left hand on the right ankle. The left hip bone, waist and lower side ribs should go down faster than the left hand. Do not put any weight on the hand but keep the weight of the body on the pelvis and upper thighs. Keep the outer edge of the heel and the little toe of the left foot firmly on the earth.
- Extend the right arm straight up towards the sky with the palm of the hand facing forward. Keep the head and neck in line with the spine and look up at the right hand.
- The spine should be in line with the line between the feet, and should divide the back in two equal parts. The left and right side of the waist and rib cage should be equally long and parallel to each other.
- On each mula bandha inhalation elongate the body in two opposite directions, splitting in the hip joints. The lower abdomen and spine elongate towards the back of the head, while the right buttock bone, coccyx and left leg extend towards the left heel.
- On each exhalation rotate the right side of the trunk backwards and the right thigh, knee and shin outwards, keeping the inner edge of the right foot on the earth. Do not swing the right hand backwards, but keep it pointing straight up towards the sky, and keep the outward rotation of the left thigh and knee.
- Hold for one minute and then proceed to 12.

12. Parivrtta Ardha Chandrasana

parvrtta=turned around; ardha=half;
chandra=moon

- On an exhalation bend the right leg and place the left hand on the earth, in line with the feet and about half a meter from the right foot.
- Place the right hand on the right hip, bring the weight of the body forward over the right foot and then straighten the right leg, lifting the left leg up till it is in line with the trunk. The toes point down to the earth.
- Extend the right arm upwards, pointing it straight up to the sky with the palm of the hand facing forward. The left arm is parallel to the right leg, so that both the arms are in one line. Keep the head in line with the spine and look up at the right hand. Root the

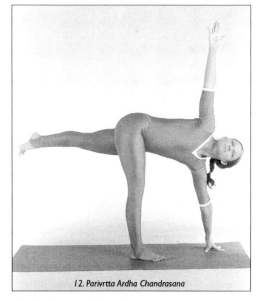

12. Parivrtta Ardha Chandrasana

right foot and perform pada bandha to activate the mula bandha.
- On each mula bandha inhalation lift the pelvis up from the right femur head and

elongate the body in two opposite directions, splitting in the hip joints. The lower abdomen and spine elongate towards the back of the head, while the right buttock bone, coccyx and left leg extend towards the left heel.

- On each exhalation rotate the right side of the trunk backwards and the right thigh, knee and shin outwards, keeping the inner edge of the right foot on the earth. Do not swing the right hand backwards, but keep it pointing straight up towards the sky.
- Hold for one minute and then bend the right leg on an exhalation to return to parivrtta trikonasana (11). Repeat 11 and 12 on the other side.

13. Virabhadrasana II

Virabhadra is the name of a hero

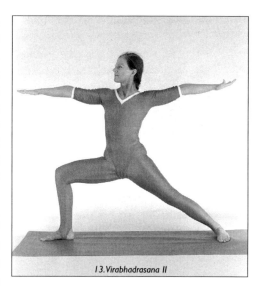

13. Virabhadrasana II

- Stand in tadasana and spread the legs.
- The distance between the feet is one and a half times the length of one leg. Turn the left foot forty-five degrees in and the right foot ninety degrees out to the right. The heel of the right foot should be in line with the center of the inner arch of the left foot. Turn the right shin, knee and thigh to face the same direction as the right foot. The pelvis also turns slightly to the right.
- Turn the left shin, knee and thigh out. This lifts the inner knee and ankle of the left leg and brings the weight on the outer edge of the left foot. For the action in the arches, ankles and knees follow the instructions given in tadasana. Root the feet and perform pada bandha to activate the mula bandha.
- On a mula bandha inhalation elongate both legs and lift the pelvis and trunk up from the femur heads. Lift the arms sideways, in line with the shoulders and parallel to the earth. The palms of the hands face the earth.
- On the exhalation bend the right knee at an angle of ninety degrees, so that the thigh is parallel to the earth. The knee is in line with the right groin and foot and the weight of the body is even on both feet.
- Keep the trunk vertical, at an angle of ninety degrees with the right thigh. On each inhalation elongate the body in opposite directions, splitting in the hip joints. The lower abdomen and spine elongate upwards towards the back of the head, the coccyx and right buttock bone drop further down and the left leg elongates towards the left heel.
- On each exhalation maintain the length of the trunk. Keep the head and neck in line with the spine and look at the right hand.
- Hold for one minute and then proceed to 14.

14.Utthita Parsvakonasana

utthita=extended; parsva=sideways; kona=angle

- On an inhalation elongate the biceps muscle of the right thigh from the knee to the buttock bone and extend that bone towards the left heel, so that the coccyx points towards that heel. At the same time elongate the right side of the body from the right groin to the tips of the fingers and roll the right side of the pelvis over the right femur head.

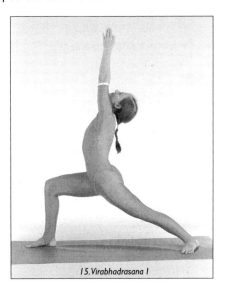
14. Utthita Parsvakonasana

- On the exhalation place the right hand on the earth on the inside of the right foot. The back of the right arm pit rests against the inside of the right knee. Extend the left arm up towards the sky with the palm of the hand facing forward.
- The right hip bone, waist and lower side ribs should go down faster than the right hand and should close with the thigh in the right groin. Do not put any weight on the right hand but keep the weight of the body on the pelvis and upper thighs. Keep the outer edge of the heel and the little toe of the left foot firmly on the earth.
- The spine should be in line with the line between the feet, and should divide the back from the waist upwards in two equal parts. The left and right side of the waist and rib cage should be equally long and parallel to each other. Keep the head and neck in line with the spine and look up at the sky.
- On each mula bandha inhalation elongate the body in two opposite directions, splitting in the hip joints. The lower abdomen and spine elongate towards the back of the head while the right buttock bone, coccyx and left leg extend towards the left heel. On each exhalation rotate the left side of the trunk backwards and the left hip and knee outwards, at the same time keeping the outward rotation of the right thigh and knee.
- Hold for one minute and then repeat 13 and 14 on the other side.

15. Virabhadrasana I

Virabhadra is the name of a hero

- Stand in tadasana and spread the legs.
- The distance between the feet is one and a half times the length of one leg. Turn the left foot forty-five degrees in and the right foot ninety degrees out to the right. The heel of the right foot should be in line with the heel of the left foot. Turn the right shin, knee and thigh to face the same direction as the right foot. The pelvis also turns slightly to the right.
- Turn the left shin, knee and thigh out. This lifts the inner knee and ankle of the left leg and brings the weight on the outer edge of the left foot. For the action in the arches,

15. Virabhadrasana I

ankles and knees follow the instructions given in tadasana.

- On a mula bandha inhalation lift the arms up over the head. This movement should start with rooting the feet and performing pada bandha in the lower spring joints. This movement, traveling upwards through the legs and the hip joints will elongate them and will activate the mula bandha. Thus the pelvis and trunk are lifted up from the femur heads. The coccyx should remain pointed down to the earth as the lower abdomen moves in and up with the mula bandha inhalation.
- Join the palms of the hands. On an inhalation elongate the legs further, lifting the pelvis and lower abdomen so that the hands and arms also go further up.
- On the exhalation rotate the pelvis and trunk towards the right, rolling over the right femur head. The line from hip bone to hip bone across the lower abdomen should be almost perpendicular to the right thigh so that the trunk from the navel upwards faces the same direction as the right foot.
- On a new inhalation lift the pelvis and trunk still further up from the femur heads. On the exhalation bend the right leg to an angle of ninety degrees, so that the thigh is parallel to the earth.
- Keep the heel and little toe of the left foot firmly on the earth and extend the right femur head slightly back towards the left heel, without bending the left knee. In this way the pelvis stays facing in the direction of the right foot.
- Keep the trunk vertical, at an angle of ninety degrees with the right thigh. On each inhalation elongate the body in opposite directions, splitting in the hip joints. The spine and arms elongate upwards, the coccyx and right buttock bone drop further down and the left leg elongates towards the left heel.
- On each exhalation maintain the length of the trunk and rotate the right side of the trunk and the right femur head further backwards.
- Hold for one minute and then proceed to 16.

16. Virabhadrasana III

Virabhadra is the name of a hero

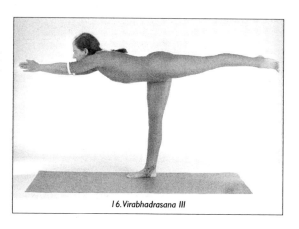

16. Virabhadrasana III

- On a mula bandha inhalation lift the pelvis up from the femur heads. On the exhalation bend forwards and place the trunk on the right thigh.
- Bring the weight of the body forward over the right foot and straighten the right leg, lifting the left leg up till it is in line with the trunk. The toes point down to the earth.
- On each inhalation lighten the weight of the trunk on the right femur head by rooting the right foot and performing pada bandha, and elongate the body in two opposite directions, splitting in the hip joints. The trunk and arms elongate forwards, while the coccyx, the right buttock bone and the left leg extend backward towards the left heel.
- Keep the hands, head, shoulders, spine, hips and left leg on one line, parallel to the earth and look at the hands.

- Hold for ten seconds. On an exhalation bend the right leg and return to virabhadrasana I (15). Repeat 15 and 16 on the other side.

17. Parivrtta Parsvakonasana

parivrtta=turned around;
parsva=sideways; kona=angle

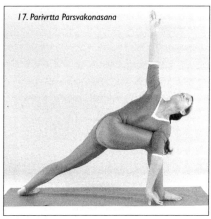

17. Parivrtta Parsvakonasana

- Stand in tadasana and spread the legs.
- The distance between the feet is one and a half times the length of one leg. Turn the left foot forty-five degrees in and the right foot ninety degrees out to the right. The heel of the right foot should be in line with the heel of the left foot. Turn the right shin, knee and thigh to face the same direction as the right foot. The pelvis also turns slightly to the right.
- Turn the left shin, knee and thigh out. This lifts the inner knee and ankle of the left leg and brings the weight on the outer edge of the left foot. For the action in the arches, ankles and knees follow the instructions given in tadasana. Root the feet and perform pada bandha to activate the mula bandha.

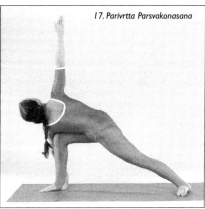

17. Parivrtta Parsvakonasana

- On a mula bandha inhalation elongate the legs and lift the pelvis and trunk up from the femur heads. Lift the arms sideways, in line with the shoulders and parallel to the earth. The palms of the hands face the earth.
- On the exhalation rotate towards the right, rolling over the right femur head. The line from hip bone to hip bone across the lower abdomen should be almost perpendicular to the right thigh, so that the trunk from the navel upwards faces the same direction as the right foot.
- On a new inhalation lift again up from the femur heads and on the exhalation bend the right knee to an angle of ninety degrees, so that the thigh is parallel to the earth. Elongate the biceps muscle of the right thigh from the knee to the buttock bone and extend that bone towards the left heel, so that the coccyx points towards that heel.
- At the same time elongate the whole left side of the body from the left groin to the tips of the fingers and, rotating the stomach and chest still further towards the right, place the left hand on the earth on the outside of the right foot. Turn the arm in the same way as in savasana, so that the back of the left shoulder near the shoulder blade presses against the outside of the right knee. Do not put any weight on the hand but keep the weight of the body on the pelvis and upper thighs. Keep the left heel on the earth. If you cannot do that, lift it just enough to facilitate the rotation of the body, and then put it back on the earth again after reaching the final position.
- The spine should be in line with the line between the feet, and should divide the back from the waist upwards in two equal parts. The left and right side of the waist and rib

cage should be equally long and parallel to each other. Extend the right arm up to the sky with the palm of the hand facing forward. Keep the head and neck in line with the spine and look up at the sky.

- On each mula bandha inhalation elongate the body in two opposite directions, splitting in the hip joints. The lower abdomen and spine elongate towards the back of the head, while the right buttock bone, coccyx and left leg extend towards the left heel.
- On each exhalation rotate the right side of the trunk backwards and the right thigh, knee and shin outwards, keeping the inner edge of the right foot on the earth. At the same time keep the outward rotation of the left thigh and knee and the left heel on the earth.
- Hold for one minute and then repeat on the other side.

18. Utthita Hasta Padangusthasana

utthita=extended; hasta=hand; padangustha=big toe

a. *Holding the foot with the same side hand*

- Stand in tadasana.
- Place the left hand on the hip, bend the right leg and hold the big toe with the index and middle fingers of the right hand. Extend the leg forward and raise it as high as possible, keeping the left leg and the trunk straight. Root the left foot and perform pada bandha to activate the mula bandha.
- On each mula bandha inhalation elongate the left leg and lift the pelvis and trunk up from the left

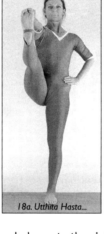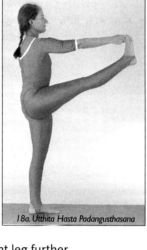

18a. Utthita Hasta...   18a. Utthita Hasta Padangusthasana

femur head. On each exhalation raise and elongate the right leg further.
- Hold for one minute and then proceed to 18b.

b. *Holding the foot with the same side hand and bringing it to the side*

- Take the right foot to the right side.
- On each mula bandha inhalation elongate the left leg and lift the pelvis and trunk up from the left femur head. On each exhalation take the right leg further to the side, without turning the pelvis.
- Hold for ten seconds and then repeat 18a and b on the other side.

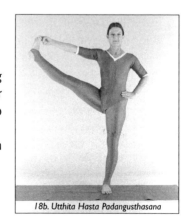

18b. Utthita Hasta Padangusthasana

c. Holding the foot with the opposite hand
- Stand in tadasana.
- Place the right hand on the hip, bend the right leg and hold the ball of the foot with the left hand. Extend the leg forward and raise it as high as possible, keeping the left leg and the trunk straight. Root the left foot and perform pada bandha to activate the mula bandha.
- On each mula bandha inhalation elongate the left leg and lift the pelvis and trunk up from the left femur head. On each exhalation raise the right leg further.
- Hold for one minute and then proceed to 18d.

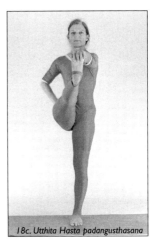

18c. Utthita Hasta padangusthasana

d. Holding the foot with the opposite hand and turning the trunk and head to the side of the raised leg
- On an exhalation turn the trunk and head towards the right till the shoulders are in line with the right leg.
- On each mula bandha inhalation elongate the left leg and lift the pelvis and trunk up from the left femur head. On each exhalation raise and elongate the right leg further and turn the trunk and head further towards the right.

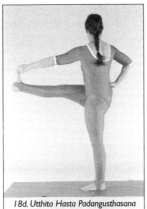

18d. Utthita Hasta Padangusthasana

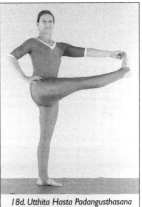

18d. Utthita Hasta Padangusthasana

- Hold for ten seconds and then repeat 18c and d on the other side.

e. Holding the foot with both hands and bringing the head to shin
- Stand in tadasana.
- Bend the right leg and hold the foot with both hands. Extend the leg forward and raise it as high as possible, keeping the left leg and the trunk straight.
- On an exhalation bring the head to the shin, keeping the back as straight as possible. Root the left foot and perform pada bandha to activate the mula bandha.
- On each mula bandha inhalation elongate the left leg and lift the pelvis and trunk up from the left femur head. On each exhalation raise the right leg further.
- Hold for ten seconds and then repeat on the other side.

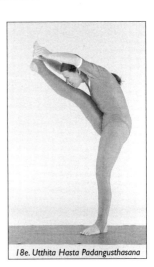

18e. Utthita Hasta Padangusthasana

19. Urdhva Prasarita Ekapadasana

urdhva=above, upwards;
prasarita=extended;
eka=one; pada=leg, foot

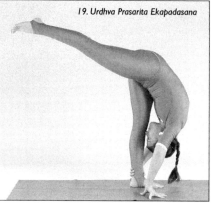

19. Urdhva Prasarita Ekapadasana

- Stand in tadasana.
- On an exhalation bend forward, place the right hand on the earth and lift the right leg up backwards, without turning the right hip back. Keep both legs straight and both hips at the same height.
- Hold the left ankle with the left hand and on an exhalation bring the head to the shin.
- On each mula bandha inhalation lift the pelvis up from the left femur head so that the spine elongates still further towards the head.
- On each exhalation slide the head further down on the left shin.
- Hold for ten seconds and then repeat on the other side.

20. Prasarita Padottanasana

prasarita=spread, extended; pada=leg, foot;
uttana=intense stretch

a. The hands on the earth, the head up

- Stand in tadasana and spread the legs.
- The distance between the feet is one and a half times the length of one leg. Turn both feet slightly in, rooting them and performing pada bandha to activate the mula bandha.
- On a mula bandha inhalation elongate both legs and lift the pelvis and trunk up from the femur heads.

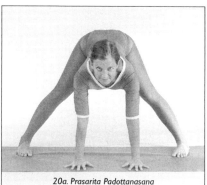

20a. Prasarita Padottanasana

- On the exhalation rotate the pelvis forward and place the hands on the earth in front of you. Keep the arms straight and the fingers pointing forward. Do not put any weight on the hands.
- Keep the hips in line with the feet and lift the head, elongating the back of the thigh upwards towards the sky.
- On each mula bandha inhalation elongate the body in two opposite directions, splitting in the hip joints. The lower abdomen and spine elongate towards the back of the head, while the buttock bones extend backwards.
- Hold for one minute and then proceed to 20b.

b. The hands and head on the earth in between the feet

- Elongating the back of the thighs still further upwards, place the hands and head in between the feet on the earth. The hands are at shoulder width and the fingers point straight forwards. The elbows are in line with the hands and armpits.
- The distance between the feet should be such that the head barely touches the earth. If the distance is too short, the back will bend.
- Hold for one minute and then proceed to 20c.

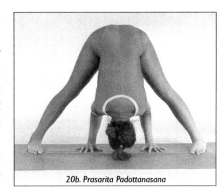

20b. Prasarita Padottanasana

c. Holding the ankles with the hands, keeping the head on the earth in between feet

- Hold the outer ankles with the hands, keeping the hips in line with the feet and the head on the earth in between the feet.
- Hold for one minute and then proceed to 20d.

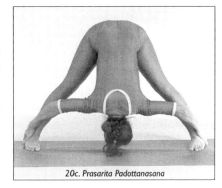

20c. Prasarita Padottanasana

d. Namasté II, the head on the earth in between the feet

- On an inhalation raise the head and trunk. Join the palms on the back in namasté II and press the knuckles of the index fingers together by taking the elbows back.
- On the exhalation take the head down again in between the feet. Keep the elbows up towards the sky and the palms of the hands firmly pressed together.
- Hold for one minute and then come up on an inhalation.

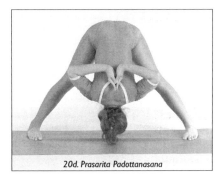

20d. Prasarita Padottanasana

21. Padangusthasana

padangustha=big toe

a. *The head up*

- Stand in tadasana.
- On a mula bandha inhalation elongate the legs and lift the trunk and pelvis up from the femur heads. On the exhalation rotate the pelvis forward and hold the big toes with the index and middle fingers of both hands.
- On each inhalation lift the head and chest further up, so that the arms are straight and the spine is elongated.
- Hold for one minute and then proceed to 21b.

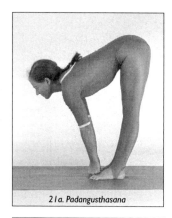

21a. Padangusthasana

b. *The head on the shins*

- On an exhalation bend the arms and rest the head on the shins.
- Hold for one minute and then come up on an inhalation.

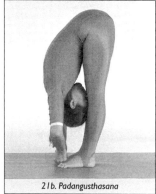

21b. Padangusthasana

22. Padahastasana

pada=leg, foot; hasta=hand

a. *The head up*

- Stand in tadasana.
- On a mula bandha inhalation elongate the legs and lift the trunk and pelvis up from the femur heads. On the exhalation rotate the pelvis forward and place the hands underneath the soles of the feet.
- On each inhalation lift the head and chest further up, so that the arms are straight and the spine is elongated.
- Hold for one minute and then proceed to 22b.

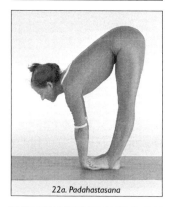

22a. Padahastasana

b. *The head on the shins*

- On an exhalation bend the arms and rest the head on the shins.
- Hold for one minute and then come up on an inhalation.

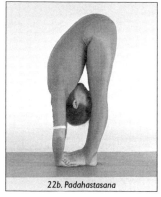

22b. Padahastasana

23. Uttanasana

uttana=intense stretch

a. The hands on the earth, the head up
- Stand in tadasana.
- On a mula bandha inhalation elongate the legs and lift the trunk and pelvis up from the femur heads. On the exhalation rotate the pelvis forward and place the hands next to the feet on the earth.
- On each inhalation lift the head and chest further up so that the arms are straight and the spine is elongated.
- Hold for one minute and then proceed to 23b.

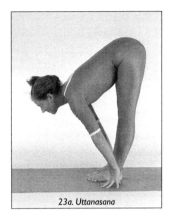

23a. Uttanasana

b. The hands on the earth, the head on the shins
- On an exhalation take the hands further back and rest the head on the shins.
- Hold for one minute and then proceed to 23c.

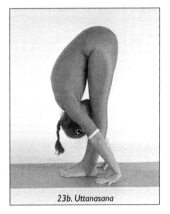

23b. Uttanasana

c. Holding the ankles, the head on the shins
- On an exhalation hold the hands behind the ankles.
- Hold for one minute and then come up on an inhalation.

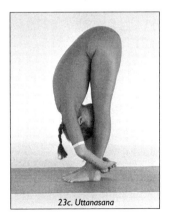

23c. Uttanasana

Part 4 Sitting Poses

Sitting Poses			
a.	Padmasana cycle	c.	Virasana cycle
b.	Vajrasana cycle	d.	Baddha Konasana cycle

Padmasana
padma=lotus

Technique
Do not try to do the full position right away, but work through the intermediate poses sukhasana and siddhasana. Many people damage their knees in this pose, because they force them. The knees are one of the most delicate joints of the body, and if they are damaged, it is usually for life, not temporarily as with other parts of the body. So work slowly, without force; pain, especially here, is a danger signal.

The legs
Sit with your legs cross-legged. This position is called **sukhasana** or the *easy pose.* Take the right foot in both hands, holding it from underneath, and lift it as high as you can (picture 5a (1)). The right hand supports the ankle and the left hand the arch. Turn the sole of the foot towards your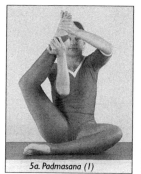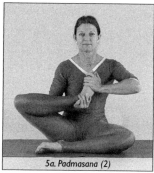

5a. Padmasana (1)

5a. Padmasana (2)

face, at face level, and rotate the knee forwards as much as you can. Keeping the head up and the back as straight as possible, bring the arch of the foot to the forehead, rotating the leg in the hip joint, *not* in the knee. Turn the sole of the foot towards you as if you want to read it: the more you turn it, the more the leg rotates in the right hip joint. At the same time rotate the right knee forward.

After touching the forehead, lower the foot and place the sole lengthwise on the sternum (picture 5a (2)); then lower it completely and place it in the left groin. The right knee rests on the left foot. This position is called siddhasana or the pose of the siddha (an accomplished yogi).

If the right knee does not reach the left foot, practice bringing it down, until it rests on it with ease. Then proceed. Before lifting the left leg to cross it over the right, lean the body backwards, till you are balancing on the back of the buttock bones. Then lift the left foot up in the same way as the right one, holding the hands underneath the foot, with the left hand supporting the ankle and the right hand the arch (picture 5a (3)). Lift the foot up to face level and turn the sole of the foot towards you. Then place it length-wise on the sternum, so that the leg rotates in the left hip rather than in the knee. Finally, lower the foot and place it in the right groin (picture

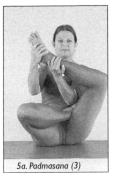
5a. Padmasana (3)

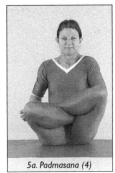
5a. Padmasana (4)

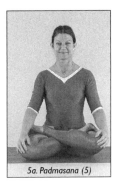
5a. Padmasana (5)

5a (4)). Then bring the body forward again so that the knees come down to the earth (picture 5a (5)). This position is called **padmasana** or the *lotus pose*. Both knees point forward at an angle of about forty-five degrees, and the left shin is crossed over the right. Try to bring the left knee down as well.

The pelvis

Pull the buttock muscles sideways and backwards with the hands, so that you sit on the points of the buttock bones, not on the flesh. The weight of the trunk is evenly distributed between the buttock bones, so that the pelvis is straight, not tilted to one side. Check the two frontal hip bones with your fingers: they should be equally high and evenly forward. The shoulder joints are in line with the hip joints, so that the trunk is at right angles to the earth; thus the weight of the trunk is transmitted to the buttock bones in a straight line. The body balances finely tuned on the gravitational line in order to sit with lightness and ease, it should not lean forward nor backward. If the body leans backward, it hangs from the frontal muscles in order not to fall over backwards; if the body leans forward, the muscles in the back are tensed in order to keep the body from falling forwards. With the spine aligned on the gravitational line, the body does not need much effort to keep straight. This means that the frontal side and the backside of the body are parallel to each other.

Keeping these joints in line, the next step, as in tadasana, is to assess the position of the pelvis. Here too, the pelvis can assume three positions. The correct one is the neutral position, in which the pelvis is vertical: the trunk rests on the points of the buttock bones, making an angle of ninety degrees with the thighs in the hip joints, and the two frontal hip bones are in vertical alignment with the groins. This position is quite rare. With most people the pelvis is rotated backwards and the trunk rests on the back of the buttock bones, or even on the coccyx.

This causes the whole back to bend, forcing the spinal vertebrae out of alignment, so that neither the spine nor the pelvis makes an angle of ninety degrees with the thighs in the hip joints. With some over-supple people, on the other hand, one sees the opposite: the pelvis is rotated too far forward, with the result that the lumbar spine curves in too much. In this case the pelvis makes an angle of less than ninety degrees with the thighs in the hip joints, and the muscles of the abdomen lose their tone; at the same time, as the coccyx is tipped back and up in the direction of the lumbar spine, the muscles in the lower back become short, narrow and tight.

You can check the position of the pelvis in the following way. Choose an outer corner where two walls meet, and sit with the back against it, resting the sacrum and the back of the head against it. If the lumbar and thoracic spine touch the corner, instead of the sacrum, the pelvis is rotated backwards: this causes the whole spinal column to bend. If, on the other hand, only the sacrum is in contact with the corner and there is a wide gap in the small of the back, between the waist and the corner, the pelvis is rotated too far forwards: this causes the lumbar spine to curve in too much. In both cases the pelvis has to be brought to a vertical position. When the pelvis is vertical, the trunk rests on the points of the buttock bones and the two frontal hip bones are in line with the groins; the spine is aligned on the corner and leaves only a space of about one inch between the lumbar spine and the corner.

Then, action has to be brought into the sacro-iliac joints. Constrict the tensor fascia lata and the adductors of the thighs slightly inwards towards each other, keep the two frontal hip bones in line with the groins and lift them up towards the ribs, so that they move forward into the arches of the feet. At the same time, root the coccyx by making the movement of counter-nutation of the sacrum and coccyx in relation to the pelvis: the coccyx roots down into the earth and moves forwards towards the pubic bone; simultaneously the upper rim of the sacrum moves also forwards. As a result of these movements, the sacro-iliac joints open, the sacrum becomes vertical, and moves forwards into the space between the two ilea, thus wedging them slightly apart. The entire pelvis widens laterally, moves vertically forwards against the femur heads and lifts up from the femur heads. As the distance between the two frontal hip bones widens, the lower abdomen moves in and up towards the navel; this tones the muscles of the lower abdomen and strengthens the internal organs. At the same time, the lumbar spine moves back to come almost in line with the, now vertical, sacrum.

As described in tadasana, the result of these movements is that the body is centered in the center of gravity (in the pelvis); do not collapse the chest or the abdominal area between the navel and the lower ribs. Keeping the shoulder joints in line with the hip joints, root the buttock bones and on each mula bandha inhalation, elongate the spinal column upwards, and on each exhalation maintain the height of the body. Do not bend the spine in the thoracic and lumbar area: the groove of the spine should be even, from base to top, and run straight upwards.

In the action of rebouncing, something has to go down for something else to go up. For example, when you jump, the feet push down onto the earth; they go down heavily with the force of gravity, so that the rest of the body can move up against gravity (the Normal Force of Newton). To get the rebounce action in the pelvis, the outer hips and inner thighs have to constrict inwards towards each other, and the buttock bones and coccyx have to root into the earth, going down with the force of gravity. Thus the rest of the pelvis, the lower abdomen and the trunk can move up against gravity, rebouncing the weight of the body back up. The only muscles that are actively used are the tensor fascia lata, the adductors and the muscles in the lower abdomen. The rest of the body – the solar plexus, chest and shoulders – are relaxed.

Most of us live from the waist up, while the trunk, from the waist down, is forgotten. The area below the navel should be full, and the trunk from the navel upwards should be empty. When the pelvis rebounces the weight of the body back upwards, the spinal vertebrae continue that movement, the trunk should not sag into the pelvis. Negating gravity, the spine elongates upwards, so that the trunk is light.

When you practice this on an outer corner between two walls, the sacrum and back of the head are in contact with the corner, but not the thoracic vertebrae. Without pushing the chest forward, you have to move the thoracic vertebrae into the body.

To open the upper part of the chest, do as follows:
a. Keep the ears in line with the shoulder and hip joints.
b. Keep the lower ribs down and in.
c. Elongate the neck up, as if balancing a book on the head. Keep the face vertical, do not tilt the chin up.

As described in tadasana, the spine should show an even groove, from the sacrum to the first thoracic vertebra, and should be straight: draw the spine upwards, out of the muscular periphery of the body, like drawing a sword out of its scabbard. Keep the hands loosely folded in front of the lower abdomen on the shins, or, palms facing up, on the knees, without putting any weight on them. The arms hang passively from the shoulder joints, and the shoulders and shoulder blades widen laterally and move down towards the waist. The head balances evenly on the spinal column: if it moves too far forward, the muscles at the back of the upper trunk and neck will be tense to prevent it from falling forwards. Keep the ears in line with the shoulder joints and hip joints, and the face vertical; do not push the chin up, but do not pull it in too much either. The cervical spine also follows the gravitational line, so that the neck elongates upwards. Change the crossing of the legs; then repeat the pose on the other side.

The above description is the physically technical description of how to sit straight, holding the body lightly up from the center of gravity, with the spine erect. The beauty of the body is when it is light. Everybody knows how to be heavy, but find out how light the body can be. This lightness depends only on the skeleton, not on the muscles. The body is light when the skeletal frame lifts up, and the muscles hang loosely from this frame: keeping the spine on the central gravitational line of the body, the muscular system has to relax: muscles relaxed, skeleton firm. Shift the weight of your awareness onto the back of the body – not the physical weight of your body, but the internal weight of your awareness. People do not realize that awareness, consciousness, has bulk and weight. It can move around and throw light on different areas of the body. Usually the internal weight of the awareness is on the frontal side of the body, on the face, the throat, the sternum, the solar plexus, creating tensions. This is where we feel most at home, and thus the neck and shoulders are pulled forwards chronically, and the back stoops. Moving the internal weight backwards automatically straightens and elongates the body, and releases the tensions at the frontal side of the body. This does not mean, however, that the spine bends backwards; rather, the spine is straight, and the internal weight 'leans' against the spine. This automatically broadens the whole back, and this, in turn, allows the spine to elongate upwards. In this action there is no muscular effort involved.

You can do the same thing in the region of the head and neck. Here too we usually keep all the tensions on the frontal side, especially on the face. This drags the head and neck forward. Moving the internal weight backwards, from the face into the back of the head and neck, will bring the head automatically in alignment with the chest. The neck broadens and elongates, without any muscular effort, so that the head comes out of the trunk like a turtle drawing its head out of its shell; when the turtle pulls its head out, the shell stays where it is. So here too, the chest stays where it is when the head elongates upwards through internal weight shifting. Try to experiment with the feeling of making an 'X-ray' of your body, keeping the skeletal structure sharply outlined, but both the muscular structure and the skin in a semi-transparent state. Then, in that semi-transparent state, carefully and deliberately expand the Energy Body, the Body of Light, till it transcends the skin.

4a Padmasana cycle

These positions can be done in *four different modes*:

a. **Performing each position separately** and holding it for one minute. To release the knees, you can do one minute of paschimottanasana in between poses.

b. *Vinyasa*
Connecting *two or more positions* by flowing from one into the other, using the breathing.

c. *Mala*
Connecting *all the positions* through surya namaskar, using the breathing, and holding each of the padmasana poses for the duration of three breaths.

d. **Taking only a few positions** and holding them for *five minutes* each. Here too you can release the knees by doing one minute of paschimottanasana in between poses.

Padmasana cycle

1. *Sukhasana*
2. *Lolasana*
3. *Swastikasana*
4. *Siddhasana*
5. *Padmasana*
   a. *Padmasana*
   b. *Parvatasana*
   c. *Gomukhasana*
   d. *Namasté II*
6. *Yoga Mudrasana I*
   a. *Supta Parvatasana*
   b. *Supta Gomukhasana*
   c. *Supta Namasté II*
7. *Supta Padmasana*

8. *Matsyasana I*
   a. *Matsyasana I*
   b. *Paryankasana I*
   c. *Paryankasana II*
9. *Matsyasana II*
   a. *Adhomukha Matsyasana II*
   b. *Urdhvamukha Matsyasana II*
10. *Parivrtta Padmasana*
11. *Tolasana*
12. *Kukkutasana*
13. *Garbha Pindasana*
14. *Goraksasana*
15. *Baddha Padmasana*
16. *Yoga Mudrasana II*

1. Sukhasana

sukha=easy

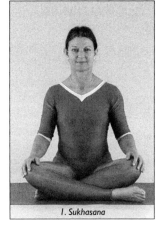

I. Sukhasana

- Sit on a blanket with the legs crossed. In all the following positions the thighs are in an exorotation position in the hip joints.
- Pull the buttock muscles backwards with the hands, so that you are sitting on the buttock bones, not on the flesh. The body weight is divided evenly between the buttock bones.
- The pelvis is in a vertical position, with the two frontal hip bones in vertical alignment above the groins. The groove of the spine is even from base to top, and runs straight upwards. Place the hands on the thighs.
- Root the two buttock bones, the coccyx and the pubic bone into the earth with the support of the pada bandha.
- On each mula bandha inhalation, elongate the spinal column upwards. On each exhalation, maintain the height of the body.
- Hold for one minute; then change the crossing of the legs.

2. Lolasana

lola=dangling

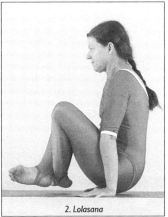

2. Lolasana

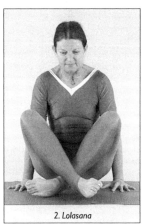

2. Lolasana

- Sit in sukhasana (1) and then proceed:
- Place the hands next to the hips on the blanket, with the fingers pointing forwards.
- On an exhalation, lift the whole body up, supporting yourself only on the hands, till the arms are straight.
- Root the hands into the earth, and perform hasta bandha to elongate the arms. Pull the knees up towards the abdomen and look straight forward.
- Hold for ten seconds; then change the crossing of the legs.

3. Swastikasana
swastika=auspicious

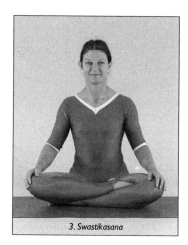

3. Swastikasana

- Sit in sukhasana (1) and then proceed:
- Widen the knees and lift one foot up. Insert the toes, pointing downwards, between the calf and biceps muscle of the other leg, turning the heel upwards.
- Pull the buttock muscles backwards with the hands, so that you are sitting on the buttock bones, not on the flesh. The body weight is divided evenly between the buttock bones.
- The pelvis is in a vertical position, with the two frontal hip bones in vertical alignment above the groins. The groove of the spine is even from base to top, and runs straight upwards. Place the hands on the thighs.
- On each mula bandha inhalation, root the buttock bones, the coccyx and the pubic bone into the earth, with the support of the pada bandha, and elongate the spinal column upwards. On each exhalation, maintain the height of the body.
- Hold for one minute; then change the crossing of the legs.

4. Siddhasana
siddha=sage

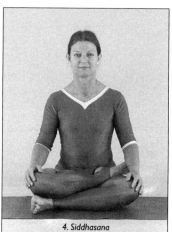

4. Siddhasana

- Sit in sukhasana (1) and then proceed:
- Lift the right foot up as described in padmasana (see page 72) and place it in the groin of the left leg, turning the sole of the foot upwards. In this pose the knees are closer together than in the previous one, and the right knee rests on the left foot.
- Pull the buttock muscles backwards with the hands, so that you are sitting on the buttock bones, not on the flesh. The body weight is divided evenly between the buttock bones.
- The pelvis is in a vertical position, with the two frontal hip bones in vertical alignment above the groins. The groove of the spine is even from base to top, and runs straight upwards. Place the hands on the thighs.
- Root the two buttock bones, the coccyx and the pubic bone into the earth with the support of the pada bandha.
- On each mula bandha inhalation, elongate the spinal column upwards. On each exhalation, maintain the height of the body.
- Hold for one minute; then change the crossing of the legs.

5. Padmasana

padma=lotus

5a. Padmasana

- For a complete explanation of this pose, see page 72.

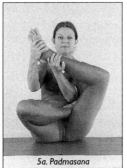

5a. Padmasana

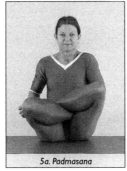

5a. Padmasana

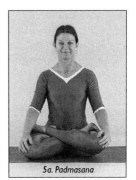

5a. Padmasana

5b. Parvatasana

parvata=mountain

- Sit in siddhasana (4) or padmasana (5) and then proceed:
- On a mula bandha inhalation, raise the arms over the head. Rooting the buttock bones, the coccyx and the pubic bone into the earth with the support of the pada bandha, constrict the outer hips and inner thighs inwards towards each other, and lift the pelvis and trunk up from the femur heads (mula bandha).
- Keep the front and back of the trunk parallel to each other, and the hands, shoulder joints and hip joints in vertical alignment.
- Clasp the hands over the head and turn the palms facing upwards, extending the knuckles of the fingers up to the sky.
- Hold for one minute; then change the crossing of the feet and the interlock of the hands.

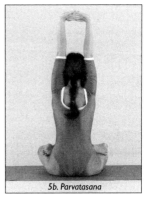

5b. Parvatasana

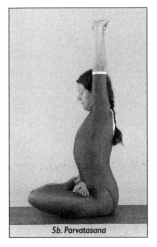

5b. Parvatasana

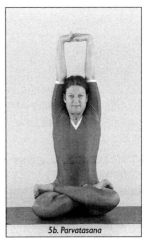

5b. Parvatasana

5c. Gomukhasana

go=cow; mukha=face

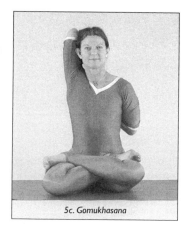

5c. Gomukhasana

- Sit in siddhasana (4) or padmasana (5) and then proceed:
- Elongate the left arm sideways and bring the hand onto the back in a circular movement. With the thumb and index finger of the right hand clasp the left wrist, push the left hand away from the back, and then up in between the shoulder blades, so that the knuckle of the little finger of the left hand rests on the spine.
- On a mula bandha inhalation, elongate the right arm up over the head, out of the right hip joint. On the exhalation, bend the elbow and clasp the left hand on the back. Keep the inner upper arm next to the ear. On each inhalation, elongate the right elbow further up, so that the hand can go further down.
- Take the left elbow back, but do not push the ribs forward. Keep the frontal ribs down and in, and the lower abdomen in and up.

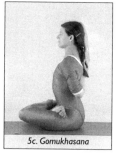

5c. Gomukhasana

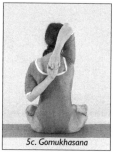

5c. Gomukhasana

- Hold for one minute; then change hands and the crossing of the feet.

5d. Namasté II

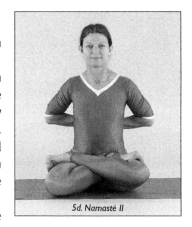

5d. Namasté II

- Sit in siddhasana (4) or padmasana (5) and then proceed:
- Elongate both arms forward, and then take them back in a circular movement to join the palms at the back. Bend the elbows, turn the fingers so that they point to the spine, and then turn them upwards. Slide the edge of the little fingers up on the spine, till the hands are in between the shoulder blades. Join the palms of the hands firmly together by taking the elbows back.
- Roll the shoulders and upper arms back, so that the shoulder blades go down and the knuckles of the index fingers are pressed together.
- Do not push the ribs forward, but keep the frontal ribs down and in, and the lower abdomen in and up.
- Hold for one minute; then release the arms and change the crossing of the feet.

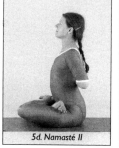

5d. Namasté II

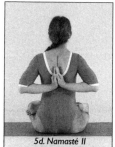

5d. Namasté II

6. Yoga Mudrasana I

mudra=closing, sealing

In poses 6 and 7 and their variations, the pelvis is rotated forward around the femur heads as in forward bendings.

6a. Supta Parvatasana
supta=lying down;
parvata=mountain

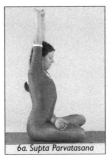
6a. Supta Parvatasana
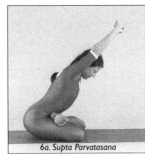
6a. Supta Parvatasana

- Sit in parvatasana (5b) and then proceed:
- On a mula bandha inhalation, lift the pelvis and trunk up from the femur heads, rooting the buttock bones into the earth with the support of the pada bandha. On the exhalation, bend forward till the whole trunk, from the groins to the sternum, rests on the crossed legs, and the head and hands rest on the blanket.

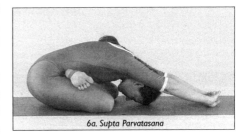
6a. Supta Parvatasana

- The trunk arrives on the legs before the head and hands arrive on the blanket. Do not lift the buttock bones up, but extend them backwards, spreading them at the same time so that the lumbar spine moves in.
- On each inhalation, extend the groins, the buttock bones and the back of the thighs further backwards. At the same time, elongate the lower abdomen, rib cage, spine, head and hands further forwards.
- On each exhalation, lower the trunk and head further with gravity onto the legs and earth.
- Hold for one minute; then come up on an inhalation, and change the crossing of the legs.

6b. Supta Gomukhasana
supta=lying down; go=cow; mukha=face

- Sit in gomukhasana (5c) and then proceed:
- On a mula bandha inhalation, lift the pelvis and trunk up from the femur heads, rooting the buttock bones into the earth with the

6b. Supta Gomukhasana

support of the pada bandha. On the exhalation, bend forward till the whole trunk, from the groins to the sternum, rests on the crossed legs and the head rests on the blanket.
- The trunk arrives on the legs before the head arrives on the blanket. Do not lift the buttock bones up, but extend them backwards, spreading them at the same time, so that the lumbar spine moves in.

- On each inhalation, extend the groins, the buttock bones and the back of the thighs further backwards. At the same time elongate the lower abdomen, rib cage, spine and head further forwards.
- On each exhalation, lower the trunk and head further with gravity onto the legs and earth, keeping both elbows up towards the sky.
- Hold for one minute. Then come up on an inhalation, raising first the head, then the chest, and then the abdomen. Change hands and the crossing of the legs.

6c. *Supta Namasté II*
supta=lying down

- Sit in namasté II (5d) and then proceed:
- On a mula bandha inhalation, lift the pelvis and trunk up from the femur heads, rooting the buttock bones into the earth with the support of the pada bandha. On the exhalation, bend forward till the whole trunk, from the groins to the sternum, rests on the crossed legs, and the head rests on the blanket.

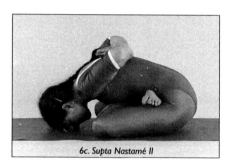
6c. Supta Nastamé II

- The trunk arrives on the legs before the head arrives on the blanket. Do not lift the buttock bones up, but extend them backwards, spreading them at the same time so that the lumbar spine moves in.
- On each inhalation, extend the groins, the buttock bones and the back of the thighs further backwards. At the same time, elongate the lower abdomen, rib cage, spine and head further forwards.
- On each exhalation, lower the trunk and head further with gravity onto the legs and earth, keeping the elbows up towards the sky.
- Hold for one minute. Then come up on an inhalation, raising first the head, then the chest, and then the abdomen. Change the crossing of the legs.

7. Supta Padmasana
supta=lying down; padma=lotus

This is yoga mudrasana I (6) performed while lying on the back, so the same rules apply.

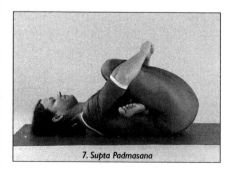
7. Supta Padmasana

- Sit in siddhasana (4) or padmasana (5) and then proceed:
- Keep the hands behind you on the blanket and, lifting the pelvis, so that you are standing on the knees, rotate it backwards, so that the coccyx rolls towards the pubic bone and the two frontal hip bones move up towards the ribs. Then lower yourself onto the elbows, and finally onto the blanket.
- Bring the knees to the chest and clasp the arms around the crossed knees.

- On each mula bandha inhalation, elongate the groins, the buttock bones and the back of the thighs backwards, away from the trunk, and the lower abdomen and rib cage forwards towards the head.
- The mula bandha inhalation always starts in the lower abdomen. Zigzagging along the spinal column through the kidney region (widening that region) and the upper chest (lifting the upper ribs), it ends up in the back of the head. Thus the back of the head is elongated away from the shoulders, and the groins are elongated away from the lower abdomen. The whole back rests evenly on the blanket, and the sacro-iliac joints, kidneys and shoulder blades are widened.
- Roll the shoulders back to the earth. On each inhalation, elongate the spinal column further, and on each exhalation, flatten the back further onto the blanket.
- Hold for one minute; then change the crossing of the legs.

8. Matsyasana I

matsya=fish

In poses 8 and 9 and their variations, the pelvis is rotated backwards around the femur heads as in back bendings.

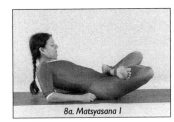

8a. Matsyasana I

8a. Matsyasana I

- Sit in siddhasana (4) or padmasana (5) and then proceed:
- Keep the hands behind you on the blanket and, lifting the pelvis, so that you are standing on the knees, rotate it backwards, so that the coccyx rolls towards the pubic bone and the two frontal hip bones move up towards the ribs. Then lower yourself onto the elbows, and finally onto the blanket. Keep the knees down.

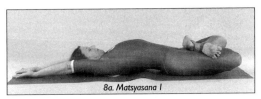

8a. Matsyasana I

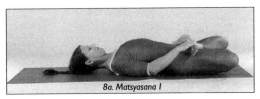

8a. Matsyasana I

- Keep the backward rotation of the pelvis, so that the lower abdomen moves in the direction of the ribs, and slide the back of the chest up in the direction of the head. In this way the whole lumbar region is elongated and brought down onto the blanket.
- Extend the thighs out of the groins, and pull the two frontal hip bones up towards the ribs: double action, down and up, so that the groins in the middle are opened.
- On a mula bandha inhalation, extend the arms over the head on the blanket, without curving the lumbar up.
- On each inhalation, extend the thighs further downwards, out of the hip joints, and the spine and arms further upwards.
- On each exhalation, press the lumbar further onto the blanket, maintaining the length of the body.
- Hold for one minute; then proceed to 8b.

8b. Paryankasana I
paryanka=couch

- Place the elbows next to the trunk on the blanket and hold the arches of the feet with the hands.
- Arch the back and chest, and rest the crown of the head on the blanket.
- Hold for thirty seconds; then proceed to 8c.

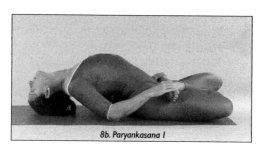
8b. Paryankasana I

8c. Paryankasana II

- Clasp the elbows over the head and elongate the upper arms out of the shoulders, so that the elbows go further down to the earth.
- Hold for thirty seconds; then change the crossing of the legs and repeat 8a, b and c.

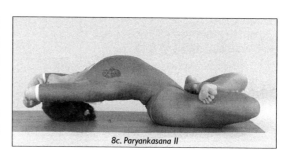
8c. Paryankasana II

9. Matsyasana II
matsya=fish

9a. Adhomukha Matsyasana II
adho=downwards;
mukha=face;
matsya=fish

This is basically the same position as matsyasana I (8a), performed upside down, so the same rules apply.

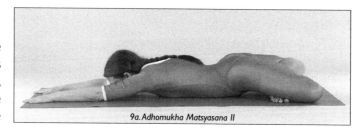
9a. Adhomukha Matsyasana II

- Sit in padmasana (5) and then proceed:
- Stand up on your knees and then lower yourself forward onto the stomach. Pull the two frontal hip bones up towards the rib cage, so that the lumbar spine elongates, and extend the thighs backwards out of the groins: double action forwards and backwards, so that the groins in the middle are opened.
- Keep the backward rotation of the pelvis, so that the lower abdomen moves in the direction of the ribs, and pull the chest in the direction of the head.
- Extend the arms over the head on the blanket and rest on the forehead.
- Hold for one minute; then proceed to 9b.

9b. *Urdhvamukha Matsyasana II*
urdhva=upwards; mukha=face;
matsya=fish

- Bend the arms. Place the hands and lower arms next to the head on the blanket, and raise the head and chest till you are resting on the bent elbows.

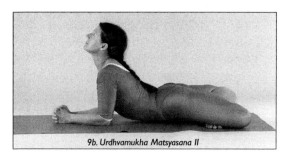
9b. Urdhvamukha Matsyasana II

- On each mula bandha inhalation, pull the lower abdomen further forwards towards the rib cage, and the ribs towards the head. Then straighten the elbows. The back is arched as in bhujangasana I (see page 209).
- Hold for one minute; then change the crossing of the legs and repeat 9a and b.

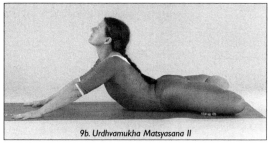
9b. Urdhvamukha Matsyasana II

10. Parivrtta Padmasana
parivrtta=turned around; padma=lotus

- Sit in padmasana (5) with the right foot crossed over the left. The knees should be fairly close together, so that both feet stick out on the sides of the thighs.
- On a mula bandha inhalation, elongate the right arm up to the sky. Lift the pelvis up from the femur heads and elongate the whole body upwards, rooting the buttock bones and the knees into the earth.
- On the exhalation, rotate the trunk towards the right, swing the right arm around the back and hold the right foot. Curl the toes of the foot around the fingers, so that the foot holds the hand as much as the hand the foot.

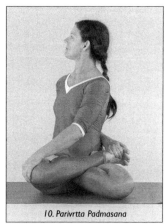
10. Parivrtta Padmasana

- Place the left hand on the right knee and turn the head towards the right.
- On each mula bandha inhalation, elongate the spinal column further upwards, rooting the buttock bones and the knees.
- On each exhalation, rotate the trunk, chest, shoulders and head further towards the right, till the chest and shoulders are perpendicular to the line between the knees.
- Hold for one minute; then change the crossing of the legs.

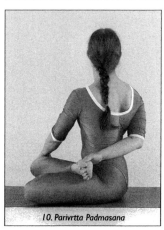
10. Parivrtta Padmasana

11. Tolasana

tola=a pair of scales

- Sit in padmasana (5).
- Place the hands next to the thighs on the blanket, with the fingers pointing forwards.
- On an exhalation, lift the whole body up from the blanket, supporting yourself only on the hands, till the arms are straight. Root the hands into the earth, performing hasta bandha to elongate the arms.
- Pull the knees up towards the ribs with the support of the pada bandha, and look straight forward.
- Hold for ten seconds; then change the crossing of the legs.

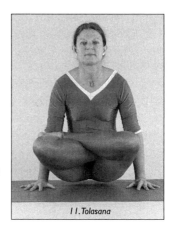

11.Tolasana

12. Kukkutasana

kukkuta=cock

- Sit in padmasana (5).
- Lift the knees up and insert the lower arms in the triangular spaces between the dorsal side of the feet, the calf muscles and the thigh muscles. Place the hands on the blanket, with the fingers pointing forwards.
- On an exhalation, lift the whole body up from the blanket, supporting yourself only on the hands, till the arms are straight. Root the hands into the earth, performing hasta bandha to elongate the arms.
- Pull the knees up towards the ribs with the support of the pada bandha, and look straight forward.
- Hold for ten seconds; then proceed to 13.

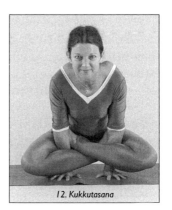

12. Kukkutasana

13. Garbha Pindasana

garbha=womb;
pinda=embryo

- Lower the buttock bones onto the earth again. Lift the crossed knees, and slide the arms still further through the legs so that the elbows also go through.
- Then bend the elbows and bring the hands to the ears, balancing the

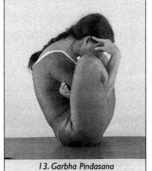

13. Garbha Pindasana

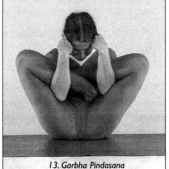

13. Garbha Pindasana

body only on the buttock bones. The spine is bent and the head is brought forward to the knees.

- Hold for ten seconds; then change the crossing of the legs and repeat 12 and 13.

14. Goraksasana

Goraksa=cowherd

This is basically the same pose as matsyasana I (8a), so the same rules apply.

- Sit in padmasana (5).
- Push up till you are standing on the knees.
- Lift the hands up from the blanket, till the thighs and trunk are vertical and you are balancing only on the knees.
- Join the palms of the hands in front of the sternum in namasté I and look straight forward.
- Hold for ten seconds; then change the crossing of the legs.

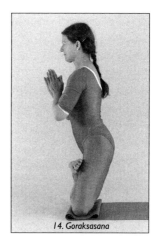

14. Goraksasana

15. Baddha Padmasana

baddha=bound; padma=lotus

- Sit in padmasana (5). To perform this pose, the knees have to be very close together.
- Wrap the arms around the back and hold the feet, the right hand holding the right foot and the left hand holding the left foot. Hold the top (left) foot first and then the bottom (right) one.
- Hold for thirty seconds; then proceed to 16.

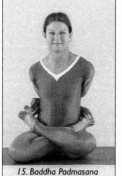

15. Baddha Padmasana

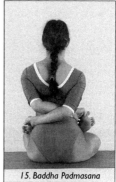

15. Baddha Padmasana

16. Yoga Mudrasana II

mudra=closing, sealing

- On a mula bandha inhalation, lift the pelvis and trunk up from the femur heads, rooting the buttock bones into the earth with the support of the pada bandha. On the exhalation, bend forward till the whole trunk, from the groins to the sternum, rests on the crossed legs and the head rests on the blanket.
- The trunk arrives on the legs before the head

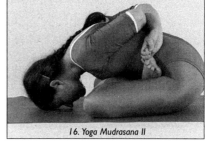

16. Yoga Mudrasana II

 arrives on the blanket. Do not lift the buttock bones up, but extend them backwards, spreading them at the same time, so that the lumbar spine moves in.
- On each inhalation, extend the groins, the buttock bones and the back of the thighs further backwards. At the same time, elongate the lower abdomen, rib cage, spine and head further forwards.
- On each exhalation, lower the trunk and head further with gravity onto the legs and earth.
- Hold for thirty seconds. Then come up on an inhalation, raising first the head, then the chest, and then the abdomen. Change the crossing of the legs and the arms and repeat 15 and 16.

4b Vajrasana cycle

These positions can be done in *four different modes*:

a. **Performing each position separately** and holding it for one minute. To release the knees, you can do one minute of paschimottanasana in between poses.

b. *Vinyasa*
Connecting two or more positions by flowing from one into the other, using the breathing.

c. *Mala*
Connecting all the positions through surya namaskar, using the breathing, and holding each of the vajrasana poses for the duration of three breaths.

d. **Taking only a few positions** and holding them for *five minutes* each. Here too you can release the knees by doing one minute of paschimottanasana in between poses.

Vajrasana cycle

1. Vajrasana I
   a. Vajrasana I
   b. Parvatasana
   c. Gomukhasana
   d. Namasté II
2. Vajrasana II
   a. Vajrasana II
   b. Supta Parvatasana
   c. Supta Gomukhasana
   d. Supta Namasté II
3. Supta Vajrasana
   a. Dvipada Supta Vajrasana
   b. Ekapada Supta Vajrasana
4. Utkatasana II

---

1. Vajrasana I

vajra=thunderbolt, the weapon of Indra

1a. Vajrasana I

- Kneel on a blanket with the knees and feet together, and then sit down on the heels, keeping the heels united. This is a neutral position of the thighs in the hip joints. Make sure that the feet and knees are even.
- Pull the buttock muscles backwards with the hands, so that the buttock bones are above the arches, not on the heels. The body weight is divided evenly between the heels.
- The pelvis is in a vertical position, with the two frontal hip bones in vertical alignment above the groins. The groove of the spine is even from base to top, and runs straight upwards. Place the hands on the thighs.
- On each mula bandha inhalation, root the shins and the back of the feet into the earth, with the support of the pada bandha, and elongate the spinal column upwards. On each exhalation, maintain the height of the body.
- Hold for one minute.

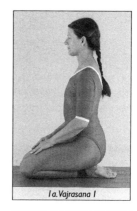
1a. Vajrasana I

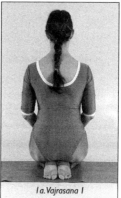
1a. Vajrasana I

1b. Parvatasana

parvata=mountain

- Sit in vajrasana I (1a) and then proceed:
- On a mula bandha inhalation, raise the arms over the head. Rooting the shins and the back of the feet into the earth with the support of the pada bandha, and the buttock bones into the heels, constrict the outer hips and inner thighs inwards towards each other, and lift the pelvis and trunk up from the femur heads (mula bandha).
- Keep the front and back of the trunk parallel to each other, and the hands, shoulder joints and hip joints in vertical alignment.

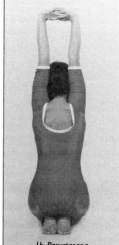
1b. Parvatasana   *1b. Parvatasana*

- Clasp the hands over the head and turn the palms facing upwards, extending the knuckles of the fingers up to the sky.
- Hold for one minute; then change the interlock of the hands.

1c. Gomukhasana
go=cow; mukha=face

- Sit in vajrasana I (1a) and then proceed:
- Elongate the left arm sideways and bring the hand onto the back in a circular movement. With the thumb and index finger of the right hand clasp the left wrist, push the left hand away from the back, and then up in between the shoulder blades, so that the knuckle of the little finger of the left hand rests on the spine.
- On a mula bandha inhalation, elongate the right arm up over the head, out of the right hip joint. On the exhalation, bend the elbow and clasp the left hand on the back. Keep the inner upper arm next to the ear. On each inhalation, elongate the right elbow further up, so that the hand can go further down.
- Take the left elbow back, but do not push the ribs forward. Keep the frontal ribs down and in, and the lower abdomen in and up.
- Hold for one minute; then change hands.

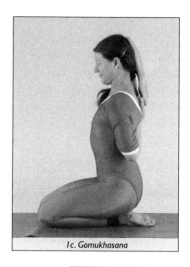

1c. Gomukhasana

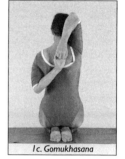

1c. Gomukhasana

1d. Namasté II

- Sit in vajrasana I (1a) and then proceed:
- Elongate both arms forward, and then take them back in a circular movement to join the palms at the back. Bend the elbows, turn the fingers so that they point to the spine, and then turn them upwards. Slide the edge of the little fingers up on the spine, till the hands are in between the shoulder blades. Join the palms of the hands firmly together by taking the elbows back.
- Roll the shoulders and upper arms back, so that the shoulder blades go down, and the knuckles of the index fingers are pressed together.
- Do not push the ribs forward, but keep the frontal ribs down and in, and the lower abdomen in and up.
- Hold for one minute; then release the arms.

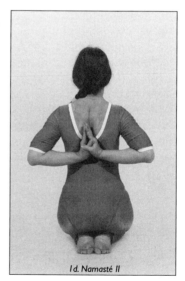

1d. Namasté II

2. Vajrasana II

In pose 2 through 4 and their variations, the pelvis is rotated forward around the femur heads as in forward bendings.

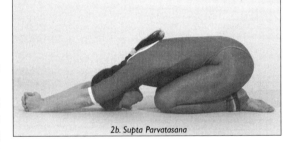

2a. Vajrasana II

2a. Virasana II

- Sit in vajrasana I (1a), hold the heels with the hands, and then proceed:
- On a mula bandha inhalation, lift the pelvis and trunk up from the femur heads, rooting the buttock bones into the heels, the shins and the back of the feet into the earth with the support of the pada bandha. On the exhalation, bend forward till the whole trunk, from the groins to the sternum, rests on the thighs, and the head rests on the blanket.
- The trunk arrives on the thighs before the head arrives on the blanket. Do not lift the buttock bones up from the heels, but extend them backwards, spreading them at the same time so that the lumbar spine moves in.
- On each inhalation, extend the buttock bones and the back of the thighs further backwards. At the same time elongate the lower abdomen, rib cage, spine and head further forwards.
- On each exhalation, lower the trunk and head further with gravity onto the thighs and earth.
- Hold for one minute; then come up on an inhalation, raising first the head, then the chest, and then the abdomen.

2b. Supta Parvatasana
   supta=lying down;
   parvata=mountain

- Sit in parvatasana (1b) and then proceed:
- On a mula bandha inhalation, lift the pelvis and trunk up from the femur heads, rooting the buttock bones into the heels, and the shins and the back of the feet into the earth with the support of the pada bandha. On the exhalation, bend forward till the whole trunk, from the groins to the sternum, rests on the thighs, and the head and hands rest on the blanket.

2b. Supta Parvatasana

- The trunk arrives on the thighs before the head and hands arrive on the blanket. Do not lift the buttock bones up from the heels, but extend them backwards, spreading them at the same time so that the lumbar spine moves in.
- On each inhalation, extend the groins, the buttock bones and the back of the thighs further backwards. At the same time elongate the lower abdomen, rib cage, spine, head and hands further forwards.
- On each exhalation, lower the trunk and head further with gravity onto the thighs and earth.
- Hold for one minute; then come up on an inhalation.

2c. *Supta Gomukhasana*
*supta=lying down; go=cow;
mukha=face*

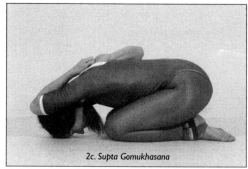
2c. Supta Gomukhasana

- Sit in gomukhasana (1c) and then proceed:
- On a mula bandha inhalation, lift the pelvis and trunk up from the femur heads, rooting the buttock bones into the heels, and the shins and the back of the feet into the earth with the support of the pada bandha. On the exhalation, bend forward till the whole trunk, from the groins to the sternum, rests on the thighs, and the head rests on the blanket.
- The trunk arrives on the thighs before the head arrives on the blanket. Do not lift the buttock bones up, but extend them backwards, spreading them at the same time, so that the lumbar spine moves in.
- On each inhalation, extend the buttock bones and the back of the thighs further backwards. At the same time elongate the lower abdomen, rib cage, spine and head further forwards.
- On each exhalation, lower the trunk and head further with gravity onto the thighs and earth, keeping both elbows up towards the sky.
- Hold for one minute. Then come up on an inhalation, raising first the head, then the chest, and then the abdomen. Change hands.

2d. *Supta Namasté II*
supta=lying down

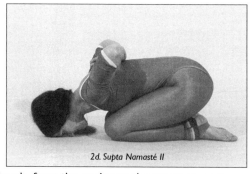
2d. Supta Namasté II

- Sit in namasté II (1d) and then proceed:
- On a mula bandha inhalation, lift the pelvis and trunk up from the femur heads, rooting the buttock bones into the heels, and the shins and the back of the feet into the earth with the support of the pada bandha. On the exhalation, bend forward till the whole trunk, from the groins to the sternum, rests on the thighs, and the head rests on the blanket.
- The trunk arrives on the thighs before the head arrives on the blanket. Do not lift the buttock bones up, but extend them backwards, spreading them at the same time so that the lumbar spine moves in.
- On each inhalation, extend the buttock bones and the back of the thighs further backwards. At the same time elongate the lower abdomen, rib cage, spine and head further forwards.
- On each exhalation, lower the trunk and head further with gravity onto the thighs and earth, keeping the elbows up towards the sky.
- Hold for one minute; then come up on an inhalation, raising first the head, then the chest, and then the abdomen.

3. Supta Vajrasana

supta=lying down

3a. Dvipada Supta Vajrasana

*dvi=two; pada=leg,foot; supta=lying
down; vajra=thunderbolt, the weapon of
Indra*

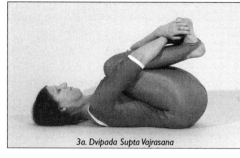

3a. Dvipada Supta Vajrasana

This is vajrasana II (2a) performed while
lying on the back, so the same rules apply.

- Lie on the back on the blanket. Bend
  the legs and bring the knees to the chest.
- Clasp the knees between the crossed arms and hold the feet, the right hand holding
  the outer edge of the left foot and the left hand the outer edge of the right foot.
- On each mula bandha inhalation, elongate the groins, the buttock bones and the back
  of the thighs backwards, away from the trunk, and the lower abdomen and rib cage
  forwards towards the head.
- The mula bandha inhalation always starts in the lower abdomen. Zigzagging along the
  spinal column through the kidney region (widening that region) and the upper chest
  (lifting the upper ribs), it ends up in the back of the head. Thus the back of the head is
  elongated away from the shoulders, and the groins are elongated away from the lower
  abdomen. The whole back rests evenly on the blanket, and the sacro-iliac joints,
  kidneys and shoulder blades are widened.
- Roll the shoulders back to the earth. On each inhalation, elongate the spinal column
  further, and on each exhalation, flatten the back further onto the blanket.
- Hold for one minute; then change the crossing of the arms.

3b. Ekapada Supta Vajrasana

*eka=one; pada=leg, foot;
supta= lying down;
vajra=thunderbolt,
the weapon of Indra*

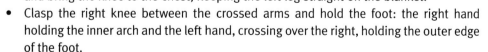

3b. Ekapada Supta Vajrasana

This is basically the same
position as the previous one,
performed with one leg only,
so the same rules apply.

- Lie on the back on the
  blanket. Bend the right leg
  and bring the knee to the chest, keeping the left leg straight on the blanket.
- Clasp the right knee between the crossed arms and hold the foot: the right hand
  holding the inner arch and the left hand, crossing over the right, holding the outer edge
  of the foot.
- On each mula bandha inhalation, elongate the right groin, the right buttock bone and
  the back of the right thigh backwards, away from the trunk, and the lower abdomen
  and rib cage forwards towards the head.
- The mula bandha inhalation always starts in the lower abdomen. Zigzagging along the
  spinal column through the kidney region (widening that region) and the upper chest
  (lifting the upper ribs), it ends up in the back of the head. Thus the back of the head

is elongated away from the shoulders, and the right groin is elongated away from the lower abdomen. The whole back rests evenly on the blanket, and the sacro-iliac joints, kidneys and shoulder blades are widened.

- Roll the shoulders back to the earth. On each inhalation, elongate the spinal column further, and on each exhalation, flatten the back further onto the blanket.
- Hold for one minute; then change legs and the crossing of the arms.

4. Utkatasana II
utkata=powerful, fierce

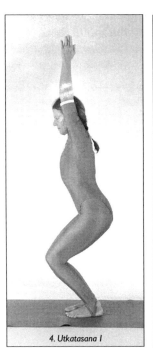 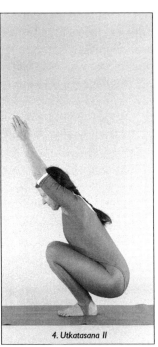

4. Utkatasana I   4. Utkatasana II

This is basically the same position as supta parvatasana (2b) performed while squatting, so the same rules apply.

- Stand in tadasana.
- On a mula bandha inhalation, elongate the arms up over the head. On the exhalation, proceed to utkatasana I (see page 57), inclining the trunk forwards at an angle of about thirty degrees.
- Inhale, and on the next exhalation bend the knees completely and squat down. Keep the inner knees together, and the heels on the earth. The arms form one continuous line with the chest and pelvis, and the trunk is now inclined forwards at an angle of forty-five degrees.
- Root the feet into the earth and perform pada bandha to support the action in the pelvis.
- On each mula bandha inhalation, elongate the buttock bones and the back of the thighs backwards, away from the trunk, and at the same time the lower abdomen, rib cage, spine, head and hands up towards the sky.
- On each exhalation, maintain that height.
- Hold for one minute; then stand up again.

4c Virasana cycle

These positions can be done in *four different modes*:

a. *Performing each position separately* and holding it for one minute. To release the knees, you can do one minute of paschimottanasana in between poses.

b. *Vinyasa*
Connecting two or more positions by flowing from one into the other, using the breathing.

c. *Mala*
Connecting all the positions through surya namaskar, using the breathing, and holding each of the virasana poses for the duration of three breaths.

d. *Taking only a few positions* and holding them for *five minutes* each. Here too you can release the knees by doing one minute of paschimottanasana in between poses

---

Virasana cycle

1. *Virasana I*
    a. *Virasana I*
    b. *Parvatasana*
    c. *Gomukhasana*
    d. *Namasté II*
    e. *Upavistha Virasana I*

2. *Virasana II*
    a. *Virasana II*
    b. *Supta Parvatasana*
    c. *Supta Gomukhasana*
    d. *Supta Namasté II*
    e. *Upavistha Virasana II*

3. *Supta Virasana*
    a. *Dvipada Supta Virasana*
    b. *Ekapada Supta Virasana*
    c. *Paryankasana I*
    d. *Paryankasana II*

4. *Bhekasana*

---

1. Virasana I

vira=hero

1a. Virasana I

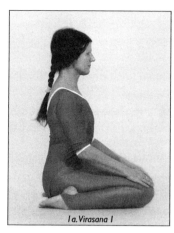

1a. Virasana I

- Kneel down on a blanket with the knees together and the feet spread. Sit down in between the feet, turning the calf muscles out: this is an endorotation of the thighs in the hip joints. Make sure that the feet and knees are even.
- With the fingers, turn the toes one by one towards the coccyx, so that the inner (big) arches of the feet follow the outer contours of the hips, and the big toes form a continuous line with the curve of the arches.
- Pull the buttock muscles backwards with the hands, so that you are sitting on the buttock bones, not on the flesh. The body weight is divided evenly between the buttock bones.
- The pelvis is in a vertical position, with the two frontal hip bones in vertical alignment above the groins. The groove of the spine is even, from base to top, and runs straight upwards. Place the hands on the thighs.
- On each mula bandha inhalation, root the buttock bones, the shins and the back of the feet into the earth, with the support of the pada bandha, and elongate the spinal column upwards. On each exhalation, maintain the height of the body.
- Hold for one minute.

1b. Parvatasana

parvata=mountain

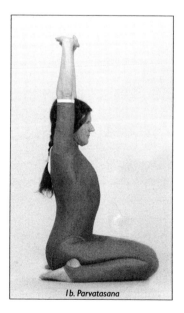

1b. Parvatasana

- Sit in virasana I (1a) and then proceed:
- On a mula bandha inhalation, raise the arms over the head. Rooting the buttock bones, the shins and the back of the feet into the earth with the support of the pada bandha, constrict the outer hips and inner thighs inwards towards each other, and lift the pelvis and trunk up from the femur heads (mula bandha).
- Keep the front and back of the trunk parallel to each other, and the hands, shoulder joints and hip joints in vertical alignment.
- Clasp the hands over the head and turn the palms facing upwards, extending the knuckles of the fingers up to the sky.
- Hold for one minute; then change the interlock of the hands.

1c.   Gomukhasana

go=cow; mukha=face

- Sit in virasana I (1a) and then proceed:
- Elongate the left arm sideways and bring the hand onto the back in a circular movement. With the thumb and index finger of the right hand clasp the left wrist, push the left hand away from the back, and then up in between the shoulder blades, so that the knuckle of the little finger of the left hand rests on the spine.
- On a mula bandha inhalation, elongate the right arm up over the head, out of the right hip joint. On the exhalation, bend the elbow and clasp the left hand on the back. Keep the inner upper arm next to the ear. On each inhalation, elongate the right elbow further up, so that the hand can go further down.

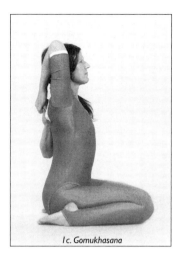

1c. Gomukhasana

- Take the left elbow back, but do not push the ribs forward. Keep the frontal ribs down and in, and the lower abdomen in and up.
- Hold for one minute; then change hands.

1d.   Namasté II

- Sit in virasana I (1a) and then proceed:
- Elongate both arms forward, and then take them back in a circular movement to join the palms at the back. Bend the elbows, turn the fingers so that they point to the spine, and then turn them upwards. Slide the edge of the little fingers up on the spine, till the hands are in between the shoulder blades. Join the palms of the hands firmly together by taking the elbows back.
- Roll the shoulders and upper arms back, so that the shoulder blades go down and the knuckles of the index fingers are pressed together.
- Do not push the ribs forward, but keep the frontal ribs down and in, and the lower abdomen in and up.

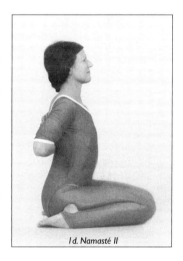

1d. Namasté II

- Hold for one minute; then release the arms.

1e. Upavistha Virasana I
upavistha=seated; vira=hero

This is a variation of virasana I (1a). In this pose the knees are spread and the tips of the big toes touch each other at the back, close to the coccyx. The inner arches of the feet adhere to the backside of the buttocks, and the big toes form a continuous line with the curve of the arches. Do not sit on the heels, but in front of them on the earth. For the rest follow the instructions given for virasana I (1a).

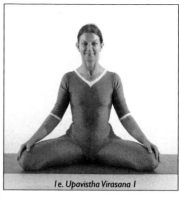
1e. Upavistha Virasana I

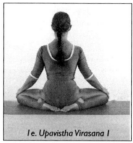
1e. Upavistha Virasana I

2. Virasana II

In pose 2 and its variations, the pelvis is rotated forward around the femur heads as in forward bendings.

2a. Virasana II
- Sit in virasana I (1a), hold the heels with the hands, and then proceed:
- On a mula bandha inhalation, lift the pelvis and trunk up from the femur heads, rooting the buttock bones, the shins and the back of the feet into the earth with the

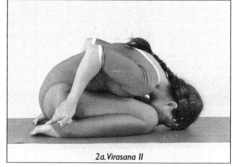
2a. Virasana II

support of the pada bandha. On the exhalation, bend forward till the whole trunk, from the groins to the sternum, rests on the thighs, and the head rests on the blanket.
- The trunk arrives on the thighs before the head arrives on the blanket. Do not lift the buttock bones up, but extend them backwards, spreading them at the same time so that the lumbar spine moves in.
- On each inhalation, extend the groins, the buttock bones and the back of the thighs further backwards. At the same time elongate the lower abdomen, rib cage, spine and head further forwards.
- On each exhalation, lower the trunk and head further with gravity onto the thighs and earth.
- Hold for one minute; then come up on an inhalation, raising first the head, then the chest, and then the abdomen.

2b. Supta Parvatasana

supta=lying down;
parvata=mountain

- Sit in parvatasana (1b) and then proceed:
- On a mula bandha inhalation, lift the pelvis and trunk up from the femur heads, rooting the buttock bones, the shins and the back of the feet into the

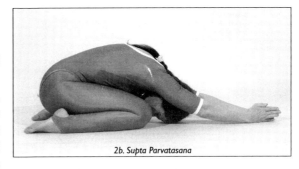

2b. Supta Parvatasana

earth with the support of the pada bandha. On the exhalation, bend forward till the whole trunk, from the groins to the sternum, rests on the thighs, and the head and hands rest on the blanket.
- The trunk arrives on the thighs before the head and hands arrive on the blanket. Do not lift the buttock bones up, but extend them backwards, spreading them at the same time so that the lumbar spine moves in.
- On each inhalation, extend the groins, the buttock bones and the back of the thighs further backwards. At the same time elongate the lower abdomen, rib cage, spine, head and hands further forwards.
- On each exhalation, lower the trunk and head further with gravity onto the thighs and earth.
- Hold for one minute; the   me up on an inhalation.

2c. Supta Gomukhasana

supta=lying down; go=cow;
mukha=face

- Sit in gomukhasana (1c) and then proceed:
- On a mula bandha inhalation, lift the pelvis and trunk up from the femur heads, rooting the buttock bones, the

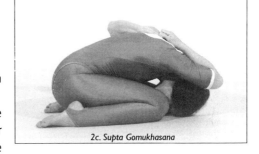

2c. Supta Gomukhasana

shins and the back of the feet into the earth with the support of the pada bandha. On the exhalation, bend forward till the whole trunk, from the groins to the sternum, rests on the thighs, and the head rests on the blanket.
- The trunk arrives on the thighs before the head arrives on the blanket. Do not lift the buttock bones up, but extend them backwards, spreading them at the same time, so that the lumbar spine moves in.
- On each inhalation, extend the groins, the buttock bones and the back of the thighs further backwards. At the same time elongate the lower abdomen, rib cage, spine and head further forwards.
- On each exhalation, lower the trunk and head further with gravity onto the thighs and earth, keeping both elbows up towards the sky.
- Hold for one minute. Then come up on an inhalation, raising first the head, then the chest, and then the abdomen. Change hands.

2d. *Supta Namasté II*
supta=lying down

- Sit in namasté II (1d) and then proceed:
- On a mula bandha inhalation, lift the pelvis and trunk up from the femur heads, rooting the buttock bones, the shins and the back of the feet into the earth with the support of the pada bandha. On the exhalation, bend

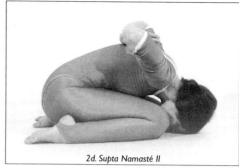

2d. Supta Namasté II

forward till the whole trunk, from the groins to the sternum, rests on the thighs, and the head rests on the blanket.
- The trunk arrives on the thighs before the head arrives on the blanket. Do not lift the buttock bones up, but extend them backwards, spreading them at the same time so that the lumbar spine moves in.
- On each inhalation, extend the groins, the buttock bones and the back of the thighs further backwards. At the same time elongate the lower abdomen, rib cage, spine and head further forwards.
- On each exhalation, lower the trunk and head further with gravity onto the thighs and earth, keeping the elbows up towards the sky.
- Hold for one minute; then come up on an inhalation, raising first the head, then the chest, and then the abdomen.

2e. *Upavistha Virasana II*
upavistha=seated;
vira=hero

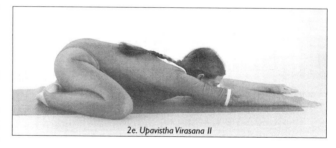

2e. Upavistha Virasana II

- Sit in upavistha virasana I (1e) and proceed:
- On a mula bandha inhalation, lift the pelvis and trunk up from the femur heads, rooting the buttock bones, the shins and the back of the feet into the earth with the support of the pada bandha. On the exhalation, bend forward till the chest and head rest on the blanket in between the thighs. Extend the arms forwards on the blanket.
- Do not lift the buttock bones up, but extend them backwards, spreading them at the same time so that the lumbar spine moves in.
- On each inhalation, extend the groins and buttock bones further backwards. At the same time elongate the lower abdomen, rib cage, spine, head and arms further forwards.
- On each exhalation, lower the trunk and head further with gravity onto the earth.
- Hold for one minute; then come up on an inhalation.

3. Supta Virasana

In pose 3 and its variations, the pelvis is rotated backwards around the femur heads as in back bendings.

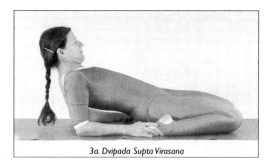
3a. Dvipada Supta Virasana

3a. Dvipada Supta Virasana
supta=lying down; vira=hero

- Sit in virasana I (1a) and then proceed:
- Keep the hands behind you on the blanket and, lifting the pelvis so that you are standing on the shins, rotate the pelvis backwards, so that the coccyx rolls towards the pubic bone and the two frontal hip bones move up towards the ribs. Then lower yourself onto the elbows, and finally onto the blanket. Keep the knees together and down.
- Keep the backward rotation of the pelvis, so that the lower abdomen moves in the direction of the ribs, and slide the back of the chest

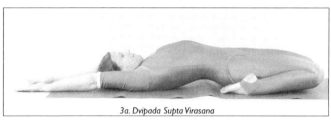
3a. Dvipada Supta Virasana

upwards in the direction of the head. In this way the whole lumbar region is elongated and brought down towards the blanket.
- Extend the thighs out of the groins and pull the two frontal hip bones up towards the ribs: double action down and up, so that the groins in the middle are opened.
- On a mula bandha inhalation, extend the arms over the head on the blanket, without curving the lumbar up.
- On each inhalation, extend the thighs further downwards out of the hip joints, and the spine and arms further upwards.
- On each exhalation, press the lumbar further towards the blanket, maintaining the length of the body.
- Hold for one minute; then proceed to 3b.

3b. Ekapada Supta Virasana
eka=one; pada=leg, foot;
supta=lying down; vira=hero
- Unfold the right leg and extend it up to the sky, holding it with both hands.
- Hold for thirty seconds; then change legs.

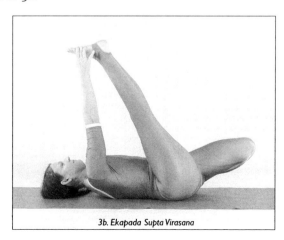
3b. Ekapada Supta Virasana

3c. *Paryankasana I*
paryanka=couch

- Lie down in supta virasana (3a) and then proceed:
- Place the elbows next to the trunk on the blanket, and hold the arches of the feet with the hands.
- Arch the back and chest and rest the crown of the head on the blanket.
- Hold for thirty seconds; then proceed to 3d.

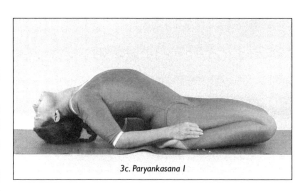

3c. Paryankasana I

3d. *Paryankasana II*

- Clasp the elbows over the head and elongate the upper arms out of the shoulders, so that the elbows go further down to the earth.
- Hold for thirty seconds.

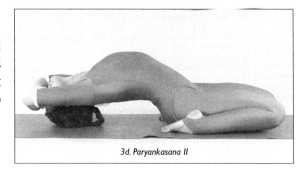

3d. Paryankasana II

4. **Bhekasana**
bheka=frog

This is paryankasana I (3c) performed while lying on the stomach.

- Lie down on the stomach on the blanket and fold the legs as in virasana I (1a)
- Place the hands on the dorsal side of the feet, with the fingers pointing forward and the

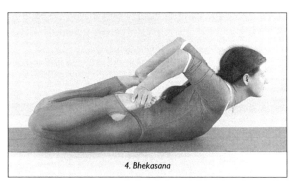

4. Bhekasana

elbows pointing up towards the sky (like locust legs). Push the feet down and raise the head and chest up.
- Hold for a few seconds.

4d Baddha Konasana cycle

These positions can be done in four different modes:

a. **Performing each position separately** and holding it for one minute. To release the knees, you can do one minute of paschimottanasana in between poses.

b. **Vinyasa**
Connecting two or more positions by flowing from one into the other, using the breathing.

c. **Mala**
Connecting all the positions through surya namaskar, using the breathing, and holding each of the baddha konasana poses for the duration of three breaths.

d. **Taking only a few positions** and holding them for *five minutes* each. Here too you can release the knees by doing one minute of paschimottanasana in between poses

<table>
<tr><td colspan="2" align="center">*Baddha Konasana cycle*</td></tr>
<tr><td>

1. *Baddha Konasana I*
    a. *Baddha Konasana I*
    b. *Parvatasana*
    c. *Gomukhasana*
    d. *Namasté II*

2. *Baddha Konasana II*
    a. *Baddha Konasana II*
    b. *Supta Parvatasana*
    c. *Supta Gomukhasana*
    d. *Supta Namasté II*

</td><td>

3. *Kandasana*

4. *Mulabandhasana*

5. *Supta Baddha Konasana*

</td></tr>
</table>

1. Baddha Konasana I

baddha=bound; kona=angle

In all the following positions the thighs are in an exorotation position in the hip joints.

1a. *Baddha Konasana I*

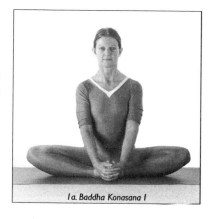

- Sit on a blanket with the knees spread sideways and the soles of the feet united. Hold the feet with the hands and pull the heels as close to the pubic bone as possible. Bring the knees down to the blanket by extending the thighs sideways out of the hip joints.
- Pull the buttock muscles backwards with the hands, so that you are sitting on the buttock bones, not on the flesh. The body weight is divided evenly between the buttock bones. Then hold the feet with the hands again.

1a. Baddha Konasana I

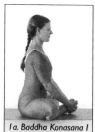

- The pelvis is in a vertical position, with the two frontal hip bones in vertical alignment above the groins. The groove of the spine is even from base to top and runs straight upwards. On each mula bandha inhalation, root the buttock bones and the outer edges of the feet into the earth with the support of the pada bandha, and elongate the spinal column upwards. On each exhalation, maintain the height of the body.

1a. Baddha Konasana I

- Hold for one minute.

1b. *Parvatasana*

parvata=mountain

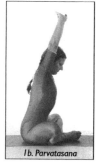

- Sit in baddha konasana I (1a) and then proceed:
- On a mula bandha inhalation, raise the arms over the head. Rooting the buttock bones and the outer edges of the feet into the earth with the support of the pada bandha, constrict the outer hips inwards towards each other, extend the thighs and knees sideways out of the hip joints, and lift the pelvis and trunk up from the femur heads (mula bandha).

1b. Parvatasana

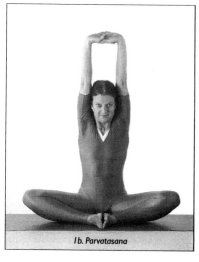

- Keep the front and back of the trunk parallel to each other, and the hands, shoulder joints and hip joints in vertical alignment.
- Clasp the hands over the head and turn the palms facing upwards, extending the knuckles of the fingers up to the sky.
- Hold for one minute; then change the hands interlock.

1b. Parvatasana

1c. Gomukhasana
go=cow; mukha=face

- Sit in baddha konasana I (1a) and then proceed:
- Elongate the left arm sideways and bring the hand onto the back in a circular movement. With the thumb and index finger of the right hand clasp the left wrist, push the left hand away from the back, and then up, in between the shoulder blades, so that the knuckle of the little finger of the left hand rests on the spine.

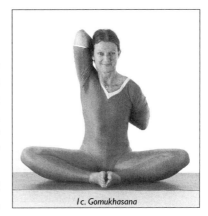

I c. Gomukhasana

- On a mula bandha inhalation, elongate the right arm up over the head, out of the right hip joint. On the exhalation, bend the elbow and clasp the left hand on the back. Keep the inner upper arm next to the ear. On each inhalation, elongate the right elbow further up, so that the hand can go further down.

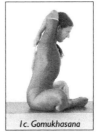

I c. Gomukhasana

- Take the left elbow back, but do not push the ribs forward. Keep the frontal ribs down and in, and the lower abdomen in and up.
- Hold for one minute; then change hands.

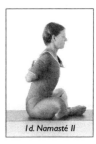

I d. Namasté II

1d. Namasté II

- Sit in baddha konasana I (1a) and then proceed:
- Elongate both arms sideways and then take them back in a circular movement to join the palms at the back. Bend the elbows, turn the fingers so that they point to the spine, and then turn them upwards. Slide the edge of the little fingers up on the spine, till the hands are in between the shoulder blades. Join the palms of the hands firmly together by taking the elbows back.

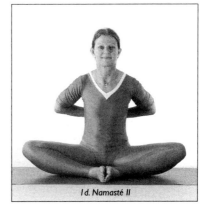

I d. Namasté II

- Roll the shoulders and upper arms back, so that the shoulder blades go down and the knuckles of the index fingers are pressed together.
- Do not push the ribs forward, but keep the frontal ribs down and in, and the lower abdomen in and up.
- Hold for one minute; then release the arms.

2. Baddha Konasana II

In pose 2 and its variations, the pelvis is rotated forward around the femur heads as in forward bendings.

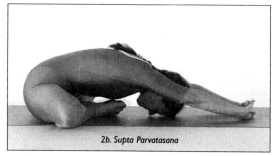

2a. Baddha Konasana II

2a. Baddha Konasana II

- Sit in baddha konasana I (1a), hold the feet with the hands, and then proceed:
- On a mula bandha inhalation, lift the pelvis and trunk up from the femur heads, rooting the buttock bones and the outer edges of the feet into the earth with the support of the pada bandha,and elongating the thighs and knees sideways out of the hip joints. On the exhalation, bend forward till the sternum rests on the feet, and the head rests on the blanket. The sternum arrives on the feet before the head arrives on the blanket. Do not lift the buttock bones up, but extend them backwards, spreading them at the same time so that the lumbar spine moves in.
- On each inhalation, extend the groins and buttock bones further backwards and the thighs further sideways. At the same time elongate the lower abdomen, rib cage, spine and head further forwards.
- On each exhalation, lower the chest and head further with gravity onto the feet and earth.
- Hold for one minute; then come up on an inhalation, raising first the head, then the chest, and then the abdomen.

2b. Supta Parvatasana

2b. Supta Parvatasana
supta=lying down;
parvata=mountain

- Sit in parvatasana (1b) and then proceed:
- On a mula bandha inhalation, lift the pelvis and trunk up from the femur heads, rooting the buttock bones and the outer edges of the feet into the earth with the support of the pada bandha and elongating the thighs and knees sideways out of the hip joints. On the exhalation, bend forward till the sternum rests on the feet, and the head and hands rest on the blanket. The sternum arrives on the feet before the head and hands arrive on the blanket. Do not lift the buttock bones up, but extend them backwards, spreading them at the same time so that the lumbar spine moves in.
- On each inhalation, extend the groins and buttock bones further backwards and the thighs further sideways. At the same time elongate the lower abdomen, rib cage, spine, head and hands further forwards.
- On each exhalation, lower the chest and head further with gravity onto the feet and earth.
- Hold for one minute; then come up on an inhalation.

2c. Supta Gomukhasana
supta=lying down; go=cow;
mukha=face

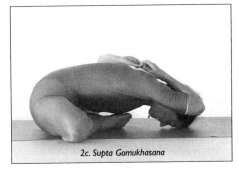

2c. Supta Gomukhasana

- Sit in gomukhasana (1c) and then proceed:
- On a mula bandha inhalation, lift the pelvis and trunk up from the femur heads, rooting the buttock bones and the outer edges of the feet into the earth with the support of the pada bandha and elongating the thighs and knees sideways out of the hip joints. On the exhalation, bend forward till the sternum rests on the feet and the head rests on the blanket. The sternum arrives on the feet before the head arrives on the blanket. Do not lift the buttock bones up, but extend them backwards, spreading them at the same time, so that the lumbar spine moves in.
- On each inhalation, extend the groins and buttock bones further backwards and the thighs further sideways. At the same time elongate the lower abdomen, rib cage, spine and head further forwards.
- On each exhalation, lower the chest and head further with gravity onto the feet and earth, keeping both elbows up towards the sky.
- Hold for one minute. Then come up on an inhalation, raising first the head, then the chest, and then the abdomen. Change hands.

2d. Supta Namasté II
supta=lying down

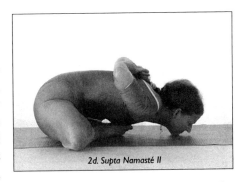

2d. Supta Namasté II

- Sit in namasté II (1d) and then proceed:
- On a mula bandha inhalation, lift the pelvis and trunk up from the femur heads, rooting the buttock bones and the outer edges of the feet into the earth with the support of the pada bandha and elongating the thighs and knees sideways out of the hip joints. On the exhalation, bend forward till the sternum rests on the feet and the head rests on the blanket. The sternum arrives on the feet before the head arrives on the blanket. Do not lift the buttock bones up, but extend them backwards, spreading them at the same time so that the lumbar spine moves in.
- On each inhalation, extend the groins and buttock bones further backwards and the thighs further sideways. At the same time elongate the lower abdomen, rib cage, spine and head further forwards.
- On each exhalation, lower the chest and head further with gravity onto the feet and earth, keeping the elbows up towards the sky.
- Hold for one minute; then come up on an inhalation, raising first the head, then the chest, and then the abdomen.

3. Kandasana

kanda=root, base of the trunk

- Sit in baddha konasana I (1a) and then proceed:
- Hold the feet, keeping the thumbs on the inner arches, and the fingers covering the dorsal side of the feet.
- Lean the body backwards and lift the feet and legs till the feet are at the height of the sternum.
- Rotate the soles of the feet towards you and place them on the sternum.
- Rotate the knees forwards as much as you can, keeping the balance on the buttock bones.
- Hold for a few seconds.

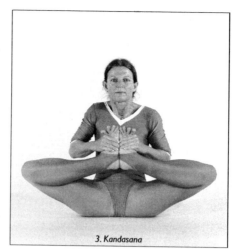

3. Kandasana

4. Mulabandhasana

mula=root, base, first chakra;
bandha=fetter

- Sit in baddha konasana I (1a) and then proceed:
- Raise the heels, insert the arms underneath the ankles and clasp the fingers around the metatarsals of the big toes.
- Turn the heels further upwards and pull the toes under them, towards the pubic bone, till the feet rest vertically on the toes, close to the pubic bone.
- Hold for a few seconds.

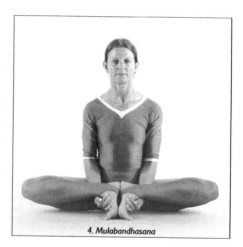

4. Mulabandhasana

5. Supta Baddha Konasana

supta=lying down; baddha=bound; kona=angle

In this pose the pelvis is rotated backwards around the femur heads as in back bendings.

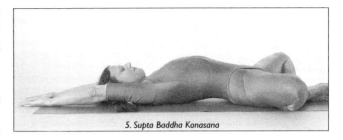

5. Supta Baddha Konasana

- Sit in baddha konasana I (1a) and then proceed:
- Keep the hands behind you on the blanket and, lifting the pelvis so that you are standing on the outer edges of the feet, rotate the pelvis backwards, so that the coccyx rolls towards the pubic bone and the two frontal hip bones move up towards the ribs. Then lower yourself onto the elbows, and finally onto the blanket. Keep the knees down.
- Keep the backward rotation of the pelvis, so that the lower abdomen moves in the direction of the ribs, and slide the back of the chest upwards in the direction of the head. In this way the whole lumbar region is elongated and brought down towards the blanket.
- Extend the thighs sideways out of the groins, and pull the two frontal hip bones up towards the ribs: double action, down and up, so that the groins in the middle are opened.
- On a mula bandha inhalation, extend the arms over the head on the blanket, without curving the lumbar up.
- On each inhalation, extend the thighs further sideways and downwards out of the hip joints, and the spine and arms further upwards.
- On each exhalation, press the lumbar further towards the blanket, maintaining the length of the body.
- Hold for one minute.

Part 5 Navalama/Boat Poses

These positions are done in the *vinyasa* mode, that is, going from one pose directly into the next one, using the breathing.

Navalama

1. *Dandasana*
2. *Paripurna Navasana*
3. *Ardha Navasana*
4. *Parvata Savasana*
5. *Supta Dandasana*

---

1. **Dandasana**
danda=staff

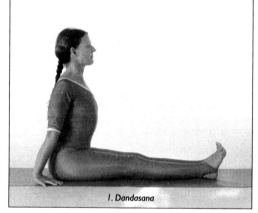

I. Dandasana

- Sit on a blanket with the legs extended straight in front of you as in paschimottanasana (see page 121).
- Place the hands next to the hips on the blanket with the fingers pointing forwards towards the feet.
- On each mula bandha inhalation, root the buttock bones, the back of the legs and the hands into the earth, performing hasta bandha, and elongate the spinal column up towards the sky. Keep the feet together and the arches strong (pada bandha).
- Hold for three breaths. On an exhalation proceed to 2.

2. Paripurna Navasana

paripurna=entire, complete;
nava=boat

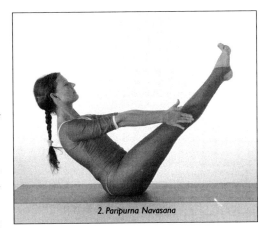

2. *Paripurna Navasana*

- Lean the trunk backwards and raise the legs up to an angle of forty-five degrees. Extend the arms forwards, parallel to the earth, with the palms of the hands parallel to the outer knees.
- Keep the back straight and the head and neck in line with the trunk. The trunk makes an angle of ninety degrees with the legs.
- Hold for three breaths. On an exhalation proceed to 3.

3. Ardha Navasana

ardha=half; nava=boat

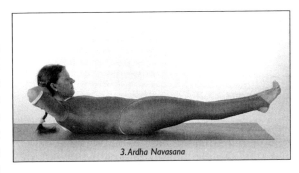

3. *Ardha Navasana*

- Clasp the hands behind the neck and lower the back and legs simultaneously, till the heels are about five inches above the blanket and the lumbar region and lower chest rest on the blanket. Keep the shoulder blades, shoulders and head off the blanket, and the elbows back.
- Hold for three breaths. On an exhalation proceed to 4.

4. Parvata Savasana

parvata=mountain;
sava=corpse

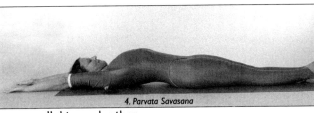

4. *Parvata Savasana*

- Lower the body completely onto the blanket and extend the arms over the head. Rest the back of the hands on the blanket, keeping the arms parallel to each other.
- On each mula bandha inhalation, elongate the arms out of the lower abdomen and sacro-iliac joints. On each exhalation, press the lumbar region more towards the blanket.
- Hold for three breaths. On an exhalation proceed to 5.

5. Supta Dandasana

supta=lying down; danda=staff

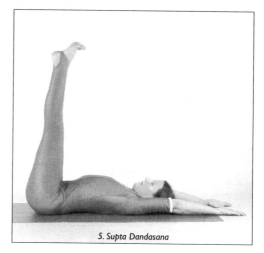

5. Supta Dandasana

- Raise the legs up to ninety degrees; keeping the knees straight and the arches strong.
- On each mula bandha inhalation, elongate the shoulders and arms further up towards the hands, and the groins further away from the lower abdomen, so that the sacrum remains flat on the blanket.
- Hold for three breaths. On an exhalation, return to dandasana, bringing the legs down onto the blanket, and raising the trunk and arms in one smooth movement.

Part 6 Leg Stretches

These positions are done in the *vinyasa* mode, that is, going from one pose directly into the next one, using the breathing.

<table>
<tr><td colspan="2" align="center">*Leg Stretches*</td></tr>
<tr><td>1. *Urdhva Prasarita Padasana*</td><td>6. *Supta Padangusthasana II*</td></tr>
<tr><td>2. *Jathara Parivartanasana*</td><td>7. *Supta Padangusthasana III*</td></tr>
<tr><td>3. *Urdhvamukha Paschimottanasana II*</td><td>8. *Anantasana*</td></tr>
<tr><td>4. *Urdhvamukha Prasarita Padottanasana II*</td><td>9. *Hanumanasana*</td></tr>
<tr><td></td><td>10. *Samakonasana*</td></tr>
<tr><td>5. *Supta Padangusthasana I*</td><td>11. *Nakrasana*</td></tr>
</table>

1. Urdhva Prasarita Padasana
urdhva=upwards; prasarita=extended; pada=leg, foot
- Lie on the back on a blanket with the legs together, extend the arms sideways at an angle of ninety degrees to the trunk, with the palms facing upward.
- On an exhalation, raise the legs to ninety degrees. Simultaneously extend the metatarsals of the big toes up towards the sky, the coccyx down towards the earth, and elongate the neck.
- Hold for one minute; then proceed to 2.

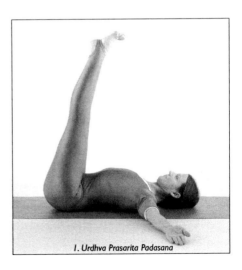

I. Urdhva Prasarita Padasana

2. Jathara Parivartanasana

jathara=stomach;
parivartana=turning, rolling

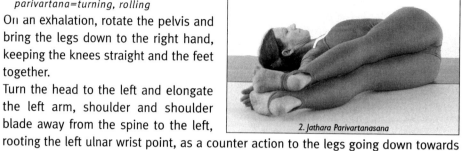

2. Jathara Parivartanasana

- On an exhalation, rotate the pelvis and bring the legs down to the right hand, keeping the knees straight and the feet together.
- Turn the head to the left and elongate the left arm, shoulder and shoulder blade away from the spine to the left, rooting the left ulnar wrist point, as a counter action to the legs going down towards the right.
- Inhale while the feet are on the right hand.
- On the exhalation lift the legs and take them over to the left hand, rotating the pelvis to the left and the head to the right.

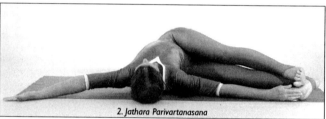

2. Jathara Parivartanasana

- Elongate the right arm, shoulder and shoulder blade away from the spine to the right, rooting the right ulnar wrist point, as a counter action to the legs going down towards the left.
- Repeat three times; then return to urdhva prasarita padasana (1) and proceed to 3.

3. Urdhvamukha Paschimottanasana II

urdhva=upwards; mukha=face;
paschima=the West, the back of the body;
uttana=intense stretch

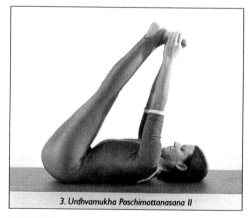

3. Urdhvamukha Paschimottanasana II

- On an exhalation hold the outer edges of the feet with the hands. Keep the knees straight and the back of the head and the sacrum on the blanket: elongate the back of the head upwards and the groins downwards, so that the whole spine is elongated.
- On an exhalation, raise the pelvis and bring the legs over the head, till they are parallel to the earth. Lift the head and bring the forehead to the shins.
- Hold for one minute; then lower the pelvis and head onto the blanket and proceed to 4.

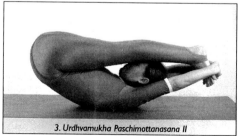

3. Urdhvamukha Paschimottanasana II

4. Urdhvamukha Prasarita Padottanasana II

urdhva=upwards; mukha=face;
prasarita=extended; pada=leg,foot;
uttana=intense stretch

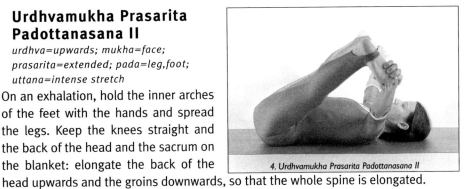

4. *Urdhvamukha Prasarita Padottanasana II*

- On an exhalation, hold the inner arches of the feet with the hands and spread the legs. Keep the knees straight and the back of the head and the sacrum on the blanket: elongate the back of the head upwards and the groins downwards, so that the whole spine is elongated.
- Turn the legs slightly outwards, elongate them out of the hip joints and lower the feet as much as you can, keeping the pelvis flat on the blanket.
- Hold for one minute; then return to urdhva prasarita padasana (1) and proceed to 5.

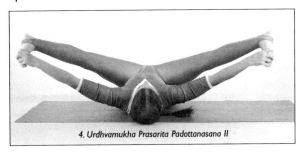

4. *Urdhvamukha Prasarita Padottanasana II*

5. Supta Padangusthasana I

supta=lying down;
padangustha=big toe

- On an exhalation, extend the left leg onto the blanket and hold the right foot with both hands. Keep both knees straight and the back of the head and the sacrum on the blanket: elongate the back of the head upwards and the groins downwards, so that the whole spine is elongated.

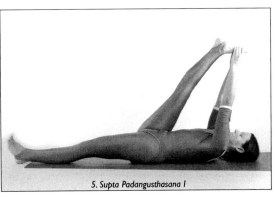

5. *Supta Padangusthasana I*

- On the next exhalation bring the right foot over the head, keeping the knee straight and the hips even; do not turn the right hip up.
- Keep the left foot strong (pada bandha) and the left knee straight; the back of the left leg and the left heel remain on the blanket.
- On each mula bandha inhalation, elongate the right groin away from the right ribs, and roll the right femur head backwards towards the left heel. On each exhalation, bring the right foot further over the head to the earth.
- Hold for one minute; then proceed to 6

6. Supta Padangusthasana II

supta=lying down;
padangustha=big toe

- Release the left hand and extend the left arm sideways on the blanket, at an angle of ninety degrees with the chest. Root the left ulnar wrist point into the blanket.

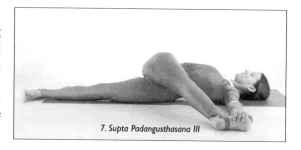

6. Supta Padangusthasana II

- Hold the inner arch of the right foot with the right hand and, on an exhalation, bring the foot down to the right side. Keep the left hip and heel down on the blanket and the left leg straight, performing pada bandha on the left foot to support the action in the pelvis.
- On each mula bandha inhalation, elongate the left leg and the spinal column, and on each exhalation take the right foot further down to the side.
- Turn the head to the left and elongate the left arm, shoulder and shoulder blade away from the spine to the left, rooting the left ulnar wrist point, as a counter action to the right leg going down towards the right.
- Hold for one minute; then proceed to 7.

7. Supta Padangusthasana III

supta=lying down;
padangustha=big toe

- On an exhalation lift the right leg up again. Release the right hand and hold the outer edge of the right foot with the left hand. Extend the right arm sideways on the blanket, at an angle of ninety degrees to the chest, and root the ulnar wrist point into the blanket.

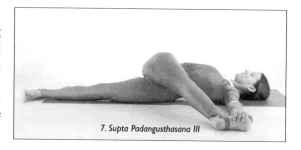

7. Supta Padangusthasana III

- On the next exhalation take the right foot down to the left, rolling the hips to the left, so that you are resting on the left hip and the outer side of the left leg and foot. Keep the left foot strong (pada bandha) and the left knee straight.

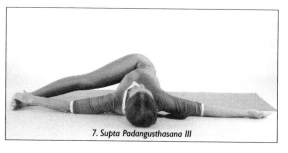

7. Supta Padangusthasana III

- Turn the head to the right and elongate the right arm, shoulder and shoulder blade away from the spine to the right, rooting the right ulnar wrist point, as a counter action to the right leg going down towards the left.
- On each mula bandha inhalation, elongate the right groin away from the right ribs and roll the right femur backwards towards the left heel.
- Hold for one minute; then repeat 5, 6 and 7 with the left leg.

8. Anantasana
ananta=infinite

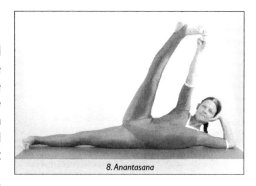

8. Anantasana

- Lie down on the left side of the trunk and the left leg. Extend the left arm in line with the side of the chest, so that the whole body makes one line, from the fingers of the left hand to the outer arch of the left foot. Bend the left arm and rest the left ear on the palm of the left hand.
- Bend the right leg. With the index and middle fingers of the right hand hold the big toe of the right foot and extend the leg up to the sky.
- Keep the body in alignment and stay on the side of the left hip; do not roll onto the backside of the pelvis.
- Rooting the whole left side of the body, especially the outer edge of the left foot (pada bandha) and the left ankle to keep

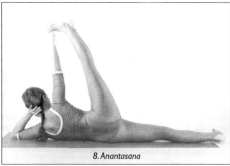

8. Anantasana

the balance and lightness of the body, elongate the right leg up to the sky, out of the right hip joint.
- Hold for one minute.

9. Hanumanasana
Hanuman is the monkey god.
This pose is the Western 'split'.

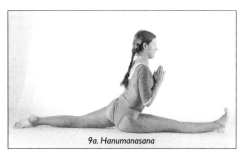

9a. Hanumanasana

9a. Hanumanasana
- Kneel on hands and knees on a blanket, and then proceed:
- Bring the right leg forward between the hands, pointing the toes of the right foot up. Slide the right heel forward on the blanket, till the knee is straight and the calf muscle and thigh rest on the blanket. At the same time, lift the left knee and slide the left foot backwards on the blanket, till the left knee is straight and the shin bone and quadriceps muscle are resting on the blanket.
- Do not turn the left hip back, but roll it forwards, so that the left knee rests on the center of the knee on the blanket. The foot too should rest on the center of the dorsal side.
- Keep the pelvis and trunk as vertical as possible and the head, chest and pelvis facing in the direction of the right foot. Join the palms in front of the sternum in Namasté I and look straight forward.
- Hold for one minute; then proceed to 9b.

9b. Hanumanasana, arms upwards

- On a mula bandha inhalation, elongate the arms up over the head and join the palms. Then proceed to 9c.

9c. Hanumanasana, bending forward

- On the exhalation, bend forward and clasp the hands beyond the right foot as in janu sirsasana (see page 123). As in all forward bendings, it is the hand on the side of the straight (forward) leg which holds the opposite hand.

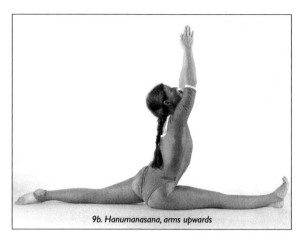
9b. Hanumanasana, arms upwards

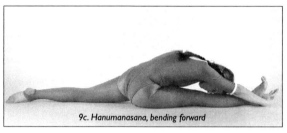
9c. Hanumanasana, bending forward

- Rest the head on the shin. On each inhalation, slide the head further forwards towards the right foot. On each exhalation, lower the trunk and head further with gravity onto the leg, keeping the back of the chest and the shoulder blades parallel to the earth.
- Hold for a few seconds; then repeat 9a, b and c on the other side.

10. Samakonasana

sama=even, same;
kona=angle

- Sit on the blanket with the legs spread as in dvipada upavistha konasana (see page 136), and then proceed:
- Keep the feet vertical with the toes pointing straight up to the sky, and place the hands next to the hips on the blanket, with the fingers pointing forwards.

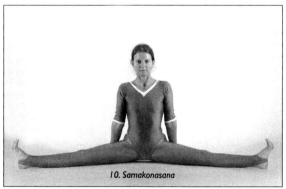
10. Samakonasana

Lift the pelvis and, sliding the legs and heels sideways out of the hip joints, bring the pelvis forwards while elongating the legs sideways, so that the angle between the two thighs increases.
- Keep the pelvis and trunk vertical and the face looking straight forward.
- Repeat lifting the pelvis and bringing it forward while sliding the legs out, till the legs form one continuous line with each other sideways (the sideways 'split').
- Hold for one minute; then proceed to 11.

11. Nakrasana

nakra=crocodile

- Place the hands in front of you on the blanket with the fingers pointing forward.
- Rotate the pelvis forward and, shifting the weight of the body onto the hands, lift the pelvis and walk forwards on the hands while elongating the legs sideways, out of the hip joints, so that the heels slide away from the trunk. The legs will start to rotate inwards, till they slide backwards by themselves and you end up lying on the stomach with the legs extended backwards.

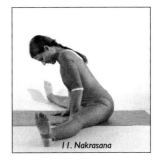

11. Nakrasana

This position involves a complete rotation of the thighs in the hip joints. Do not attempt to do this pose until you have gained sufficient suppleness in dvipada upavistha konasana (see page 136).

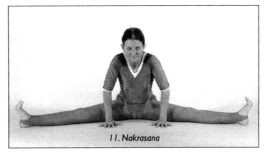

11. Nakrasana

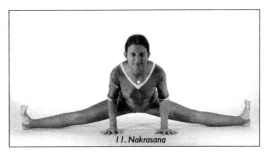

11. Nakrasana

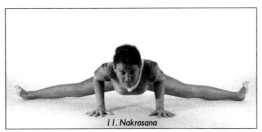

11. Nakrasana

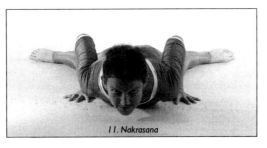

11. Nakrasana

Part 7 Forward Bendings

These positions can be done in four different modes:

a. ***Performing each position separately*** and holding it for one minute.

b. *Vinyasa*
Connecting two or more positions by flowing from one into the other, using the breathing.

c. *Mala*
Connecting all the positions through surya namaskar, using the breathing, and holding each of the forward bendings for the duration of three breaths.

d. ***Taking only a few positions*** and holding them for *five minutes* each.

Forward Bendings

1. Paschimottanasana
2. Parivrtta Paschimottanasana
3. Janu Sirsasana
   a. Maha Mudra
   b. Janu Sirsasana
4. Parivrtta Janu Sirsasana
5. Ardha Baddha Padma Paschimottanasana
6. Triangmukhaikapada Paschimottanasana I
7. Triangmukhaikapada Paschimottanasana II
8. Parivrtta Triangmukhaikapada Paschimottanasana II
9. Krounchasana
10. Akarna Dhanurasana
11. Marichyasana I
12. Marichyasana II
13. Ubhaya Padangusthasana
    a. Ubhaya Padangusthasana
    b. Urdhvamukha Prasarita Padottanasana I
14. Urdhvamukha Paschimottanasana I
15. Upavistha Konasana
    a. Dvipada Upavistha Konasana
    b. Ekapada Upavistha Konasana
    c. Parivrttaikapada Upavistha Konasana
16. Baddha Konasana II
17. Malasana
18. Kurmasana
19. Ekapada Sirsasana cycle
    a. Ekapada Sirsasana
    b. Kala Bhairavasana
    c. Bhairavasana
    d. Skandasana
    e. Chakorasana I
    f. Ruchikasana
    g. Durvasasana
20. Yoga Nidrasana
21. Dvipada Sirsasana
    a. Dvipada Sirsasana
    b. Chakorasana II

1. Paschimottanasana

*paschima=the West, the back of the
body; uttana=intense stretch*

Paschimottanasana is described in detail,
as it forms the basic pose for all the
following forward bending positions (see
also "Comparative Studies of Various
Asanas", page 239).

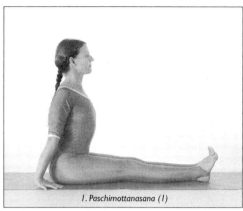

1. Paschimottanasana (1)

First part

- Sit on a blanket with the legs extended
  straight in front of you. Keep the knees
  straight with the knee caps facing the sky; do not turn the legs in or out. The back of
  the knees are in contact with the blanket.
- The feet are at equal distances from the trunk. Elongate the heels and big toe bones
  away from you, and pull the little toe bones towards you, so that the feet are vertical
  and all the toes are in line. Perform pada bandha in order to support the action in the
  pelvis.
- Pull the buttock muscles sideways and back with the hands, so that you sit on the
  buttock bones, not on the flesh. The weight of the trunk is evenly distributed between
  both buttock bones.
- The shoulder joints are in line with the hip joints and the back is vertical, so that the
  trunk is at a right angle to the legs. Thus the weight of the trunk is transmitted to the
  buttock bones in a straight line.
- The pelvis is vertical, so that the body rests on the points of the buttock bones, and is
  at right angles to the thighs in the hip joints, with the two frontal hip bones in line with
  the groins. Many people have the pelvis rotated backwards in paschimottanasana,
  with the trunk resting on the back of the buttock bones or even on the coccyx, and this
  causes the back to bend, forcing the spinal vertebrae out of alignment. In this case one
  has to work at rotating the pelvis forward around the femur heads until it is vertical.
- With the pelvis in a vertical position, action has to be brought in the sacro-iliac joints.
  Constrict the outer hips and the adductor muscles on the inside of the thighs inwards
  towards each other and, keeping the two frontal hip bones in vertical alignment with
  the groins, lift them up and move them slightly forward, while rooting the buttock
  bones. The upper rim of the sacrum too is brought forward, together with the two
  frontal hip bones. At the same time, you have to also root the coccyx and move it
  forwards towards the pubic bone.
- As a result the entire pelvis widens laterally, is brought vertically forward towards the
  femur heads and lifted up from those femur heads, and the lower abdomen moves in
  and up towards the navel (mula bandha). This whole movement is the rebounce action:
  the coccyx and buttock bones root into the earth, going down with the force of gravity,
  so that the rest of the pelvis, the lower abdomen and the trunk elongate upwards
  against gravity.
- This whole movement is, of course, done on the mula bandha breathing, which creates
  the lightness in the spine that accompanies the anatomical movements.

Second part

- On an exhalation, rotate the pelvis forward to an angle of about forty-five degrees. Hold the outer edges of the feet with the hands, without moving the inner ankles apart and without bending the knees. Root the back of the thighs and the buttock bones into the earth without tightening the frontal part of the thighs.

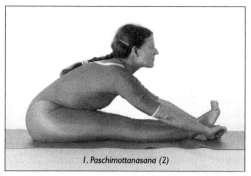
1. Paschimottanasana (2)

- As the pelvis rotates forwards, do not draw the coccyx up towards the lumbar spine, but root it, elongating the back of the thighs, the buttock bones and the coccyx backwards. At the same time, lift the rest of the pelvis up from the femur heads and bring it forwards. Thus the pelvis is extended in opposite directions and widens at the back and the front: dual movement.
- One mistake is that the two frontal hip bones stay back when the body bends forwards, which means that the pelvis remains tilted backwards. This causes the body to bend in the lumbar vertebrae instead of in the groins. Another mistake is that the two frontal hip bones move forwards and down, which means that the whole pelvis, including the sacrum and the coccyx, is rotated forwards. Thus the coccyx is tipped back and up towards the lumbar spine, which collapses inward. This has a weakening effect on the lumbar spine.
- In the correct movement, the two frontal hip bones move forward and up as the pelvis rotates forwards. The abdomen below the navel moves forwards faster than the part above the navel, and the two frontal hip bones come to rest on the thighs before the ribs do.
- When the pelvis widens, the lower back widens too, and the lumbar spine elongates out of the pelvis by itself, giving the thrust for the entire spine to elongate forwards and up. No part of the trunk should aid the spine in elongating: the rib cage remains passive, and the spine and head are drawn out of the trunk like a sword out of its scabbard.
- When the lumbar spine elongates out of the pelvis, the thoracic spine continues that movement, so that the groove of the spine is visible from the sacrum up to the first thoracic vertebra, and has the same depth everywhere.

Third part

- When you have reached the maximum elongation from the sacrum to the back of the head, and from the pubic bone to the throat, place the head on the shins. The closer the forehead moves towards the feet, the better.

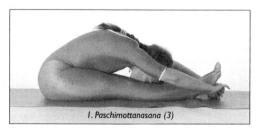
1. Paschimottanasana (3)

- Turn the palm of the right hand forward. With the thumb and the four fingers form a ring and place the dorsal side of the wrist in the outer arch of the right foot. Turn the palm of the left hand forwards as well and insert the fingers of the left hand in the ring formed by the right hand. In this way there is the possibility of future elongation. Many people just clasp the fingers beyond the soles of the feet as in head balance, which means that there is no room for future elongation. In the way described above, the left hand can keep on sliding forward within the ring formed by the right hand, till the fingers of the right hand hold the left wrist, or even further. To maintain the evenness of the body, change hands every now and then.

- Many people pull the trunk forward with the hands, arms and shoulders. Thus they often pull only the chest, leaving the pelvis behind. The driving force for the trunk to elongate forwards lies in the pelvis: rubbing forwards on the buttock bones and rooting them, draw the two frontal hip bones forwards along the thighs towards the knees.
- The spinal column elongates forwards horizontally, but the chest remains passive: as the spine elongates forwards, the lower ribs too are drawn forwards along the thighs towards the knees as a result of the movement of pelvis and spine. Again, these movements should be done on the mula bandha breathing, elongating forwards on each inhalation, and lowering he trunk on each exhalation. Keep the shoulder blades, shoulders, arms and hands relaxed.
- Hold for one to ten minutes; then come up on an inhalation.

2. Parivrtta Paschimottanasana

parivrtta=turned around; paschima=the West, the back of the body; uttana=intense stretch

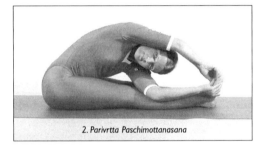

2. Parivrtta Paschimottanasana

- Sit in paschimottanasana (1).
- On an exhalation, turn to the right. Rotate the left arm as in savasana and hold with the left hand the outer edge of the right foot. With the right hand hold the outer edge of the left foot. Turn the trunk further to the right, insert the head in between the arms, and look up at the sky.
- Hold for one minute; then repeat on the other side .

3. Janu Sirsasana

janu=knee; sirsa=head

As janu sirsasana is one of the more complex positions in yoga, it is described here in great detail (see also Part Two: "Comparative Studies of Various Asanas: Front face – Back face", page 251).

3a. Maha Mudra

maha=great, noble; mudra=shutting, closing.

First part
- Sit on a blanket with the legs extended straight in front of you. Keep the knees straight with the knee caps facing the sky; do not turn the legs in or out. The back of the knees are in contact with the blanket.
- Bend the left leg and place the sole of the left foot against the inner side of the right thigh, near the pubic bone. Do not let the foot slip underneath the right thigh; it barely touches it. The left (bent) knee rests on the blanket. The left thigh is at right angles to

the right thigh and the left frontal hip bone is slightly further back than the right one.

- The right leg extends straight out of the right hip joint, with the right foot in line with the right frontal hip bone. The knee is straight and the knee cap faces the sky; the back of the knee is in contact with the blanket. Elongate the heel and big toe bone away from you, and pull the little toe bone towards you, so that the foot is vertical and all the toes are in line. Perform pada bandha with the right foot to support the action in the pelvis.

Second part
- On a mula bandha inhalation, lift the pelvis up from the femur heads and bring the weight of the body onto the right buttock bone, so that the left buttock bone is slightly lifted. Turn the pelvis and chest to the right, till the shoulders are perpendicular to the right leg. Root the right buttock bone into the earth, and elongate the spinal column upwards out of the sacro-iliac joints.

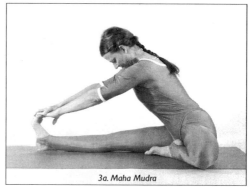
3a. Maha Mudra

- On the exhalation, rotate the pelvis forwards to an angle of about forty-five degrees, and with both hands hold the right foot, keeping that foot vertical. This position is called **maha mudra**.
- As the left frontal hip bone is further back than the right one, the spine (trunk) is not perpendicular to the right leg. You have to rotate the trunk towards the right, until the frontal central line (navel-sternum-throat) is in line with the right leg. The left thigh rotates inwards towards the left foot, and the left frontal hip bone rotates towards the navel, while the right one rotates away from the navel towards the right: the left side of waist and rib cage rotate towards the frontal central line, while the right side rotates away from that line towards the right. Beginners often rotate only the shoulders and ribs, but the movement should come from the pelvis.
- Do not pull the knee cap up, but release the tension at the front of the thigh and root the back of the knee into the earth. Extend the back of the leg from the knee to the heel forwards, elongating the heel away from you, and from the knee to the buttock bone backwards. The weight of the body is mainly on the right buttock bone: the left buttock bone is slightly lifted off the blanket, while the left thigh and hip bone rotate inwards.
- The spine, from the sacrum up to the cervical spine, is straight: if there is a deviation to the left it means that the trunk has not been fully rotated. It is very important for the spine to be straight from the beginning, because if there is a curvature to the left, there will be a great strain on the left side of the spine and on the left sacro-iliac joint in the third part of the pose. When the spine is straight and in the center of the back, the width of the rib cage and waist on the left and right side of the spine is equal; if the left side of the back is broader, the spine has curved to the left. Both sides of the back should be evenly long, straight, and parallel to each other.

3b. Janu Sirsasana

Third part

- When you have reached maximum elongation from the sacrum to the back of the head, and from the pubic bone to the throat, place the head on the shin of the right leg. Keep the right foot vertical. The closer the forehead moves towards the right foot, the better. This position is called **janu sirsasana**.

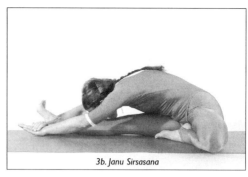

3b. Janu Sirsasana

- Turn the palm of the right hand forward, with the thumb and the four fingers form a ring and place the dorsal side of the wrist in the outer arch of the right foot. Turn the palm of the left hand forward as well and insert the fingers of the left hand in the ring formed by the right hand. In this way there is the possibility of future elongation. Many people just clasp the fingers beyond the sole of the foot as in head balance, which means that there is no room for future elongation. In the way described above the left hand can keep on sliding forwards within the ring formed by the right hand, till the fingers of the right hand hold the left wrist or even further. It is important to note that, with the right leg extended forward, it is the right hand which forms the ring for the left hand to slide through. This is because, by placing the back side of the right wrist in the small arch, that pressure stabilizes the right foot in its vertical position.
- The lower abdomen arrives first on the right thigh, then the navel; the navel comes to rest exactly on the midline of the right thigh. If this is not the case, but the navel stays on the inner side of the thigh, it means that you have not perfected the first part of this pose.
- After the navel, the sternum has to come to rest on the thigh, close to the knee on the midline of the thigh, not on the inner side. The head is the last to come and rest on the shin. You can either place the forehead on the shin, or, if you are more supple, the chin, so that the eyes look at the right foot. In both cases the neck, shoulders, shoulder blades and arms remain relaxed.
- On each mula bandha inhalation, slide the head (and of course the whole trunk) closer to the right foot.
- Hold for one minute; then repeat on the other side.

4. Parivrtta Janu Sirsasana

parivrtta=turned around; janu=knee;
sirsa=head

Sit in maha mudra (3a) with the right leg extended straight in front of you and proceed:

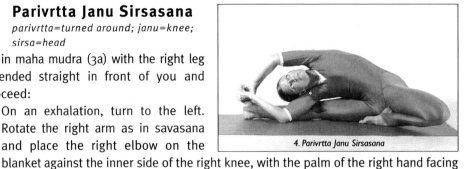

4. Parivrtta Janu Sirsasana

- On an exhalation, turn to the left. Rotate the right arm as in savasana and place the right elbow on the blanket against the inner side of the right knee, with the palm of the right hand facing up to the sky. Turn the whole trunk (pelvis, chest, shoulders and head) to the left.
- Hold with the right hand the inner arch of the right foot. Extend the left arm up to the sky and elongate it out of the left hip joint; then hold the outer edge of the left foot with the left hand. Insert the head in between the arms and turn completely to the left, till the shoulders are vertically aligned above the right thigh. Look up at the sky.
- Extend the left thigh out of the left hip joint, keeping the left knee down on the blanket.
- On each mula bandha inhalation, elongate the whole right side of the trunk, from the right groin to the right armpit, forwards towards the right foot. Slide the right elbow closer to the right foot, so that the whole right side of the trunk rests on the thigh.
- On each exhalation, continue the rotation of the trunk to the left.
- Hold for one minute; then repeat on the other side.

5. Ardha Baddha Padma Paschimottanasana

ardha=half; baddha=bound;
padma=lotus; paschima=the West
the back of the body;
uttana=intense stretch

- Sit on a blanket with the legs extended straight in front of you. Keep the knees straight with the knee caps facing the sky; do not turn the legs in or out. The back of the knees are in contact with the blanket.

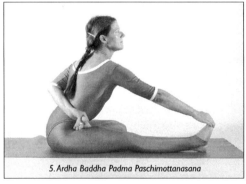

5. Ardha Baddha Padma Paschimottanasana

- Bend the left leg and place the left foot in the groin of the right leg in the same way as for padmasana (see page 72). The left (bent) knee is close to the right (straight) knee, so that the left thigh makes an angle of forty-five degrees or less with the right one. (Note that in janu sirsasana (3b) the left thigh makes an angle of ninety degrees with the right one.) In this way the pelvis is straight and the line between the two frontal hip bones, across the lower abdomen, is at right angles to the straight leg (which in janu sirsasana is not the case).

- The right leg extends straight out of the right hip joint, with the right foot in line with the right frontal hip bone. The knee is straight, and the knee cap faces the sky; the back of the knee is in contact with the blanket. Elongate the heel and big toe bone away from you, and pull the little toe bone towards you, so that the foot is vertical and all the toes are in line. Perform pada bandha with the right foot to support the action in the pelvis.

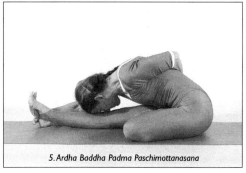
5. Ardha Baddha Padma Paschimottanasana

- The weight of the body is divided equally between both buttock bones, and the left knee rests on the blanket.
- On an exhalation, rotate the left arm around the back in a large, circular movement and hold the metatarsals of the left foot. As the fingers curl around the metatarsals, the toes should also curl around the fingers, so that the foot holds the hand as much as the hand holds the foot. Keep the left shoulder, rib cage, frontal hip bone and groin forward, facing in the direction of the right foot, and keep the left knee close to the right one, and on the blanket.
- On a mula bandha inhalation, lift the pelvis up from the femur heads, rooting the buttock bones into the earth and elongating the spinal column upwards out of the sacro-iliac joints.
- On the exhalation, rotate the pelvis forward to about forty-five degrees, and with the right hand hold the right foot, keeping the foot vertical.
- As the pelvis lifts up and moves forwards, the right frontal hip bone moves into the arch of the left foot, so that the heel of the left foot is embedded deep within the flesh of the lower abdomen, between the pubic bone and the navel.
- Do not pull the right knee cap up, but release the tension at the front of the thigh and root the back of the knee into the earth. Extend the back of the leg from the knee to the heel forwards, elongating the heel away from you, and from the knee to the buttock bone backwards.
- After reaching maximum elongation of the spinal column, lower the trunk onto the right leg. This should be done in stages, using the mula bandha breathing. On each inhalation, elongate forwards and on each exhalation, lower the trunk further. Lift the lower abdomen up and bring the lower ribs forwards over the foot onto the right thigh.
- The head is the last to come and rest on the shin beyond the knee. You can either place the forehead on the shin or, if you are more supple, the chin, so that the eyes look at the right foot. In both cases the neck, shoulders, shoulder blades and right arm remain relaxed. On each mula bandha inhalation, slide the head (and of course the whole trunk) closer to the right foot.
- Hold for one minute; then repeat on the other side.

6. Triangmukhaikapada Paschimottanasana I

tri=three; anqa=limb; mukha=face;
eka=one; pada=leg,foot;
paschima=the West, the back of the
body; uttana=intense stretch

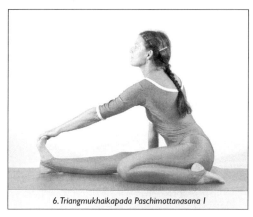

6. Triangmukhaikapada Paschimottanasana I

- Sit on a blanket with the legs extended straight in front of you. Keep the knees straight with the knee caps facing the sky; do not turn the legs in or out. The back of the knees are in contact with the blanket.

- Bend the left leg backwards and place the left foot along the outside of the left hip as in virasana I (see page 96). The arch of the left foot follows the curve of the left hip, so that the toes point towards the coccyx. The left knee stays next to the right knee, so that the inner knees and thighs remain in contact with each other. The right frontal hip bone has the same height

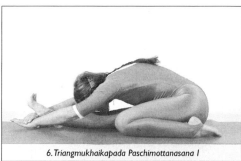

6. Triangmukhaikapada Paschimottanasana I

as the left one, and the weight of the body is evenly distributed between both buttock bones. The pelvis is straight and the line between the two frontal hip bones, across the lower abdomen, is at right angles to the straight leg.

- The right leg extends straight out of the right hip joint, with the right foot in line with the right frontal hip bone. The knee is straight, and the knee cap faces the sky; the back of the knee is in contact with the blanket. Elongate the heel and big toe bone away from you, and pull the little toe bone towards you, so that the foot is vertical and all the toes are in line. Perform pada bandha with the right foot to support the action in the pelvis.

- On a mula bandha inhalation, lift the pelvis up from the femur heads, rooting the buttock bones into the earth and elongating the spinal column upwards out of the sacro-iliac joints.

- On the exhalation, rotate the pelvis forward to an angle of about forty-five degrees, and with the left hand hold the outer edge of the right foot, keeping that foot vertical. The right hand rests lightly on the blanket on the right side of the right leg, do not put any weight on that hand.

- Do not pull the right knee cap up, but release the tension at the front of the thigh and root the back of the knee into the earth. Extend the back of the leg from the knee to the heel forwards, elongating the heel away from you, and from the knee to the buttock bone backwards.

- After reaching maximum elongation of the spinal column, lower the trunk onto the right leg. This is done in stages, using the mula bandha breathing, so that on each inhalation you elongate forward, and on each exhalation you lower the trunk further, till the rib cage rests evenly on both thighs as in paschimottanasana (1). Keep the right foot vertical.

- Turn the palm of the right hand forward, with the thumb and the four fingers form a ring and place the dorsal side of the wrist in the outer arch of the right foot. Turn the palm of the left hand forward as well, and insert the fingers of the left hand in the ring formed by the right hand (see the explanation given in janu sirsasana (3)). Do not tilt the left shoulder, shoulder blade and the left side of the rib cage up, but keep the whole back parallel to the earth.
- The head is the last to come and rest on the shin beyond the knee. As this pose is more like paschimottanasana (1) than like janu sirsasana (3), the head rests against the inner side of the right shin. You can either place the forehead on the inner side of the shin or, if you are more supple, the chin, so that the eyes look at the right foot. In both cases the neck, shoulders, shoulder blades and arms remain relaxed. On each mula bandha inhalation, slide the head (and of course the whole trunk) closer to the right foot.
- Hold for one minute; then repeat on the other side.

7. Triangmukhaikapada Paschimottanasana II

tri=three; anga=limb; mukha=face;
eka=one; pada=leg,foot;
paschima=the West, the back of the
body; uttana=intense stretch

This is basically the same position as the previous one, with the difference that here the left thigh forms an angle of ninety degrees with the right one, and the big toe at the back of the pelvis touches the coccyx as in upavistha virasana I (see page 98). One could call this position a reversed janu sirsasana (3). In janu sirsasana the left thigh is exorotated as in sukhasana (see page 83), while here the left thigh is endorotated as in virasana (see page 96). Thus the technique is the same as for janu sirsasana (3). Follow the instructions given for that pose.

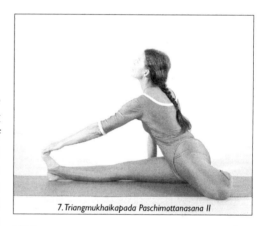
7. Triangmukhaikapada Paschimottanasana II

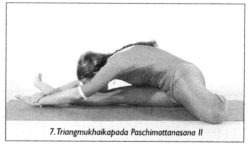
7. Triangmukhaikapada Paschimottanasana II

- Hold for one minute; then repeat on the other side.

8. Parivrtta Triangmukhaikapada Paschimottanasana II

parivrtta=turned around; tri=three;
anga=limb; mukha=face; eka=one;
pada=leg, foot; paschima=the West, the
back of the body; uttana=intense stretch

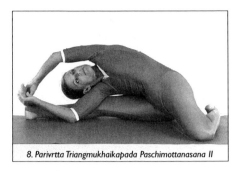

8. Parivrtta Triangmukhaikapada Paschimottanasana II

This position is basically the same as parivrtta janu sirsasana (4). The difference is that here the left leg is endorotated as in upavistha virasana I (see page 98), while in parivrtta janu sirsasana (4) the left leg is exorotated as for sukhasana (see page 77).

- Sit in triangmukhaikapada paschimottanasana II (7) with the right leg extended straight in front of you and proceed:
- On an exhalation, turn to the left. Rotate the right arm as in savasana and place the right elbow on the blanket against the inner side of the right knee, with the palm of the right hand facing up to the sky. Turn the whole trunk (pelvis, chest, shoulders and head) to the left.
- Hold with the right hand the inner arch of the right foot. Extend the left arm up to the sky and elongate it out of the left hip joint, then hold the outer edge of the left foot with the left hand. Insert the head in between the arms and turn completely to the left, till the two shoulders are vertically aligned above the right thigh. Look up at the sky.
- Extend the left thigh out of the left hip joint, keeping the left knee down on the blanket.
- On each mula bandha inhalation, elongate the whole right side of the trunk, from the right groin to the right armpit, forwards towards the right foot. Slide the right elbow closer to the right foot, so that the whole right side of the trunk rests on the thigh.
- On each exhalation, continue the rotation of the trunk to the left.
- Hold for one minute; then repeat on the other side.

9. Krounchasana

krouncha=heron

This position is basically the same as triangmukhaikapada paschimottanasana I (6). The difference is that here the right leg is extended upwards instead of resting on the earth.

- Sit on a blanket with the legs extended straight in front of you. Keep the knees straight with the knee caps facing the sky; do not turn the legs in or out. The back of the knees are in contact with the blanket.
- Bend the left leg and place the left foot along the outer side of the left hip as in virasana I (see page 96). The arch of the left foot follows the curve of the left hip, so that the toes point towards the coccyx. The left knee stays next to the right knee, so that the inner knees and thighs remain in contact with each other. The right frontal hip bone has the same height as the left one, and the weight of the body is evenly

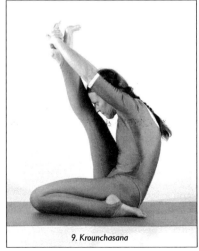

9. Krounchasana

distributed between both buttock bones. The pelvis is straight, and the line between the two frontal hip bones, across the lower abdomen, is at a right angle to the straight leg.

- Bend the right leg. Turn the palm of the right hand upward, with the thumb and the four fingers form a ring and place the dorsal side of the wrist in the outer arch of the right foot. Turn the palm of the left hand upward as well, and insert the fingers of the left hand in the ring formed by the right hand (see the explanation given in janu sirsasana (3)). Then extend the right leg up towards the sky.
- On each mula bandha inhalation, lift the pelvis up from the femur heads, rooting the buttock bones into the earth and elongating the spinal column upwards out of the sacro-iliac joints. On each exhalation, rotate the pelvis further forwards and bring the right leg and the trunk closer to each other.
- The head is the last to come and rest on the shin beyond the knee. You can either place the forehead on the inner side of the shin or, if you are more supple, the chin, so that the eyes look up at the right foot. In both cases the neck, shoulders, shoulder blades and arms remain fairly relaxed. On each mula bandha inhalation, slide the head (and of course the whole trunk) up, closer to the right foot.
- Hold for one minute; then repeat on the other side.

10. Akarna Dhanurasana

a=near to; karna=ear; dhanu=bow

This pose is a combination of paschimottanasana (1) and krounchasana (9).

- Sit on a blanket with the legs extended straight in front of you.
- Bend forward; with the index and middle finger of the left hand, hold the big toe of the left foot, and with the index and middle finger of the right hand, hold the big toe of the right foot.
- Without turning the trunk or hips, bend the right leg and lift the right foot up next to the right ear. The right knee points backwards and sideways, away from the trunk, at an angle of forty-five degrees. Then extend the right leg up as in krounchasana (9).
- Hold for one minute; then repeat on the other side.

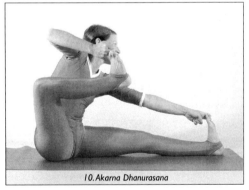

10. Akarna Dhanurasana

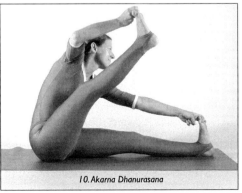

10. Akarna Dhanurasana

11. Marichyasana I

Marichi is the son of Brahman

- Sit on a blanket with the legs extended straight in front of you.
- Bend the left leg, so that the knee points up towards the sky and the left foot rests on the blanket next to the right thigh, with the toes pointing straight forward. In this position, the left buttock bone does not rest on the blanket, but the weight of the body is distributed between the right buttock bone and the left foot.

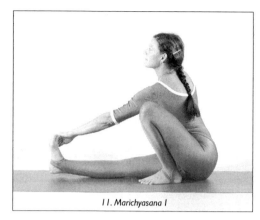

11. Marichyasana I

- The right leg extends straight out of the right hip joint, with the right foot in line with the right frontal hip bone. The knee is straight and the knee cap faces the sky. The back of the knee is in contact with the blanket. Elongate the heel and big toe bone away from you, and pull the little toe bone toward you,

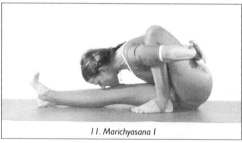

11. Marichyasana I

so that the foot is vertical and all the toes are in a line. Perform pada bandha with both feet to support the action in the pelvis.
- On a mula bandha inhalation, lift the pelvis up from the femur heads, rooting the left foot and the right buttock bone into the earth, and elongating the spinal column upwards out of the sacro-iliac joints.
- On the exhalation, rotate the pelvis forward to an angle of about forty-five degrees.
- Rotate the left frontal hip bone, the left side of the rib cage and the left shoulder forward, and place the left shoulder against the inner side of the left knee. Hold with the fingers of the left hand the outer edge of the right foot, keeping that foot vertical. The right hand rests lightly on the blanket on the right side of the right leg, do not put any weight on that hand.
- The inner side of the left knee rests against the backside of the left armpit, and the inner side of the left thigh rests against the left side of the rib cage.
- On each mula bandha inhalation, lift the pelvis up from the femur heads, rooting the right buttock bone and the left foot into the earth, and elongating the spinal column upwards out of the sacro-iliac joints.
- On each exhalation, rotate the trunk further towards the right.
- When you have reached the maximum elongation from the sacrum to the back of the head, and from the pubic bone to the throat, rotate the left arm backwards around the left knee in a large, circular movement. Do not elongate and rotate the left arm from the shoulder joint, but rather from the spinal column between the shoulder blades.
- Rotate the right arm backwards as well with a large, circular movement, and clasp the hands on the back. With the left knee bent, it is the left hand which has to hold the right hand. The reason is that in this position the left shoulder is in a slightly dangerous endorotation. By holding the right hand with the left, the muscles of the left shoulder

are tensed and are therefore better able to hold the left shoulder in a strong and stable position.

- On each mula bandha inhalation, lift the pelvis up from the femur heads, rooting the left foot and the right buttock bone into the earth and elongating the spinal column forwards out of the sacro-iliac joints. On each exhalation, rotate the pelvis further forward and bring the trunk closer to the right leg.
- The head is the last to come and rest on the shin beyond the knee. You can either place the forehead on the shin or, if you are more supple, the chin, so that the eyes look at the right foot.
- Hold for one minute; then repeat on the other side.

12. Marichyasana II

Marichi is the son of Brahman

This is a combination of padmasana (see page 72) and marichyasana I.

- Sit on a blanket with the legs extended straight in front of you.
- Place the right foot in the left groin as in padmasana (see page 72).
- Lean the body over on the right hip. Bend the left knee as in marichyasana I so that the knee points up towards the sky and the left foot rests on the blanket. The left heel touches the back of the left thigh and the toes point straight forward. In this position the left buttock bone does not rest on the blanket, but the weight of the body is distributed between the right hip and thigh, and the left foot.

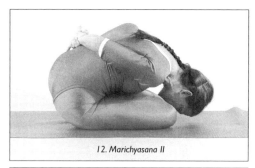

12. Marichyasana II

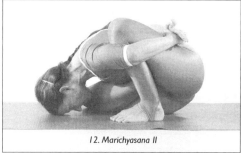

12. Marichyasana II

- On a mula bandha inhalation, lift the pelvis up from the femur heads. Root the left foot into the earth, bring the weight of the body forward onto the right thigh and knee, and elongate the spinal column upwards out of the sacro-iliac joints.
- On the exhalation, rotate the pelvis forward to an angle of about forty-five degrees.
- Rotate the left frontal hip bone, the left side of the rib cage and the left shoulder forward, and place the left shoulder against the inner side of the left knee. Elongate the left arm forward out of the left groin.
- The inner side of the left knee rests against the backside of the left armpit, and the inner side of the left thigh rests against the left side of the rib cage.
- On each mula bandha inhalation, lift the pelvis up from the femur heads, rooting the right thigh and knee and the left foot into the earth, and elongating the spinal column upwards out of the sacro-iliac joints.
- When you have reached maximum elongation from the sacrum to the back of the head, and from the pubic bone to the throat, rotate the left arm backwards around the left knee in a large, circular movement. Do not elongate and rotate the left arm from the shoulder joint, but rather from the spinal column between the shoulder blades.

- Rotate the right arm backwards as well with a large, circular movement, and clasp the hands on the back. With the left knee bent as in marichyasana I, it is the left hand which has to hold the right. The reason is that in this position the left shoulder is in a slightly dangerous endorotation. By holding with the left hand the right, the muscles of the left shoulder are tensed and therefore are better able to hold the left shoulder in a strong and stable position.
- On each mula bandha inhalation, lift the pelvis up from the femur heads, rooting the left foot and the right thigh and knee into the earth, and elongating the spinal column forwards out of the sacro-iliac joints. On each exhalation, rotate the pelvis further forward and bring the trunk closer to the right leg.
- The head is the last to come and rest on the blanket in between the left foot and the right knee.
- Hold for one minute; then repeat on the other side.

13. Ubhaya Padangusthasana
ubhaya=both; padangustha=big toe

13a. *Ubhaya Padangusthasana*

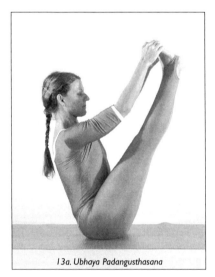

13a. Ubhaya Padangusthasana

This position is basically the same as the second part of paschimottanasana (1). The difference is that here the legs are extended up towards the sky, and the body balances on the buttock bones.
- Sit on a blanket with the legs extended straight in front of you.
- Bend the knees and hold the big toes with the index and middle fingers of the hands.
- Lean the body slightly backwards and extend the legs up towards the sky, keeping the inner ankles together. Do not bend the lumbar and thoracic spine. This position is an excellent toner for the front and back muscles of the trunk.
- On each mula bandha inhalation, lift the pelvis up from the femur heads, rooting the buttock bones into the earth and elongating the spinal column upwards out of the sacro-iliac joints. On each exhalation, rotate the pelvis further forward, so that the weight of the body rolls forwards onto the points of the buttock bones.
- Hold for one minute; then proceed to 13b.

13b. *Urdhvamukha Prasarita Padottanasana I*

urdhva=upwards; mukha=face;
prasarita=spread; pada=leg, foot;
uttana=intense stretch

This position is the same as dvipada upavistha konasana (15a). The difference is that here the legs are extended up towards the sky and the body balances on the buttock bones.

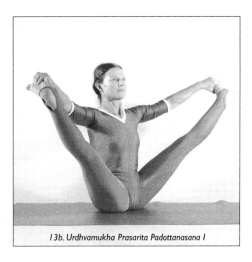

13b. Urdhvamukha Prasarita Padottanasana I

- Spread the legs, maintaining the balancing position on the buttock bones.
- Follow the same instructions as for the previous pose.
- Hold for one minute.

14. Urdhvamukha Paschimottanasana I

urdhva=upwards; mukha=face; paschima=the West,
the back of the body; uttana=intense stretch

This position is the same as the third part of paschimottanasana (1). The difference is that here the legs are extended up towards the sky and the body balances on the buttock bones.

- Sit in ubhaya padangusthasana (13a) and proceed:
- On an exhalation, close the trunk and head with the legs as described in paschimottanasana (1). As you are here working upwards against the force of gravity, it is harder to keep the back straight and elongate the spinal column upwards out of the groins and the sacro-iliac joints. Follow the instructions given for paschimottanasana (1).
- Hold for one minute.

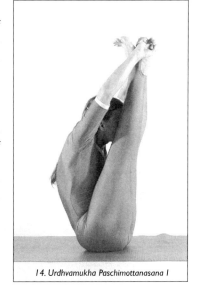

14. Urdhvamukha Paschimottanasana I

15. Upavistha Konasana

upavistha=seated;
kona=angle

15a. Dvipada Upavistha Konasana

dvi=two; pada=leg, foot; upavistha=seated; kona=angle

First part

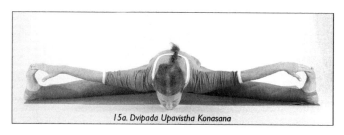

15a. Dvipada Upavistha Konasana

- Sit on a blanket with the legs extended straight in front of you.
- Spread the legs as far apart as possible. Keep the knees straight with the knee caps facing the sky; do not turn the legs in or out. The back of the knees are in contact with the blanket. Elongate the heels and big toe bones away from you, and pull the little toe bones towards you, so that the feet are vertical and the toes point straight up to the sky. Perform pada bandha to support the action in the pelvis.
- Do not pull the knee caps up, but release the tension at the front of the thighs and root the back of the knees into the earth. Extend the back of the legs from the knees to the heels forwards, elongating the heels away from you, and from the knees to the buttock bones backwards.
- Root the buttock bones and the coccyx into the earth, together with the back of the thighs, and draw the two frontal hip bones forward and up towards the ribs: rebounce action, extending the pelvis in opposite directions, down and up.

Follow the instructions given in paschimottanasana (1). The only difference is that in this position, the legs are spread.

Second part

- On an exhalation, rotate the pelvis forward and place the hands on the ankles or feet. The feet remain vertical and the backs of the knees remain in contact with the blanket.
- Follow the instructions given in paschimottanasana (1). The only difference is that in this position, the legs are spread and thus you can rotate the pelvis more than forty-five degrees forward.
- Do not allow the legs to rotate inward as the body bends forwards: the knee caps continue facing the sky. In this pose, special care must be taken not to tip the coccyx back and up towards the lumbar spine. Keep the coccyx firmly rooted by elongating the buttock bones and coccyx back and down as you draw the two frontal hip bones forward and up.

Third part

- When you have reached maximum elongation from the sacrum to the back of the head and from the pubic bone to the throat, place the head on the blanket. The further the head moves forward, the better.
- Here too the driving force for the trunk to elongate forwards lies in the pelvis. Rubbing forward on the buttock bones and rooting them, draw the two frontal hip bones forward

and elongate the spine horizontally forwards. The chest remains passive; as the spine elongates, the rib cage too moves forwards as a result of the movement of the pelvis and the spine.

- Keep the shoulder blades, shoulders, arms and hands relaxed. Eventually, you can place the chest on the blanket in between the legs. Keep the palms of the hands on the tips of the toes with the fingers straight. Slide the hands further sideways on the toes as the trunk and head slide forwards on the blanket.
- Hold for one to five minutes.

15b. *Ekapada Upavistha Konasana*

eka=one; pada=leg, foot; upavistha=seated; kona=angle

- Start with the first part of dvipada upavistha konasana (15a) and proceed:

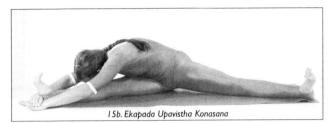
15b. Ekapada Upavistha Konasana

First part
- On a mula bandha inhalation, lift the pelvis up from the femur heads, rooting the buttock bones into the earth and elongating the spinal column upwards out of the sacro-iliac joints.
- On the exhalation, rotate the pelvis and trunk towards the right and with the left hand hold the outer edge of the right foot, keeping that foot vertical. The right hand rests lightly on the blanket on the right side of the right leg, do not put any weight on that hand.
- Rotate the trunk toward the right, until the frontal central line (navel-sternum-throat) is in line with the right leg. The left thigh rotates slightly inwards, and the left frontal hip bone rotates toward the navel, while the right frontal hip bone rotates away from the navel to the right: the left side of waist and rib cage rotates towards the right leg, while the right side rotates away from the right leg towards the right. Beginners often rotate only shoulders and ribs, but the movement should come from the pelvis.
- Do not pull the knee caps up; release the tension at the front of the thighs and root the back of the knees into the earth. At the same time, elongate the back of the legs from the buttock bones towards the heels, elongating the heels away from you. The weight of the body is mainly on the right buttock bone. The left buttock bone is slightly lifted off the blanket and the left thigh and frontal hip bone rotate slightly inwards.
- The spine from the sacrum up to the cervical spine is straight; if there is a deviation to the left it means that the trunk has not been fully rotated. It is very important for the spine to be straight from the beginning; if there is a curvature to the left, there will be a great strain on the left side of the spine and on the left sacro-iliac joint in the second part of the pose. When the spine is straight and in the center of the back, the width of rib cage and waist on the left and right side of the spine is equal; if the left side of the back is broader, the spine has curved to the left. Both sides of the back should be evenly long, straight, and parallel to each other.

Second part

- When you have reached maximum elongation from the sacrum to the back of the head, and from the pubic bone to the throat, place the head on the shin of the right leg. The closer the forehead moves towards the right foot, the better. Keep the right foot vertical.
- Turn the palm of the right hand forward, with the thumb and the four fingers form a ring and place the dorsal side of the wrist in the outer arch of the right foot. Turn the palm of the left hand forward as well, and insert the fingers of the left hand in the ring formed by the right hand. In this way there is the possibility of future elongation. It is important to note that on the right side it is the right hand which forms the ring for the left hand to slide through. This is because, by placing the back side of the right wrist in the small arch of the right foot, that pressure stabilizes the right foot in its vertical position (see the description in janu sirsasana (3)).
- The lower abdomen arrives first on the right thigh, then the navel; the navel comes to rest exactly on the midline of the right thigh. If this is not the case, but the navel stays on the inner side of the thigh, it means you have not perfected the first part of this pose.
- After the navel, the sternum comes to rest on the thigh, close to the knee on the midline of the thigh, not on the inner side. The head is the last to come and rest on the shin. You can either place the forehead on the shin, or, if you are more supple, the chin, so that the eyes look at the right foot. In both cases the neck, shoulders, shoulder blades and arms remain relaxed. On each mula bandha inhalation, slide the head (and of course the whole trunk) closer to the right foot.
- Hold for one minute; then repeat on the other side.

15c. *Parivrttaikapada Upavistha Konasana*

Parivrtta=turned around; eka=one; pada=leg,foot; upavistha=seated; kona=angle

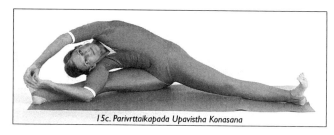

15c. Parivrttaikapada Upavistha Konasana

This position is basically the same as parivrtta janu sirsasana (4). The difference is that here both legs are straight, while in parivrtta janu sirsasana the leg towards which you are turning, is bent.

- Start with the first part of ekapada upavistha konasana (15b) towards the right leg and proceed:
- On an exhalation, turn to the left. Rotate the right arm as in savasana and place the right elbow on the blanket against the inner side of the right knee, with the palm of the right hand facing up to the sky. Turn the whole trunk (pelvis, chest, shoulders and head) to the left.
- Hold with the right hand the inner arch of the right foot. Extend the left arm up to the sky and elongate it out of the left hip joint, then hold the outer edge of the right foot with the left hand. Insert the head in between the arms and turn completely to the left, till the two shoulders are vertically aligned above the right thigh. Look up at the sky.

- Extend the left leg out of the left hip joint, keeping the left knee down on the blanket.
- On each mula bandha inhalation, elongate the whole right side of the trunk, from the right groin to the right armpit, forwards towards the right foot. Slide the right elbow closer to the right foot, so that the whole right side of the trunk rests on the thigh.
- On each exhalation, continue the rotation of the trunk to the left.
- Hold for one minute; then repeat on the other side.

16. Baddha Konasana II
baddha=bound; kona=angle
(See also page 106.)

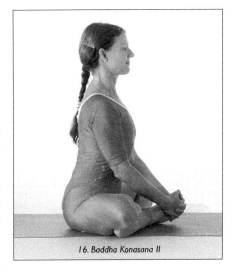
16. Baddha Konasana II

- Sit on a blanket with the knees spread sideways and the soles of the feet united. Hold with the hands the feet and pull the heels as close to the pubic bone as possible. Lower the knees to the blanket by elongating the thighs sideways out of the hip joints.
- Pull the buttock muscles backwards with the hands, so that you are sitting on the buttock bones, not on the flesh. The body weight is divided evenly between both buttock bones. Then hold the feet with the hands again.
- The pelvis is in a vertical position, with the two frontal hip bones in vertical alignment above the groins. The groove of the spine is even from base to top and runs straight upwards.

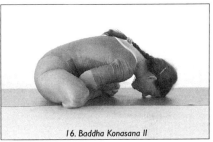
16. Baddha Konasana II

- On a mula bandha inhalation, root the buttock bones, the outer thighs and the outer edges of the feet into the earth, lift the pelvis and trunk up from the femur heads and elongate the spinal column upwards.
- On the exhalation, extend the thighs and knees sideways out of the hip joints and bend forward, till the sternum rests on the feet and the head on the blanket. The sternum arrives on the feet before the head arrives on the blanket. Do not lift the buttock bones up, but extend them backwards, spreading them at the same time.
- On each inhalation, extend the buttock bones further backwards and the thighs further sideways. At the same time, elongate the lower abdomen, rib cage, spine and head further forwards.
- On each exhalation, lower the trunk and head with gravity onto the feet and earth.
- Hold for one to five minutes; then come up on an inhalation, raising first the head, then the chest, and then the abdomen.

17. Malasana

mala=garland

- Start with utkatasana II (see page 94) and proceed:
- Widen the knees, lower the elbows onto the blanket, and then press the inner thighs against the sides of the rib cage.
- On a mula bandha inhalation, root the feet into the earth, extend the groins, the buttock bones and the back of the thighs backwards, and elongate the lower abdomen, rib cage, spine, head and hands forwards.
- On the exhalation, rotate both arms backwards with a large, circular movement, and clasp the hands on the back. Or, hold the back of the heels with the hands if you cannot clasp the hands on the back. Then lower the head onto the blanket.
- Hold for one minute; then stand up again in tadasana on an exhalation.

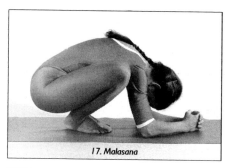

17. Malasana

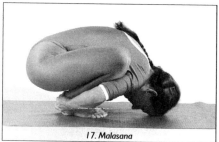

17. Malasana

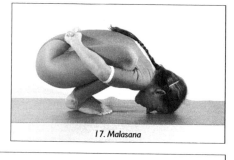

17. Malasana

18. Kurmasana

kurma=tortoise

- Sit on a blanket with the legs extended straight in front of you.
- Widen the legs, until the distance between the feet is slightly more than the width of the shoulders.
- Bend the knees. Turn the legs slightly outwards and insert the shoulders underneath the knees, till the backs of the knees rest on the deltoid muscles. Then extend the arms sideways.

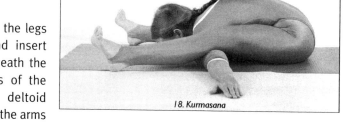

18. Kurmasana

- Roll the legs inwards again, till the knees point straight up towards the sky and the inner thighs press against the side ribs. Extend the legs till they are straight, and elongate the heels forward, keeping the feet vertical.
- Rest the head on the blanket, on either the forehead or the chin. On each mula bandha inhalation, elongate the trunk and spine forward from the groins towards the head. On each exhalation, elongate the legs further forwards, so that the knees press down more onto the deltoid muscles, and elongate the arms further sideways.
- Hold for one minute.

19. Ekapada Sirsasana cycle
eka=one; pada=leg, foot; sirsa=head

19a. Ekapada Sirsasana

- Sit on a blanket with the legs extended straight in front of you.
- Hold the right foot in both hands and lift it as for padmasana (see page 72). The right hand supports the right ankle, and the left hand holds the metatarsals of the foot.
- Lift the foot to face level and rotate the knee so that it points sideways, not backwards.
- Place the right hand on the calf muscle of the right leg, and with the thumb push the calf muscle backwards over the shoulder.
- Turn the chest and shoulders towards the left, and insert the right shoulder underneath the knee of the right leg.
- Then lift the right foot over the back of the head, till the outer ankle rests against the back of the neck.
- Lift the face to look forward, not downwards. The back will be bent, but try to keep the bending minimal. Fold the hands in namasté I in front of the sternum.
- As the tendency in this pose is to roll the pelvis backwards on the buttock bones, you have to counteract that by keeping the left leg firm and performing pada bandha with the left foot. In this way you can pull the trunk forward to the vertical line.
- On each mula bandha inhalation, elongate the trunk upwards, and on each exhalation maintain that height.
- Hold for a few seconds; then repeat on the other side.

Practice this position for a while till you feel comfortable in it. Then you can try the variations. These variations are done in the vinyasa mode, that is, proceeding directly from one to the next, using the breathing.

19b. Kala Bhairavasana

Kala Bhairava is Shiva in his aspect as destroyer of the universe

- Start with ekapada sirsasana (19a) and proceed:
- Roll onto the left hip and the outer edge of the left foot. Place the left hand behind the body on the blanket, so that the arm forms an angle of ninety degrees with the side of the trunk, and the fingers point away from the left hip. Push the body up on the left hand and the left foot.
- This pose resembles kasyapasana (see page 184). The left side of the trunk forms one continuous line with the left leg. Extend the right arm up to the sky and look straight forward.
- Root the left hand, performing hasta bandha, and the outer edge of the left foot, performing pada bandha, to lighten the body.
- Hold for a few seconds; then proceed to 19c.

19a. Ekapada Sirsasana

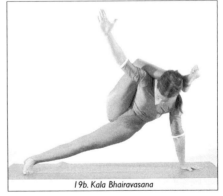
19b. Kala Bhairavasana

19c. Bhairavasana
bhairava=terrible,
formidable

- Lower the body again on the left hip and then roll onto the back.
- Press the back of the neck firmly against the outer right ankle, so that the foot does not slip over the head.

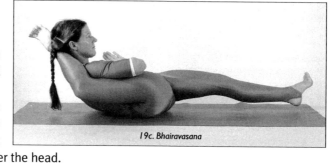
19c. Bhairavasana

- Extend the left leg on the blanket, so that the knee faces straight up towards the sky and the left heel rests on the blanket. Perform pada bandha on the left foot to keep the leg straight and firm.
- Hold for a few seconds; then proceed to 19d.

19d. Skandasana
Skanda is Kartikeya, the god of war

- Come back up again to ekapada sirsasana (19a).
- On an exhalation, bend the trunk forward, hold the left foot with the hands and bring the head to the shin.
- Hold for a few seconds; then proceed to 19e.

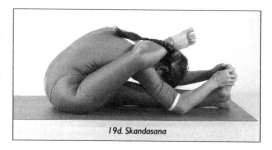
19d. Skandasana

19e. Chakorasana I
chakora is a bird

- Come back up to ekapada sirsasana (19a) and place the hands next to the hips on the blanket.
- Push the whole body up, till you are standing on the two hands only, with the left leg extended straight forward. Look straight forward.
- This pose resembles ekahasta bhujasana (see page 188). As in ekahasta bhujasana, the weight of the straight (suspended) leg is sustained by the abdominal muscles.
- On each mula bandha inhalation,

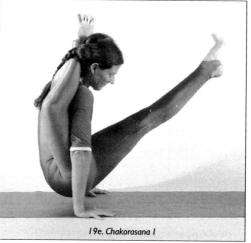
19e. Chakorasana I

root the hands and perform hasta bandha to lighten the body.
- Hold for a few seconds; then proceed to 19f.

19f. Ruchikasana
Ruchika is the name of a sage

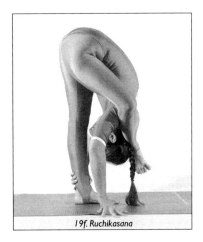

19f. Ruchikasana

- Sit down again in ekapada sirsasana (19a) and bend the left knee. Place the sole of the foot close to the left buttock bone on the blanket, with the knee pointing up towards the sky.
- Place the hands on the blanket next to you, lift the pelvis up and bring the weight of the body onto the left foot. Then stand up. Keep the right hand on the blanket next to the left foot and hold the left ankle with the left hand. Rest the head on the shin. This pose resembles ardha baddha padmottanasana.
- Hold for a few seconds; then proceed to 19g.

19g. Durvasasana
Durvasa is the name of a saint

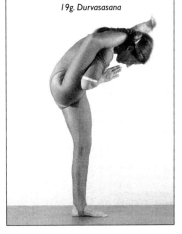

19g. Durvasasana

- On an inhalation, raise the trunk and stand straight up on the left leg.
- In this pose it is very difficult to stand straight. The main issue is to keep the balance and to lift the trunk and head as much as possible.
- Hold for a few seconds; then repeat 19a through 19g on the other side.

20. Yoga Nidrasana
nidra=sleep

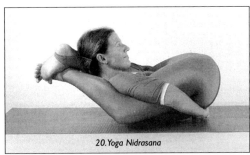

20. Yoga Nidrasana

- Lie on the back on a blanket.
- Bend the legs and spread the knees, so that the backs of the knees rest against the outer sides of the deltoid muscles. Hold the ankles with the hands, with the thumbs pointing inwards towards each other.
- Raise the head, and insert the shoulders one by one inside the knees. Cross the ankles behind the head or neck.
- Rotate the arms backwards around the thighs, and clasp the hands at the back of the pelvis.
- In this pose the back is bent. Try, however, to straighten it as much as possible, using the mula bandha breathing: on each mula bandha inhalation, widen the upper chest and shoulders, and extend the feet further backwards, so that the angle in the knees increases. On each exhalation, lower the sacrum further to the earth.

- Hold for a few seconds (you can increase the time to one minute); then change the crossing of the feet.

The following positions are done in the vinyasa mode, that is, flowing from one into the other, using the breathing:

21. Dvipada Sirsasana

dvi=two; pada=leg, foot; sirsa=head

21a. Dvipada Sirsasana

This is basically the same position as yoga nidrasana (20). The difference is that here you are not lying on the back, but are sitting on the buttock bones. Thus the added problem in this pose is that of the balance. This again depends on a finely tuned cooperation between the lower back muscles and the abdominal muscles.

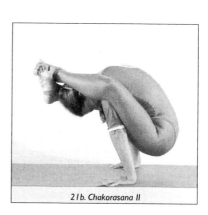
21a. Dvipada Sirsasana

- Start with ekapada sirsasana (19a), placing the right foot behind the neck.
- Bend the left leg and bring the left foot back over the head in the same way. Cross the ankles in the neck as in yoga nidrasana (20), fold the palms in front of the sternum in namasté I and look straight forward.
- Hold for a few seconds; then proceed to 21b.

21b. Chakorasana II

chakora is a bird

- Place the hands next to the hips on the blanket, slant the body a little forward and push up, till you are standing on the hands. Perform hasta bandha in order to lighten the body.
- Keep the grip between the feet and ankles strong, so that the legs will not slip off from the head.
- Hold for a few seconds; thange the crossing of the feet and repeat 21a and b.

21b. Chakorasana II

Part 8 Twisting Poses

These positions can be done in *three different modes:*

a. ***Performing each position*** separately and holding it for one minute.

b. *Vinyasa*
Connecting two or more positions by flowing from one into the other, using the breathing.

c. *Mala*
Connecting all the positions through surya namaskar, using the breathing and holding each of the twisting poses for the duration of three breaths.

Twisting poses

1. Parivrttaikapada Padmasana I
2. Parivrttaikapada Padmasana II
3. Parivrtta Padmasana
4. Bharadvajasana I
5. Bharadvajasana II
6. Vamadevasana
7. Yogadandasana
8. Marichyasana III
9. Marichyasana IV
10. Marichyasana V
11. Pasasana
12. Ardha Matsyendrasana
13. Paripurna Matsyendrasana

---

1. Parivrttaikapada Padmasana I

*parivrtta=turned around; eka=one;
pada=leg,foot; padma=lotus*

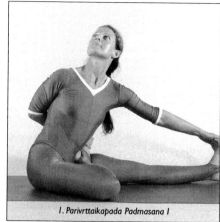

I. Parivrttaikapada Padmasana I

- Sit on a blanket with the legs extended straight in front of you.
- Take the right foot in both hands as for padmasana (see page 72) and place it in the left groin.
- On a mula bandha inhalation root the buttock bones and the right knee into the earth, lift the pelvis up from the femur heads and elongate the whole body upwards. Extend the right arm up to the sky.
- On the exhalation rotate the trunk towards the right, swing the right arm around the back and hold the right foot. Curl the toes of the foot around the fingers, so that the foot holds as much the hand as the hand the foot (pada bandha).
- Keep the left leg straight and perform pada bandha on both the feet to support the action in the pelvis. With the left hand hold the left foot from the top and turn the head towards the right.
- On each mula bandha inhalation elongate the lower abdomen and spinal column further upwards towards the back of the head, rooting the buttock bones and the right knee into the earth.
- On each exhalation rotate the trunk, chest, shoulders and head further towards the right till the chest and shoulders are aligned with the left (straight) leg.
- Hold for one minute. Then repeat on the other side

2. Parivrttaikapada Padmasana II

*parivrtta=turned around; eka=one;
pada=leg, foot; padma=lotus*

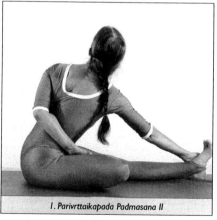

I. Parivrttaikapada Padmasana II

- Sit on a blanket with the legs extended straight in front of you.
- Take the right foot in both hands as for padmasana (see page 72) and place it in the left groin.
- On a mula bandha inhalation root the buttock bones and the right knee into the earth, lift the pelvis up from the femur heads and elongate the whole body upwards. Extend the left arm up to the sky.
- On the exhalation rotate the trunk towards the left, swing the left arm around the back, and hold the right shin.
- Keep the left leg straight and perform pada bandha on both feet to support the action in the pelvis. With the right hand hold the left foot and turn the head towards the left.

- On each mula bandha inhalation elongate the lower abdomen and spinal column further upwards towards the back of the head, rooting the buttock bones and the right knee into the earth.
- On each exhalation rotate the trunk, chest, shoulders and head further towards the left till the chest and shoulders are aligned with the left (straight) leg.
- Hold for one minute. Then repeat on the other side.

3. Parivrtta Padmasana
parivrtta=turned around; padma=lotus

3a. Parivrtta Siddhasana

For those people who cannot do full padmasana (see page 72) this twisting pose can also be done in siddhasana (see page 78).

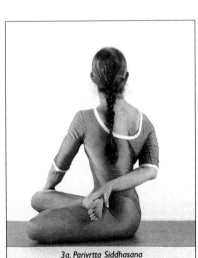

- Sit in siddhasana with the right foot on the left thigh. The knees should be fairly close together so that both feet stick out on the sides of the thighs. Thus the right knee rests on the left shin and ankle, not on the foot.
- On a mula bandha inhalation root the buttock bones and the left knee into the earth, lift the pelvis up from the femur heads and elongate the whole body upwards. Extend the right arm up to the sky.

3a. Parivrtta Siddhasana

- On the exhalation rotate the trunk towards the right, swing the right arm around the back and hold the right foot. Curl the toes of the foot around the fingers, so that the foot holds as much the hand as the hand the foot (pada bandha).
- Cross the left arm over the right thigh, turning the arm as in savasana. Place the back of the wrist against the outer right thigh and hold the left foot. Curl the toes of the foot around the fingers, so that the foot holds as much the hand as the hand the foot (pada bandha).
- Turn the head towards the right.
- On each mula bandha inhalation elongate the lower abdomen and spinal column further upwards towards the back of the head, rooting the buttock bones and the left knee into the earth.
- On each exhalation rotate the trunk, chest, shoulders and head further towards the right till the chest and shoulders are perpendicular to the line between the knees.
- Hold for one minute. Then repeat on the other side.

3a. Parivrtta Siddhasana

3b. *Parivrtta Padmasana*

This is the same position done in full padmasana.

- Sit in padmasana (see page 72) with the right leg crossing over the left. The knees should be fairly close together so that both feet stick out on the sides of the thighs.
- On a mula bandha inhalation root the buttock bones and the knees into the earth, lift the pelvis up from the femur heads and elongate the whole body upwards. Extend the right arm up to the sky.
- On the exhalation rotate the trunk towards the right, swing the right arm around the back and hold the right foot. Curl the toes of the foot

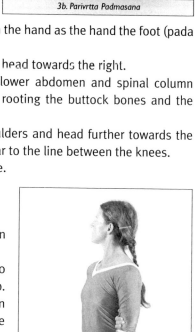

3b. Parivrtta Padmasana

around the fingers, so that the foot holds as much the hand as the hand the foot (pada bandha).
- Place the left hand on the right knee and turn the head towards the right.
- On each mula bandha inhalation elongate the lower abdomen and spinal column further upwards towards the back of the head, rooting the buttock bones and the knees into the earth.
- On each exhalation rotate the trunk, chest, shoulders and head further towards the right till the chest and shoulders are perpendicular to the line between the knees.
- Hold for one minute. Then repeat on the other side.

4. Bharadvajasana I

Bharadvaja is the father of Drona

- Sit on a blanket with the legs extended straight in front of you.
- Bend both legs to the left and place them next to the left hip, so that you are sitting on the right hip. The toes of the right foot rest on the achilles tendon of the left foot. Even though the left buttock bone does not rest on the blanket, it is important to nevertheless bring the weight of the body back onto it, so that the weight is divided evenly on both the buttock bones.
- On a mula bandha inhalation root the buttock bones and the knees into the earth, lift the pelvis up from the femur heads and elongate the whole body upwards. Extend the right arm up to the sky.
- On the exhalation rotate the trunk towards the right, swing the right arm around the back, and hold the left upper arm.
- Place the left hand on the right knee and turn the head towards the right.

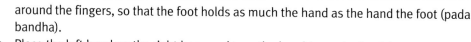
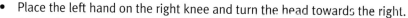

4. Bharadvajasana I

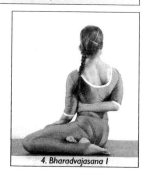

4. Bharadvajasana I

- On each mula bandha inhalation elongate the lower abdomen and spinal column further upwards towards the back of the head, rooting the buttock bones and the knees into the earth.
- On each exhalation rotate the trunk, chest, shoulders and head further towards the right till the chest and shoulders are perpendicular to the line between the knees.
- Hold for one minute. Then repeat on the other side.

5. Bharadvajasana II
Bharadvaja is the father of Drona

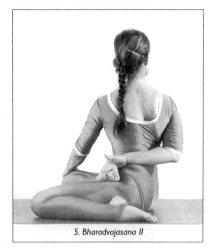

5. *Bharadvajasana II*

- Sit on a blanket with the legs extended straight in front of you.
- Bend the left leg to the left and place it next to the left hip as in virasana I (see page 96).
- Take the right foot in both hands as for padmasana (see page 72) and place it in the left groin. The left knee now points straight forward, and the right knee points at an angle of forty-five degrees to the right.
- In this position both buttock bones and both knees are on the blanket.
- On a mula bandha inhalation root the buttock bones and the knees into the earth, lift the pelvis up from the femur heads and elongate the whole body upwards. Extend the right arm up to the sky.
- On the exhalation rotate the trunk towards the right, swing the right arm around the back and hold the right foot. Curl the toes of the foot around the fingers, so that the foot holds as much the hand as the hand the foot (pada bandha).
- Place the left hand on the right knee and turn the head towards the right.
- On each mula bandha inhalation elongate the lower abdomen and spinal column further

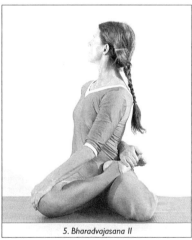

5. *Bharadvajasana II*

upwards towards the back of the head, rooting the buttock bones and the knees into the earth.
- On each exhalation rotate the trunk, chest, shoulders and head further towards the right till the chest and shoulders are perpendicular to the line between the knees.
- In this pose there is a diagonal action: the left buttock bone and the right knee have to go down simultaneously, so that the rooting is done on a diagonal line: left buttock bone-right knee, and right buttock bone-left knee.
- Hold for one minute. Then repeat on the other side.

6. Vamadevasana

Vamadeva is a name for Shiva

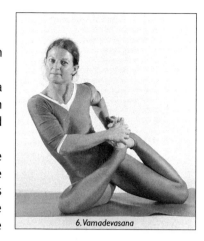

6. Vamadevasana

- Sit on a blanket with the legs extended straight In front of you.
- Bend the left leg backwards as in upavistha virasana I (see page 98) till the left thigh makes an angle of ninety degrees with the right one. Bend the right leg as for sukhasana (see page 77).
- Lift with the left hand the left foot up and rotate the left thigh inwards, turning the arm so that the fingers point forwards and the left elbow points backwards. Hold with the palm of the hand the dorsal side of the left foot. Push the foot till the left heel touches the left femur head.
- Hold with the right hand the dorsal side of the right foot and raise the foot, keeping the knee on the blanket.
- Join the heels and the soles of the two feet together on the outer left hip.
- Hold for a few seconds. Then repeat on the other side.

7. Yogadandasana

danda=staff

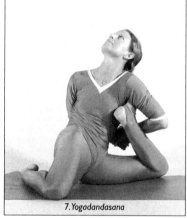

7. Yogadandasana

- Sit on a blanket with the legs extended straight in front of you.
- Bend the right leg as in virasana I (see page 96).
- Bend the left leg as for sukhasana (see page 77). Hold the left foot with both hands and raise it, turning the leg as for padmasana (see page 72).
- Flex the foot at an angle of ninety degrees to the shin. Hold with the right hand the heel and with the left hand the outer edge of the left foot. The left arm crosses over the shin bone. In this way the right hand can push and the left hand can pull the foot backwards.
- Pull the left knee back and down till the outer left thigh rests on the blanket, so that the left thigh rotates even deeper in the left hip joint. The trunk is now resting only on the left hip, while the right hip is raised.
- Release the left hand, lean on the left hip and place the triceps muscle of the left arm in the arch of the left foot.
- Push with the right hand the left foot still further backwards. At the same time turn the chest and shoulders towards the right, till the sole of the left foot rests in the left armpit.
- Rotate the left arm backwards around the foot. Swing the right arm around the back and clasp the hands on the back. The left hand holds the right one.
- Turn the head and chest to the right.
- Hold for a few seconds. Then repeat on the other side.

8. Marichyasana III

Marichi is a sage

- Sit on a blanket with the legs extended straight in front of you.
- Bend the right leg so that the knee points up towards the sky and the right foot rests on the blanket next to the left thigh. The toes point straight forward.

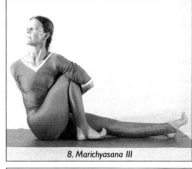

8. Marichyasana III

- The left leg extends straight out of the left hip joint with the left foot in line with the left frontal hip bone. The knee should be straight with the knee cap facing the sky and the back of the knee in contact with the blanket. Elongate the heel and big toe bone away from you and pull the little toe bone towards you, so that the foot is vertical and all the toes are in a line. Perform pada bandha with the left foot in order to support the action in the pelvis.

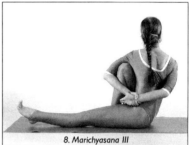

8. Marichyasana III

- On a mula bandha inhalation lift the pelvis up from the femur heads, rooting the right foot and the buttock bones into the earth and elongating the spinal column upwards.
- On the exhalation place the right hand back of you on the blanket and rotate the lower abdomen, waist, chest, shoulders and head towards the right.
- Rotate the left arm as in savasana and place the back side of the left upper arm, close to the arm pit, against the outer side of the right knee or thigh. Keep pointing the right knee straight up to the sky and use the pressure of the left arm against the right outer knee to rotate further towards the right.
- Slide the left arm still further forward on the outer right thigh till the right knee rests in the back side of the left armpit. Do not cross the right knee over the left groin, but keep the right knee, groin, foot and buttock bone all in one line.
- Rotate the left arm backwards around the right shin. Extend the right arm sideways and, with a large, circular movement, swing it backwards around the back. Do not elongate and rotate the right arm from the shoulder joint, but rather from the spinal column between the shoulder blades. Clasp the hands on the back. With the right knee bent it is the left hand which has to hold the right hand. The reason is that in this position the left shoulder is in a slightly dangerous endorotation. By holding the right hand with the left, the muscles of the left shoulder are tensed and are therefore better able to hold the left shoulder in a firm and stable position.
- On each mula bandha inhalation elongate the lower abdomen and spinal column further upwards towards the back of the head, bringing the weight of the body forward onto the right foot. Root the buttock bones and the right foot, performing pada bandha with both feet to activate the mula bandha.
- On each exhalation rotate the trunk, chest, shoulders and head further towards the right till the chest and shoulders are aligned with the left leg. Rotate the right femur head backwards towards the coccyx in order to keep the knee, groin, foot and buttock bone in one line.
- Hold for one minute. Then repeat on the other side.

9. Marichyasana IV

Marichi is a sage

This is basically the same position as marichyasana III (8). The difference is that here the left leg is bent as in virasana I (see page 96) instead of being straight as in marichyasana III (8).

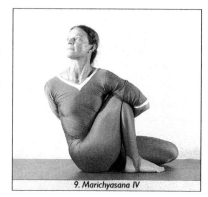

9. Marichyasana IV

- Sit on a blanket with the legs extended straight in front of you.
- Bend the left leg to the left and place the left foot next to the left hip as in virasana I (see page 96).
- Bend the right leg so that the knee points up towards the sky and the right foot rests on the blanket next to the left thigh. The toes point straight forward.
- The left thigh extends straight out of the left hip joint, so that the left knee is in line with the left frontal hip bone. The weight of the body is divided evenly on both buttock bones.
- For the rest follow the instructions given in marichyasana III (8).
- Hold for one minute. Then repeat on the other side.

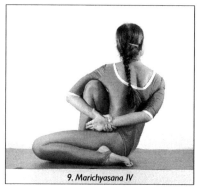

9. Marichyasana IV

10. Marichyasana V

Marichi is a sage

This is basically the same position as marichyasana III (8). The difference is that here the left leg is bent as in padmasana (see page 72) instead of being straight as in marichyasana III (8).

- Sit on a blanket with the legs extended straight in front of you.
- Take the left foot in both hands as for padmasana (see page 72) and place it in the right groin.

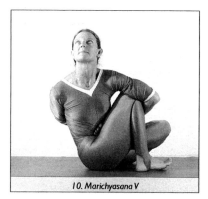

10. Marichyasana V

- Bend the right leg so that the knee points up towards the sky and the right foot rests on the blanket. The toes point straight forward.
- In this position the weight of the body is more on the left hip.
- For the rest follow the instructions given in marichyasana III (8).
- Hold for one minute. Then repeat on the other side.

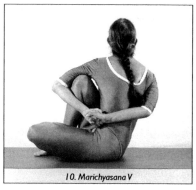

10. Marichyasana V

11. Pasasana

pasa=noose, cord

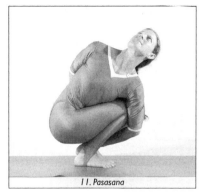

11. Pasasana

- Start with utkatasana II (see page 94) and proceed:
- On a mula bandha inhalation lift the pelvis up from the femur heads, rooting the feet into the earth and performing pada bandha. Extend the buttock bones backwards and elongate the spinal column upwards.
- On the exhalation place the right hand back of you on the blanket and rotate the lower abdomen, waist, chest, shoulders and head towards the right. Keep the knees pointing straight forward.
- Rotate the left arm as in savasana and place the back side of the left upper arm close to the armpit against the outer side of the right knee or thigh. Use the pressure of the left arm against the outside of the right knee to rotate the trunk further towards the right.
- Slide the left arm still further forward on the outer right thigh, till the right knee rests in the

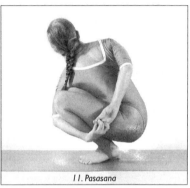

11. Pasasana

back side of the left armpit. Do not move the knees over to the left, but keep the knees, groins, feet and buttock bones all in one line, with the knees pointing straight forward.
- Rotate the left arm backwards around the right shin. Extend the right arm sideways and, with a large, circular movement, swing it around the back. Do not elongate and rotate the right arm from the shoulder joint, but rather from the spinal column between the shoulder blades. Clasp the hands on the back. When turning to the right it is the left hand which has to hold the right hand.
- On each mula bandha inhalation elongate the lower abdomen and spinal column further upwards towards the back of the head and bring the weight of the body forward onto the lower spring joints of the feet. Rooting the feet and elongating the buttock bones backwards use the spring joints to rebounce the weight of the body back upwards (pada bandha), so that the pose is stable and light at the same time.
- On each exhalation rotate the trunk, chest, shoulders and head further towards the right till the chest and shoulders are aligned with the thighs.
- Hold for one minute. Then repeat on the other side.

12. Ardha Matsyendrasana

*ardha=half; Matsyendra is one of the founders
of Hatha Vidya (matsya=fish; indra=king)*

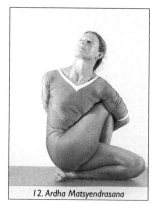

12. Ardha Matsyendrasana

- Sit on a blanket with the legs extended straight in front of you.
- Bend the left leg to the left and place the left foot next to the left hip as in virasana I (see page 96).
- Place the hands on the blanket next to you, lift the pelvis up and roll the buttock bones onto the left foot. Turn the left foot under in such a way that it makes an angle of ninety degrees with the shin. The foot rests on the outer edge, not on the dorsal side, on the blanket.
- Both the buttock bones rest on the foot, the left one on the inner heel and the right one on the metatarsal of the big toe.
- Swing the right foot over the left thigh and place the right foot next to the outer left thigh, about halfway between the knee and the hip. The toes point straight forward.
- On a mula bandha inhalation lift the pelvis up from the femur heads, rooting the right foot into the earth and the buttock bones into the left foot. Elongate the spinal column upwards.
- On the exhalation place the right hand back of you on the blanket and rotate the lower abdomen, waist, chest, shoulders and head towards the right.

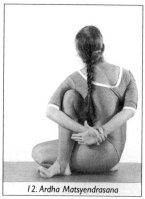

12. Ardha Matsyendrasana

- Rotate the left arm as in savasana and place the back side of the left upper arm close to the armpit against the outer right knee or thigh. Keep pointing the right knee straight up to the sky and use the pressure of the left arm against the outer side of the right knee to rotate further towards the right.
- Slide the left arm still further forward on the outer right thigh till the right knee rests in the back side of the left armpit.
- Rotate the left arm backwards around the right shin. Extend the right arm sideways and, with a large, circular movement, swing it backwards around the back. Do not elongate and rotate the right arm from the shoulder joint, but rather from the spinal column between the shoulder blades. Clasp the hands on the back. When turning towards the right it is the left hand which has to hold the right hand.
- On each mula bandha inhalation elongate the lower abdomen and spinal column further upwards towards the back of the head and root the buttock bones and the right foot. Perform pada bandha with both feet to activate the mula bandha.
- On each exhalation rotate the trunk, chest, shoulders and head further towards the right till the chest and shoulders are aligned with the left thigh. Rotate the right femur head backwards towards the coccyx in order to keep the right buttock bone firmly on the metatarsal of the left foot.
- Hold for one minute. Then repeat on the other side.

The general tendency in this pose is to slide the buttock bones off the foot. This results in a tilting of the pelvis with consequent stress on the downward sacro-iliac joint. Thus special attention has to be given to keeping both buttock bones on the foot.

13. Paripurna Matsyendrasana

paripurna=complete; Matsyendra is one of the
founders of Hatha Vidya (matsya=fish; indra=king)

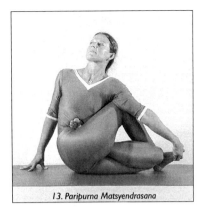

13. Paripurna Matsyendrasana

- Sit on a blanket with the legs extended straight in front of you.
- Bend the left leg and place the left foot in the right groin as for padmasana (see page 72).
- Bend the right leg and swing the right foot over the left thigh, bringing the weight of the body onto the outer left hip and raising the right hip up. Rest the right foot against the outer side of the left thigh, close to the knee. The toes point straight forward.
- On a mula bandha inhalation lift the pelvis up from the femur heads, rooting the left hip into the earth and elongating the spinal column upwards.
- On the exhalation place the right hand back of you on the blanket and rotate the lower abdomen, waist, chest, shoulders and head towards the right.
- Rotate the left arm as in savasana and place the back side of the left upper arm close to the armpit against the outer side of the right knee. Keep pointing the right knee straight up to the sky and use the pressure of the left arm against the right outer knee to rotate further towards the right.
- Slide the left arm still further forward on the outer right knee till the right knee rests in the back side of the left armpit. Then rotate the arm backwards around the shin and hold the right foot.
- On each mula bandha inhalation elongate the lower abdomen and spinal column further upwards towards the back of the head, and on each exhalation rotate the trunk, chest, shoulders and head further towards the right.
- Hold for a few seconds. Then repeat on the other side

This twisting pose is the most difficult of all. Do not force it, as you can hurt the knee. It may take a long time to master this pose.

Part 9 Sirsasana/Head Balance cycle

These positions are done in the *vinyasa* mode, that is, going from one pose directly into the next one, using the breathing.

Sirsasana cycle

1. Salamba Sirsasana I
2. Urdhva Dandasana
3. Parivrtta Sirsasana
4. Parivrttaikapada Sirsasana
5. Parsvaikapada Sirsasana
6. Ekapada Sirsasana
7. Urdhva Padma Sirsasana
8. Parivrtta Urdhva Padma Sirsasana
9. Pinda Sirsasana

10. Vajra Sirsasana
11. Parivrtta Vajra Sirsasana
12. Prasarita Padottana Sirsasana
13. Baddha Kona Sirsasana
14. Salamba Sirsasana II
15. Salamba Sirsasana III
16. Muktahasta Sirsasana
17. Baddhahasta Sirsasana

Sirsasana or *head balance* is one of the best known yoga poses and is often called the king of the postures in traditional texts. It was recommended that this pose be done every day, together with sarvangasana or shoulder balance, for a certain length of time in order to keep the body young, healthy and full of vigor.

Though standing on one's head may look spectacular, it is actually one of the easier positions. The main problem is to find the balance, but once that has been established, the body has exactly the same feeling as in tadasana. In tadasana the body is aligned on the force of gravity in spine, pelvis and legs; in head balance it is aligned in the same way. Many people stand on their heads with great muscular effort, because they are out of alignment with the force of gravity. As a result they have to use more muscles – and the wrong ones – than necessary to keep the body from falling.

Head balance is, as the name says, a balance. The legs, pelvis and spine balance on the head and the more they form a straight and continuous line with the neck, the more the body balances on the skeletal structure, not on the upholding force of the muscles.

Practice the straight head balance called *salamba sirsasana I* first, till that comes naturally, before proceeding to the variations.

1. Salamba Sirsasana I

sa=with; alamba=support; sirsa=head

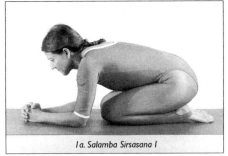

1a. Salamba Sirsasana I

- Place a folded blanket on the earth and kneel in front of it.
- Place the elbows and lower arms on the blanket, with the elbows at the same width as the arm pits. Keep them in line; do not keep one elbow further forward than the other. Interlock the fingers and thumbs, and tuck the bottom little finger into the palm of the other hand to make the rim of the hands and wrists equal (photo 1a).
- The wrist has four sides: the inner side (the palm), the back side (the dorsal side), the thumb (radial) side and the little finger (ulnar) side. It was discovered long ago in martial arts that certain points on the wrists induce strength in the arm and the whole body, while other points induce weakness. Both in karate and in sword fighting the point that is of vital importance is the one on the inner wrist, on the side of the little finger, called the ulnar wrist point. This is a key point in all martial arts. Anatomically speaking, this point connects three pair of major muscles: the latissimus dorsi, the pectoralis major and the deltoid muscles. It is the combination of these three muscles that lends strength to the arms and trunk, and enables the karate master to break the bricks, and the sword master to win a duel. In yoga too this point is of vital importance, especially in a position like head balance, as it gives the body stability and endurance.
- Keeping the fingers soft and relaxed and the ulnar wrist points rooted into the earth, place the head on the blanket between the wrists and palms of the hands. The head rests exactly on the top of the skull, halfway between the forehead and the crown, on the fontanel (the thousand-petalled lotus). The face looks straight forward, with the chin and the forehead in vertical alignment.
- Place the knees against the forehead, in between the elbows, with the toes tucked under (photo 1b). Press the elbows against the knees, so that the shoulder blades, the latissimus dorsi and the deltoid muscles widen and the upper back is opened; at the same time, move the shoulder blades towards the waist. If the shoulder blades move towards the spine, the shoulders collapse and the weight of the body will fall into the neck vertebrae.

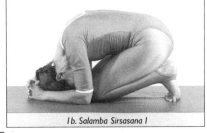

1b. Salamba Sirsasana I

- Root the top of the head into the blanket, so that the cervical and thoracic spine elongate up towards the sky. In head balance, the rebounce action of the rooting lies in the joint between the first cervical vertebra (the atlas) and the base of the skull. The more the head roots, the more this joint opens, giving the thrust for the rest of the spinal column to move up against the force of gravity. The muscles involved in this elongation of the spine are those vertical ones that run closest to the spinal vertebrae. These muscles should be alerted right from the beginning, so that the body balances in the final pose only on the spinal column and its vertical muscles, not on the shoulders and trapezius muscles, whose fibers run parallel to the earth and are therefore incapable of producing the rebounce force.

In this context it is interesting to note that the big, peripheral muscles of the body, which include the trapezius muscles, are geared for short-term, dynamic action (weight lifting and trapeze work), not for long-term, static action. In head balance, where you want to stand for at least five minutes, the body needs to utilize muscles geared for long-term, static action; these are exactly those vertical muscles that run closest to the spinal column.

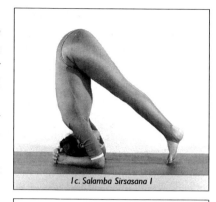

1c. Salamba Sirsasana I

- On an inhalation, raise the knees, keeping the feet on the earth (photo 1c), till the trunk is vertical and the hip joints are in line with the shoulder joints. Do not take the hips back, and do not bend the spine, but keep spine and neck erect.

- On the exhalation, continue the rooting of the head and the elongation of the cervical and thoracic spine, so that the legs are raised to the vertical in one smooth movement, hinging in the femo-iliac joints. The legs are light going up, as it is the vertical spinal muscles that do the work. Keep the knees straight and the feet together (photo 1d and 1e).

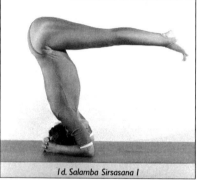

1d. Salamba Sirsasana I

- In salamba sirsasana I the ears, shoulder joints, hip joints and ankle joints are in vertical align-ment, and the entire weight of the body is borne on the head; the elbows, lower arms and hands are used only to maintain the balance. Root the ulnar wrist points into the earth, as it is from here, as well as from the head, that the energy moves up towards the feet to make the connection with the lower spring joints.

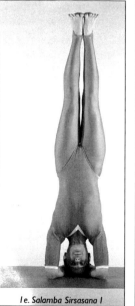

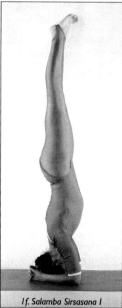

1e. Salamba Sirsasana I

1f. Salamba Sirsasana I

- Breathe slowly and easily, using each mula bandha inhalation to create the wave upwards that lightens the body, and each exhalation to consolidate that height of the body (photo 1f).

- Elongate the sides of the arm pits, so that the upper arms are almost in line with the sides of the chest; the upper arms and chest should be almost vertical. If the weight of the body is on the front of the trunk (solar plexus) and not on the back (spine and head), the lumbar spine sags, and the chest is not vertical, but slanted, as the lower part is further forward than the upper part. To make the chest vertical, the arm pits and upper ribs have to move forwards, and the lower ribs and lumbar spine backwards.
- This is the same movement as in tadasana: the straightening of chest and lumbar starts in the pelvis; the only difference is that here the body is upside down. The pelvis is vertical, with the buttock bones pointing straight up towards the sky. If it is tilted forward around the femur heads, the curve in the lumbar spine becomes too pronounced and the weight of the body falls on the front of the trunk. As a result the muscles of the abdomen lose their tone, while the muscles in the lower back become short, narrow and tight. To correct this position make the following movements: keep the ankles and hip joints in line with the shoulder joints, and the knees straight. Then rotate the pelvis backwards, so that the two frontal hip bones move towards the ribs and the coccyx rolls towards the pubic bone. At the same time, bring the lumbar vertebrae back, but not the thoracic vertebrae. In this way the weight of the body is brought onto the back (spine and head) and the head, chest and pelvis are aligned vertically.
- Thus, to create the lightness in the body in head balance, the head and the ulnar wrist points have to go down with the force of gravity (rooting), while the spinal column and the legs elongate up against the force of gravity (rebounce, The Normal Force of Newton).
  To draw the chest out of the shoulder joints, roll the deltoid, triceps and latissimus dorsi muscles forwards towards the face, slightly pressurizing the elbows inwards, and then lift the chest vertically up from the shoulder heads (note that in tadasana the pelvis is drawn upwards from the femur heads by constricting the tensor fascia lata and the adductors on the inside of the thighs inwards).
- To prevent the pelvis from resting heavily on the lumbar spine, constrict the tensor fascia lata and the adductor muscles of the thighs inwards and elongate the legs up, out of the femo-iliac joints, so that they pull the pelvis up. Keep the legs perpendicular and the knees straight, with the knee caps facing forward, and keep the arches of the feet strong, especially the upper and lower spring joints of the feet, with the toes in line as in tadasana.
- The neck has the same shape and length as in tadasana, is soft and natural, and the first cervical and the first thoracic vertebra are in vertical alignment.
- Hold for as long as you can maintain the alignment and lightness. Eventually you should be able to stay up for ten minutes.
- To come down, reverse the process and come back to your original starting point on one smooth exhalation.

When you can stay in this position for five minutes with a certain degree of comfort, you can start to practice the variations:

2. Urdhva Dandasana

urdhva=upwards; danda=staff

- Stand in salamba sirsasana I (1e) and proceed:
- On an exhalation bring the legs down to an angle of ninety degrees, so that they are parallel to the earth. Keep the back straight and continue rooting the head and the ulnar wrist points. This will help the spinal column to maintain the upward elongation. At the same time, continue rolling the deltoid, triceps and latissimus dorsi

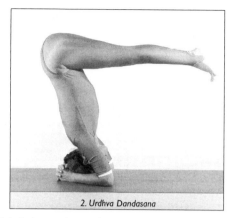

2. Urdhva Dandasana

muscles forwards, constricting the elbows slightly inwards, so that the shoulder blades remain wide.
- Hold for thirty seconds. On an exhalation, take the legs back up to salamba sirsasana I (1e), and proceed to 3.

3. Parivrtta Sirsasana

parivrtta=turned around; sirsa=head

- On an exhalation, rotate the hips towards the right. As they rotate towards the right, the right shoulder and shoulder blade should not yield. Pay special attention to rolling the right deltoid, triceps and latissimus dorsi muscles forward, so that the right elbow stays in line with the right armpit.
- The left and right side of waist and hips should remain parallel to each other; do not lower the left hip as you turn towards the right: the line between the two frontal hip bones remains parallel to the earth.
- Do not curve the lumbar spine forwards by dropping the feet backwards. The line from the bridge of the nose through the sternum, the pubic bone and the middle of the ankles remains vertical.
- Hold for one minute. On an exhalation, come back to the center and repeat on the other side.
- Come back to the center and proceed to 4.

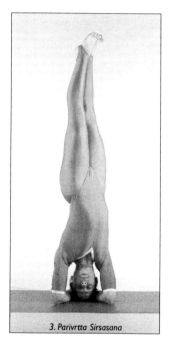

3. Parivrtta Sirsasana

4. Parivrttaikapada Sirsasana

parivrtta=turned around; eka=one; pada=leg, foot; sirsa=head

- Extend the left foot forward and the right foot back.
- On an exhalation, rotate the hips towards the right. As they rotate towards the right, the right shoulder and shoulder blade should not yield. Pay special attention to rolling the right deltoid, triceps and latissimus dorsi muscles forward, so that the right elbow stays in line with the right armpit.

- Spread the legs as much as you can, but keep the feet at the same height from the earth. This means that you have to pay more attention to the right leg, elongating it out of the right sacro-iliac joint. There is a slight curve in the lumbar spine, but do not exaggerate this: the lower abdomen remains in contact with the lower ribs. This is done through the mula bandha breathing: the lower abdomen moves back towards the sacrum and then up towards the lower thoracic diaphragm, so that the lower abdomen stays toned and the right leg elongates out of the groin, not out of the waist.
- The left and right side of waist and hips should remain parallel to each other; do not lower the left hip as you turn towards the right: the line

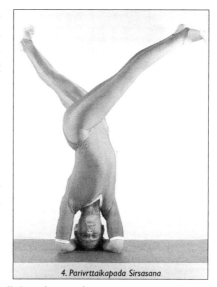

4. Parivrttaikapada Sirsasana

between the two frontal hip bones remains parallel to the earth.
- Hold for one minute. On an exhalation, come back to the center and repeat on the other side.
- Come back to the center and proceed to 5.

5. Parsvaikapada Sirsasana

parsva=sideways; eka=one; pada=leg, foot; sirsa=head

- On an exhalation, rotate the right leg out and take the foot sideways to the earth. Keep the left side of the trunk and the left leg straight; the knee cap of the left leg and the left groin continue facing straight forward (photo 5a).

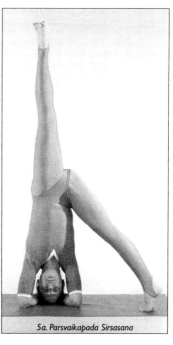

5a. Parsvaikapada Sirsasana

- To get a better movement you can hold the right foot with the right hand (photo 5b). Root the head and the left ulnar wrist point and elongate the spine upwards.
- Do not lower the right hip; the line between the two frontal hip bones remains parallel to the earth.
- Hold for thirty seconds. On an exhalation, take the leg up again and repeat on the other side.

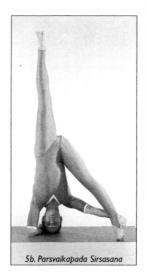

5b. Parsvaikapada Sirsasana

- Then proceed to 6.

6. Ekapada Sirsasana

eka=one; pada=leg, foot; sirsa=head

- On an exhalation take the right foot straight down, in line with the right armpit. Keep the left side of the trunk and the left leg straight; the knee cap of the left leg and the left groin continue facing straight forward (photo 6a).
- To get a better movement, you can hold the right foot with the right hand (photo 6b). Root the head and the left ulnar wrist point and elongate the spine upwards.
- Do not lower the right hip; the line between the two frontal hip bones remains parallel to the earth.
- Hold for thirty seconds.

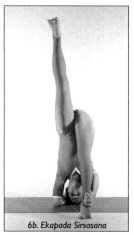

6b. Ekapada Sirsasana

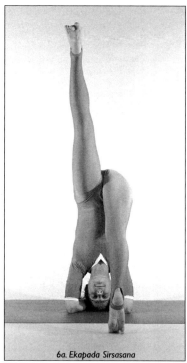

6a. Ekapada Sirsasana

On an exhalation, take the leg up again and repeat on the other side.

- Then proceed to 7.

7. Urdhva Padma Sirsasana

urdhva=upwards; padma=lotus; sirsa=head

- Cross the legs in padmasana (see page 72) and extend the knees up towards the sky. Do not curve the lumbar spine in; performing pada bandha to stabilize the hip joints, rotate the pelvis backwards, so that the coccyx rolls towards the pubic bone and the lower abdomen and the two frontal hip bones move towards the lower frontal ribs. Thus the lumbar spine is elongated.
- Extend the thighs out of the hip joints, so that the groins are opened and the knees point straight up towards the sky.
- For the rest, follow the instructions given in salamba sirsasana I (1).
- Hold for thirty seconds, and then proceed to 8.

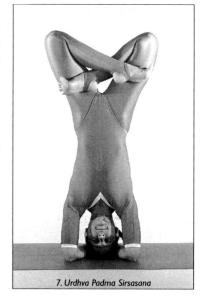

7. Urdhva Padma Sirsasana

8. Parivrtta Urdhva Padma Sirsasana

parivrtta=turned around; urdhva=upwards; padma=lotus; sirsa=head

- On an exhalation, rotate the hips towards the right. As they rotate towards the right, the right shoulder and shoulder blade should not yield. Pay special attention to rolling the right deltoid, triceps and latissimus dorsi muscles forward, so that the right elbow stays in line with the right armpit.
- The left and right side of waist and hips should remain parallel to each other; do not lower the left hip as you turn towards the right: the line between the two frontal hip bones remains parallel to the earth.

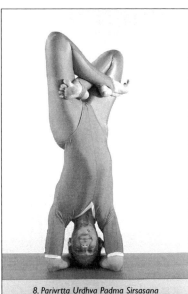
8. Parivrtta Urdhva Padma Sirsasana

- Do not curve the lumbar spine forwards by dropping the knees backwards. The line from the bridge of the nose through the sternum, the pubic bone and the crossed shin bones remains vertical.
- Hold for thirty seconds. On an exhalation come back to the center and repeat on the other side.
- Then proceed to 9.

9. Pinda Sirsasana

pinda=embryo; sirsa=head

- On an exhalation bring the knees down towards the stomach. Even though the back will bend slightly, continue rooting the head and the ulnar wrist points, so that the spinal column maintains a certain elongation.
- Hold for thirty seconds. On an exhalation come back up again. Change the crossing of the legs and repeat 7, 8 and 9.
- Straighten the legs and proceed to 10.

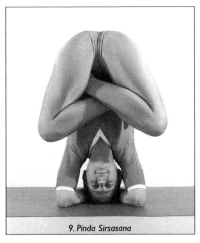
9. Pinda Sirsasana

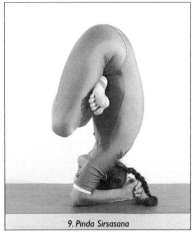
9. Pinda Sirsasana

10. Vajra Sirsasana

vajra=thunderbolt, weapon of indra;
sirsa=head

- Bend the knees backwards without curving the lumbar spine. Performing pada bandha to stabilize the hip joints, rotate the pelvis backwards, so that the coccyx rolls towards the pubic bone and the lower abdomen and the two frontal hip bones move towards the lower frontal ribs. Thus the lumbar spine is elongated.
- At the same time extend the thighs out of the hip joints, so that the groins are opened and the knees point straight up towards the sky.
- For the rest follow the instructions given in salamba sirsasana I (1).
- Hold for thirty seconds; then proceed to 11.

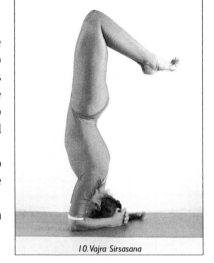

10. Vajra Sirsasana

11. Parivrtta Vajra Sirsasana

parivrtta=turned around; vajra=thunderbolt,
weapon of indra; sirsa=head

- On an exhalation rotate the hips towards the right. As they rotate towards the right, the right shoulder and shoulder blade should not yield. Pay special attention to rolling the right deltoid, triceps and latissimus dorsi muscles forward, so that the right elbow stays in line with the right armpit.
- The left and right side of waist and hips should remain parallel to each other; do not lower the left hip as you turn towards the right; the line between the two frontal hip bones remains parallel to the earth.
- Do not curve the lumbar spine forwards by dropping the knees backwards; the line from the bridge of the nose through the sternum, the pubic bone and the inner knees remains vertical.

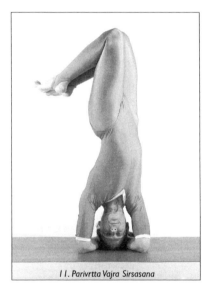

11. Parivrtta Vajra Sirsasana

- Hold for thirty seconds. On an exhalation, come back to the center and repeat on the other side.
- Come back to the center, straighten the legs and proceed to 12.

12. Prasarita Padottana Sirsasana

prasarita=spread, extended;
pada=leg, foot;
uttana=intense stretch;
sirsa=head

- Spread the legs to the maximum, keeping the feet at the same height from the earth.
- Hold for thirty seconds; then proceed to 13.

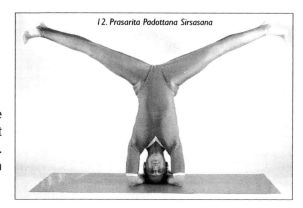
12. Prasarita Padottana Sirsasana

13. Baddha Kona Sirsasana

baddha=bound; kona=angle; sirsa=head

- Join the soles of the feet together as in baddha konasana (see page 104) and pull the heels down towards the pubic bone. The toes point straight up towards the sky.
- Hold for thirty second, and then straighten the legs.

When you have reached sufficient balance in these variations, you can try the following ones:

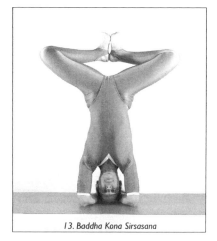
13. Baddha Kona Sirsasana

14. Salamba Sirsasana II

sa=with; alamba=support; sirsa=head

- On an exhalation, release the hands back of the head, bring them forward and place the palms of the hands on the blanket in front of you. The fingers point towards the face, and the wrists and elbows are in line with the armpits, with an angle of ninety degrees in the elbows.
- Root the head and the hands (hastha bandha): performing hasta bandha activates the arms, shoulders and shoulder blades. Elongate the elbows forward, away from the head, and keep the upper arms and elbows parallel to each other by rolling the deltoid, triceps and latissimus dorsi muscles forwards, and constricting the elbows slightly inwards towards each other.
- Hold for thirty seconds, and then proceed to 15.

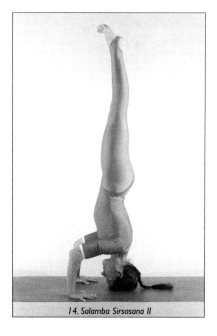
14. Salamba Sirsasana II

15. Salamba Sirsasana III

sa=with; alamba=support; sirsa=head

- Turn the hands the other way round, so that the fingers point away from the face. The wrists and elbows stay in line with the armpits, and the elbows maintain an angle of ninety degrees.
- Root the head and the hands (hastha bandha); performing hasta bandha activates the arms, shoulders and shoulder blades. Elongate the elbows forward, away from the head, and keep the upper arms and elbows parallel to each other by rolling the deltoid, triceps and latissimus dorsi muscles forwards, and constricting the elbows slightly inwards towards each other.
- Hold for thirty seconds, and then proceed to 16.

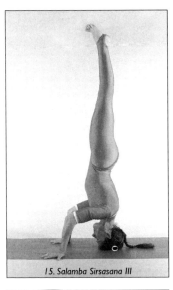

15. Salamba Sirsasana III

16. Muktahasta Sirsasana

mukta=free; hasta=hand; sirsa=head

- Extend the arms in front of you with the back of the hands resting on the blanket and the palms facing upward. The arms and hands can be slightly wider than the armpits to facilitate the balance.
- Hold for thirty seconds, and then proceed to 17.

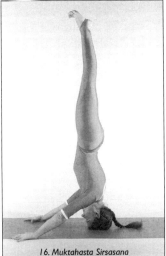

16. Muktahasta Sirsasana

17. Baddhahasta Sirsasana

baddha=bound; hasta=hand; sirsa=head

- Fold the arms in front of the face and clasp the elbows with the hands.
- Hold for thirty seconds. On an exhalation return to salamba sirsasana I.

To come down from salamba sirsasana I (1), follow the instructions for going up, in the reverse order.

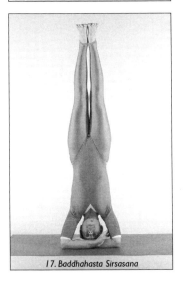

17. Baddhahasta Sirsasana

Part 10 Sarvangasana/Shoulder Balance cycle

These positions should be done in the *vinyasa* mode, that is, going from one pose directly into the next one, using the breathing.

Sarvangasana cycle

1. Halasana
2. Karnapidasana
3. Salamba Sarvangasana I
4. Parsvaikapada Sarvangasana
5. Ekapada Sarvangasana
6. Supta Konasana
7. Parsva Halasana
8. Parsva Karnapidasana
9. Parsva Sarvangasana
10. Parsva Setubandhasana

11. Setubandhasana
12. Ekapada Setubandhasana
13. Urdhva Padma Sarvangasana
14. Parsva Urdhva Padma Sarvangasana
15. Parsva Pinda Sarvangasana
16. Pinda Sarvangasana
17. Salamba Sarvangasana II
18. Niralamba Sarvangasana I
19. Niralamba Sarvangasana II

1.   Halasana

hala=plough

(See also "Comparative Studies of various Asanas", page 244)

- Lie on the back on a blanket.
- On an exhalation bring the feet over the head to the blanket. Keep the knees straight and arms extended backwards.
- Clasp the hands as for salamba sirsasana I (see page 157) and elongate the wrists away from the shoulders, so that the shoulders are pulled backwards away from the ears. Rotate the upper arms out so that the deltoid muscles roll underneath the shoulders and the biceps muscles rotate up towards the sky. Lift the shoulder blades up from the blanket in order to bring the trunk onto the tops of the shoulders.

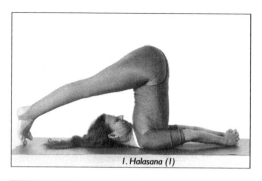

1. Halasana (1)

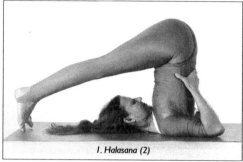

1. Halasana (2)

- Elongate the spine upwards so that all the vertebrae move into the body. The hip joints are in a vertical alignment with the shoulder joints. In order to elongate the spine upwards you have to extend the back of the thighs from the knees towards the buttock bones, spreading the buttock bones and lifting them up towards the sky. Elongate the ulnar wrist points away from you and root them into the earth. This will enable the latissimus dorsi to lift the chest up and thus to elongate the spine.
- As the spine moves in and the trunk lifts up from the shoulder heads, the sternum moves up and forwards towards the chin. Perform jalandhara bandha (see page 37) in order to avoid pressing the neck vertebrae onto the earth. Lift the corners of the jaws (not the chin) up by sliding the skull on the first vertebra and then join the chin with the sternum. In this way the first two vertebrae of the neck do not press onto the earth, but are lifted into the neck.
- Rest the feet on the tip of the toes. There should be very little weight on the feet, all the body weight is on the spine and hips. Then place the hands on the back.
- Hold for five minutes. Proceed to 2.

2.   Karnapidasana

karna=ear; pida=pressure

- On an exhalation extend the arms over the head and bend the knees next to the ears.
- The pelvis has to roll over the head and the back has to bend to bring the knees down. Keep the feet together with the toes pointing away from the head and clasp the

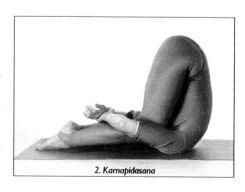

2. Karnapidasana

elbows in the knees.

- Hold for one minute.
- If you can do this easily, slide the feet further out to bring the knees down to the blanket over the head. In this way the upper spine between the shoulder blades is elongated even more.
- Extend the arms back again and clasp the hands as for salamba sirsasana I (see page 157). Roll the upper arms out and the deltoid muscles under, and then place the hands back on the back, as close to the shoulder blades as possible.
- Proceed to 3.

3. Salamba Sarvangasana I

sa=with; alamba=support;
sarva=whole; anga=body

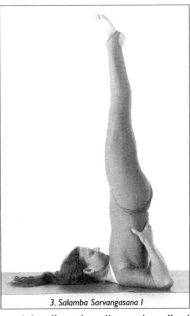

3. Salamba Sarvangasana I

- On an inhalation raise the knees and elongate the spinal column upwards. On the exhalation lift the legs up to salamba sarvangasana I, keeping the knees straight and the feet together.
- Seen from the side the ankles, knees, hip joints and shoulder joints are in a vertical alignment.
- Clasp the hands as in salamba sirsasana I (see page 157) and extend the arms backwards. Roll the upper arms out so that the biceps muscles rotate up to the sky and the deltoid muscles roll underneath the shoulder heads. Root the ulnar wrist points so that the spine in between the shoulder blades elongates upwards.
- Then place the hands back again on the back and lift the chest up from the shoulder heads. Perform jalandhara bandha as described in halasana (1), so that the neck vertebrae do not press on the blanket.
- On each mula bandha inhalation lift the chest and trunk up from the shoulder heads and elongate the legs up out of the pelvis. Keep the inner ankles together and the knees facing straight forward.
- On each exhalation maintain the height of the body.
- Hold for five minutes. On an exhalation go back to halasana (1) and down till you are lying again on the back.

When you can stay for five minutes in this position with a certain degree of comfort you can start to practice the variations:

4. Parsvaikapada Sarvangasana

parsva=sideways; eka=one; pada=leg, foot; sarva=whole; anga=body

- Stand in salamba sarvangasana I (3) and proceed:
- On an exhalation rotate the right leg outwards and take the foot down sideways to the earth.
- Keep the left side of the trunk and the left leg completely straight. The knee cap of the left leg and the left groin should stay facing straight forward.
- Do not drop the right hip. To keep the line between the two frontal hip bones parallel to the earth you have to roll the right femur head back and up towards the left heel.

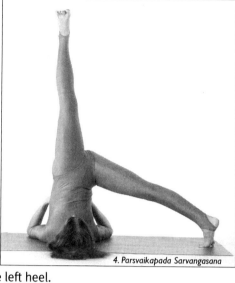

4. Parsvaikapada Sarvangasana

- Hold for thirty seconds. On an exhalation take the leg up again and repeat on the other side.
- Proceed to 5.

5. Ekapada Sarvangasana

eka=one; pada=leg, foot; sarva=whole; anga=body

- On an exhalation take the right foot straight down to the earth, in line with the right shoulder.
- Keep the left side of the trunk and the left leg completely straight. The knee cap of the left leg and the left groin should stay facing straight forward.
- Do not drop the right hip. To keep the line between the two frontal hip bones parallel to the earth you have to roll the right femur head back and up towards the left heel.
- Hold for thirty seconds. On an exhalation take the leg up again and repeat on the other side.
- Proceed to 6.

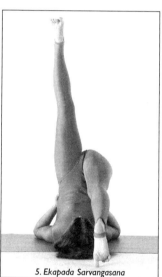

5. Ekapada Sarvangasana

6. Supta Konasana

supta=lying down; kona=angle

- On an exhalation come down to halasana (1) and spread the legs. Follow the instructions given for halasana.
- Hold for thirty seconds. Proceed to 7.

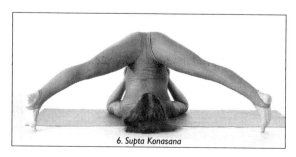

6. Supta Konasana

7. Parsva Halasana

parsva=sideways; hala=plough

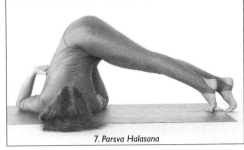
7. Parsva Halasana

- On an exhalation walk the feet towards the right, rotating the hips and spinal column, but not the shoulders. The left foot joins the right foot. Keep the feet vertical and keep only the tips of the big toes on the blanket.
- The shoulders and elbows should remain as in halasana (1), do not displace the left shoulder and elbow as you walk the feet towards the right.
- Keep the right hip up. Both buttock bones should have the same height from the earth.
- Hold for thirty seconds. Proceed to 8.

8. Parsva Karnapidasana

parsva=sideways; karna=ear; pida=pressure

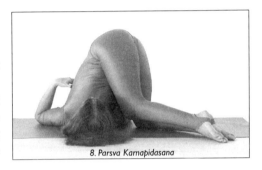
8. Parsva Karnapidasana

- On an exhalation bend the knees next to the right ear.
- The pelvis has to roll over the right shoulder and the back has to bend to bring the knees down. Keep the feet together with the toes pointing away from the head.
- Hold for thirty seconds. Then repeat 7 and 8 on the other side.
- Go up again to salamba sarvangasana I (3).
- Proceed to 9.

9. Parsva Sarvangasana

parsva=sideways; sarva=whole; anga=body

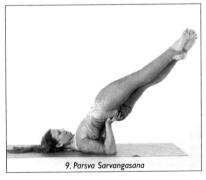
9. Parsva Sarvangasana

- Lower the pelvis and bring the legs halfway down over the head. Turn the hips towards the left and rest the sacrum on the palm of the right hand. The left hip turns backwards, and the right hip turns forwards towards the face.
- Keep the left hand as a support on the left rib cage and lower the legs backwards over the right hand. Keep the knees straight and the upper and lower spring joints of the feet active (pada bandha) and in touch with the lower abdomen, so that you do not lose the balance. Eventually the legs will be parallel to the earth.
- Extend the legs out of the groins, not out of the waist. Pull the two frontal hip bones in the direction of the lower frontal ribs, and extend the coccyx towards the heels. In this way the muscles of the lower abdomen stay toned and the lumbar spine stays long.
- Proceed to 10.

10. Parsva Setubandhasana

parsva=sideways; setu=bridge; setu bandha=the construction of a bridge

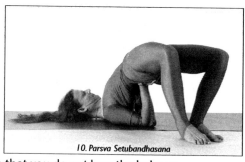

10. Parsva Setubandhasana

- Bend the knees and, keeping the feet together, extend the feet downwards till they reach the blanket. The knees can spread a little as the feet go down, but keep the upper and lower spring joints of the feet active (pada bandha) and in touch with the lower abdomen, so that you do not lose the balance.
- Keep rotating the left hip backwards and the right hip forwards towards the face, and keep the support of the left hand on the rib cage.
- If you lose control in this pose and drop onto the blanket, instead of gently landing the feet, it means that you have not used the abdominal muscles correctly. The weight of the legs was supported by the waist and lumbar spine, instead of by the groins and lower abdomen.
- Hold for a few seconds. Then come back up again, keeping the feet together.
- To bring the feet up you have to pull the pubic bone towards the navel, so that the lower abdomen brings the legs up. Join the knees and come back up to parsva sarvangasana (9).
- Return to salamba sarvangasana I (3) and repeat 9 and 10 on the left side.
- Proceed to 11.

11. Setubandhasana

setu=bridge; setu bandha=the construction of a bridge

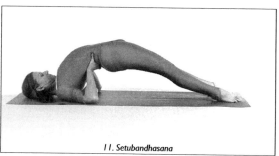

11. Setubandhasana

- To set up the right conditions for going into Setubandhasana it is best to bring the legs first down from salamba sarvangasana I (3) into karnapidasana (2).
- Keep the knees together, reaching over the head to the blanket. Place the hands close to the shoulder blades with the elbows and lower arms parallel to each other.
- Lift the knees and, keeping the knees and feet together and the legs bent, roll the trunk over the hands backwards till the feet reach the blanket back of the trunk. This is a back bending position.
- Pull the two frontal hip bones towards the lower ribs and extend the coccyx towards the heels as the feet go down, so that the legs are extended out of the groins, not out of the waist. The muscles of the lower abdomen serve as the 'brakes' for the feet to go down slowly. In all the back bendings, the two frontal hip bones and the lower ribs have to maintain their magnetic attraction towards each other in order to keep the length in the lumbar spine. If they lose this contact, the lumbar spine will be compressed in the curve.
- The knees can spread slightly when going down, but keep the feet together and the upper and lower spring joints active (pada bandha) and in contact with the lower abdomen, so that you do not lose the balance.

- Extend the legs and place the feet at hip width on the mat. The inner borders of the feet are parallel to each other and the knees are slightly wider than hip width. Keep the feet even, do not keep one foot further forward than the other.
- To create one smooth curve at the front of the body you have to separate the pelvis from the femur heads by rooting the feet (pada bandha) and by elongating the legs out of the hip joints. At the same time the coccyx has to extend out of the lumbar spine towards the heels, so that the lumbar vertebrae do not get compressed. The groins should be completely open and should form one continuous line between the upper thighs and the two frontal hip bones.
- Root the back of the head and the back of the upper arms, so that the thoracic spine in between the shoulder blades is elongated and the chest is lifted up from the shoulder heads.
- Resisting the knees slightly backwards towards the shoulders blades and the shoulder blades towards the knees, the chest and pelvis have no other choice but to go up. This gives the height and the lightness to the body.
- On each mula bandha inhalation lift the trunk by connecting the pada bandha, the mula bandha, the uddiyana bandha and the jalandhara bandha, rooting the feet, the head and the arms.
- Hold for one minute. Proceed to 12.

12. Ekapada Setubandhasana

eka=one; pada=leg,foot; setu=bridge;
setu bandha=the construction of a bridge

- When you have reached a stable position, bend the right knee and extend the right leg straight up towards the sky. Do not tilt the pelvis. The two frontal hip bones should stay parallel to each other and to the earth.
- The right leg extends upwards in a vertical alignment with the right groin, and the left foot and knee extend in alignment with the left groin.
- To get the height and lightness of

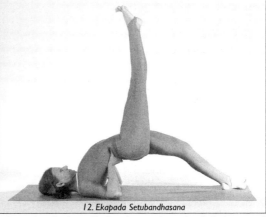

12. Ekapada Setubandhasana

the pelvis you have to root the left foot (pada bandha), elongating the left leg, and elongate the right leg upwards out of the right hip joint. This is in conformity with the principle that the part of the body which is below forms the stable base for the part of the body which is above to elongate upwards against gravity.
- Hold for a few seconds. Then repeat with the other leg.
- On an exhalation walk the feet in towards the head and jump back up to salamba sarvangasana I (3), keeping the feet together.
- Proceed to 13.

13. Urdhva Padma Sarvangasana

urdhva=upwards; padma=lotus; sarva=whole;
anga=body

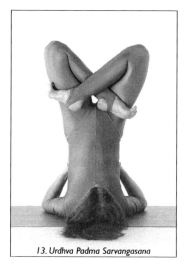

13. Urdhva Padma Sarvangasana

- Cross the legs in padmasana (see page 72) and extend the knees up towards the sky. In salamba sirsasana I you cannot use the hands to cross the legs in padmasana, but in salamba sarvangasana I you can. Therefore you can first learn urdhva padmasana in salamba sarvangasana I before you try it in salamba sirsasana I.
- Performing pada bandha in order to stabilize the hip joints rotate the pelvis backwards. The coccyx rolls towards the pubic bone and the lower abdomen and two frontal hip bones move towards the lower frontal ribs. Thus the lumbar spine is elongated.
- Extend the thighs out of the hip joints, so that the groins are opened and the knees point straight up towards the sky.
- For the rest follow the instructions given in salamba sarvangasana I (3).
- Hold for thirty seconds. Proceed to 14.

14. Parsva Urdhva Padma Sarvangasana

parsva=sideways; urdhva=upwards;
padma=lotus; sarva=whole; anga=body

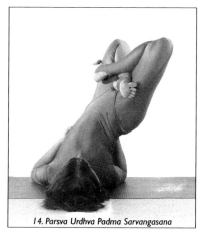

14. Parsva Urdhva Padma Sarvangasana

- Lower the pelvis and bring the crossed legs halfway down over the head. Turn the hips towards the left and rest the sacrum on the palm of the right hand. The left hip turns backwards, and the right hip turns forwards towards the face.
- Keep the left hand as a support on the left rib cage and lower the thighs backwards over the right hand. Keep the upper and lower spring joints of the feet active (pada bandha) and in touch with the lower abdomen, so that you do not lose the balance. Eventually the thighs will be parallel to the earth.
- Extend the thighs out of the groins, not out of the waist. Pull the two frontal hip bones in the direction of the lower frontal ribs, and extend the coccyx towards the heels. In this way the muscles of the lower abdomen stay toned and the lumbar spine stays long.
- Hold for thirty seconds. Then repeat on the other side.
- Come back up to urdhva padma sarvangasana (13). Proceed to 15.

15. Parsva Pinda Sarvangasana

parsva=sideways; pinda=embryo;
sarva=whole; anga=body

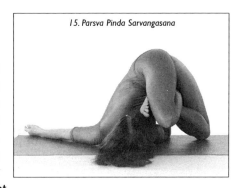

15. Parsva Pinda Sarvangasana

- Lower the pelvis and place the right hip bone on the right hand. Turn the right hip backwards and the left hip forwards towards the face. Then place the right knee next to the right upper arm on the blanket.
- Elongate the left arm sideways, out of the left shoulder joint, as a counterweight for the knees, and root the left ulnar wrist point.
- Continue the rotation of the hips and bring the left knee also down, next to the right ear.
- This whole movement is a diagonal forward bending movement, elongating and twisting across the whole spinal column.
- Hold for thirty seconds. Then repeat on the other side.
- Come back to the center. Proceed to 16.

16. Pinda Sarvangasana

pinda=embryo; sarva=whole;
anga=body

- On an exhalation bend the back, bring the crossed knees down to the forehead and clasp the arms around the knees.
- Hold for thirty seconds. Change the crossing of the legs and repeat 13, 14, 15 and 16.
- Return to salamba sarvangasana I (3). Proceed to 17.

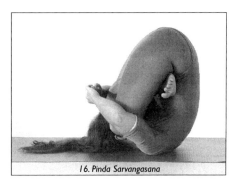

16. Pinda Sarvangasana

17. Salamba Sarvangasana II

sa=with; alamba=support;
sarva=whole; anga=body

- Clasp the hands as for salamba sirsasana I (see page 157) and extend the arms backwards.
- Extend the wrists away from the shoulders so that the shoulders are pulled backwards away from the ears. At the same time rotate the upper arms out so that the deltoid muscles roll underneath the shoulders and the biceps muscles rotate up towards the sky. Root the ulnar wrist points. This enables the latissimus dorsi to lift the chest up from the shoulder heads and thus to elongate the spine.
- Hold for thirty seconds. Proceed to 18.

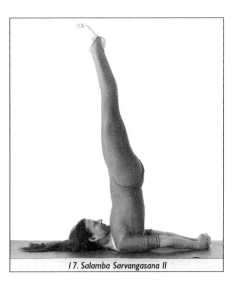

17. Salamba Sarvangasana II

18. Niralamba Sarvangasana I

nir=without; alamba=support;
sarva=whole; anga=body

- Raise the arms in an arc of a hundred and eighty degrees over the head to the blanket. Keep the arms parallel to each other and the back of the hands resting on the blanket. Keep the back as straight as possible.
- Hold for thirty seconds. Proceed to 19.

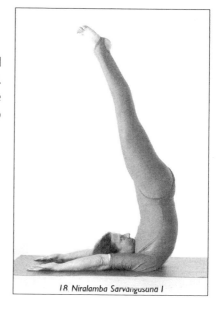

18. Niralamba Sarvangasana I

19. Niralamba Sarvangasana II

nir=without; alamba=support;
sarva=whole; anga=body

- Extend the arms up till the palms of the hands rest on the front of the thighs. The fingers point up towards the sky.
- Hold for thirty seconds.

In the last three variations the balance is the main issue, and this depends on the strength and stability of the back and abdominal muscles. Therefore it is important to include them in the daily practice.

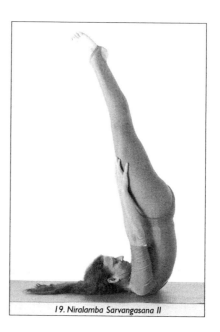

19. Niralamba Sarvangasana II

Part 11 Hand Balancings

These positions can be done in *four different modes*:

a.   ***Performing each position separately*** and holding it for thirty seconds.

b.   ***Vinyasa***
Connecting two or more positions by flowing from one into the other, using the breathing.

c.   ***Mala***
Connecting all the positions through surya namaskar in the following way, using the breathing:
- Stand in tadasana » inhale, extend the arms upwards » exhale, bend down into uttanasana, inhale, raise the head » exhale, jump back into chaturanga dandasana » inhale, go into urdhvamukha svanasana » exhale, go into adhomukha svanasana, inhale » exhale, go into vasisthasana I on the right side, stay for three breaths, inhale » exhale, return into adhomukha svanasana, inhale » exhale, go into vasisthasana I on the left side, stay for three breaths, inhale » exhale, return into adhomukha svanasana, inhale » exhale, jump forward into uttanasana » inhale, stand up again in tadasana, exhale » inhale, extend the arms upwards, etc.

d.   ***You can also start each one of positions 17 through 26*** from salamba sirsasana II, finishing by dropping back and pushing up into urdhva dhanurasana.

In tadasana and the standing poses, the rebounce force and the resulting elongation upwards with the anti-gravitational lightness and 'bounciness' come through the correct application of the pada bandha, that is, the lifting of the talocalcaneonavicular joint and the talocruralis joint, or the lower and upper 'spring' joints.

In adhomukha vrksasana and the other hand balancings, the same elongation upwards with the anti-gravitational lightness and 'bounciness' come through the correct application of the hasta bandha. Hasta bandha, as described on page 38 on the bandhas, is the act of rooting the rim of the palm into the earth, that is, the wrist and the fingers, and then 'sucking' the center of the palm upwards. One can compare this to the 'suckers' on the hands and feet of lizards, with which they scale walls and ceilings. This shoots the energy through the arms and shoulders, and thus elongates them.

Hand Balancings	
1. Adhomukha Vrksasana	14. Mayurasana
2. Padma Adhomukha Vrksasana	15. Padma Mayurasana
3. Pincha Mayurasana	16. Hamsasana
4. Padma Pincha Mayurasana	17. Bakasana
5. Vasisthasana I	18. Parsva Bakasana
6. Vasisthasana II	19. Ekapada Bakasana I
7. Kasyapasana	20. Ekapada Bakasana II
8. Visvamitrasana	21. Dvipada Koundinyasana
9. Dvihasta Bhujasana	22. Ekapada Koundinyasana
10. Titthibhasana	23. Ekapada Galavasana
11. Bhujapidasana	24. Urdhva Kukkutasana
12. Ekahasta Bhujasana	25. Galavasana
13. Astavakrasana	26. Parsva Kukkutasana

1. Adhomukha Vrksasana

adho=downwards; mukha=face; vrksa=tree

1a. Close to the wall

- Kneel down close to a wall, facing it.
- Place the hands on the earth, close to the wall. The arms are parallel to each other, with the hands in alignment with the armpits. Keep the middle fingers parallel to each other and the other fingers and the thumbs spread. Make sure that the hands are even; do not keep one hand further forward than the other. Turn the pits of the elbows forward towards the wall (savasana rotation of the arms).
- On an exhalation, lift the knees, walk the feet closer to the hands and jump up till both the heels are on the wall (change legs each time you jump up on the wall, so as not to create an imbalance in the back muscles by always using the same leg).
- The pelvis is the area in the body which contains the heaviest bone and muscle structure. If the feet jump up fast and the trunk is pulled up by that speed and the strength of the leg muscles, the pelvis will sag and the result is a 'collision' of the pelvis with the lumbar vertebrae. This will weaken the lumbar vertebrae. The correct way of jumping up into adhomukha vrksasana is by pulling the legs

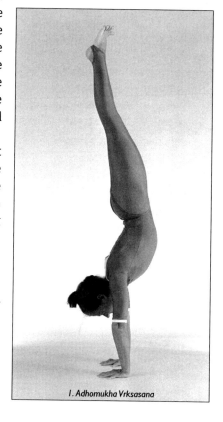

1. Adhomukha Vrksasana

and the pelvis up with the back muscles, so that those muscles will get stronger, and the pelvis does not collapse into the lumbar. The pelvis should actually arrive first on the wall, before the heels.

- Keep only the heels on the wall and bring the rest of the body in alignment, with the hip joints straight above the shoulder joints and the middle bones of the hands. Keep the arches of the feet strong (pada bandha) and the inner ankles together.
- Keep the top of the head pointing straight downwards, in between the inner arms. Keeping the head flexed backwards gives more curve in the upper thoracic spine, but makes it harder for the shoulders to elongate; on the other hand, keeping the head straight down in between the upper arms gives more freedom in the shoulder blades to slide the chest upwards, out of the shoulder joints.
- Root the hands into the earth and perform hasta bandha. This creates the rebounce force in the arms and shoulder joints, so that they elongate automatically. The weight of the body is above the middle bones of the palms, not above the bones of the wrists.
- On each mula bandha inhalation, elongate the body vertically upwards from the middle bones of the hands to the middle bones of the feet. Thus the whole body is connected into one unit through the five major bandhas: lifting the chest up from the shoulder heads, lifting the pelvis up from the lumbar spine, and lifting the legs up from the hip joints.
- On each exhalation maintain that height.
- Hold for one minute.

1b. With two legs
When you have gained confidence jumping up with one leg, you can start to practice jumping with both legs together. Here especially it is obvious that you have to pull the pelvis and legs up with the back muscles, otherwise you will never get up.
- Start as for 1a, but keep the hands slightly further away from the wall and the head flexed backwards.
- On an exhalation jump up, keeping the inner ankles and knees together and pulling the body up with the back muscles. It is very easy to check the strength of those muscles. If the knees and feet spread apart ('frog'-jumping) while jumping up, this is a clear indication of the weakness of the lumbar muscles. Thus the importance of keeping the inner knees and ankles together.
- Root the hands while jumping up, so that the shoulders do not yield: the shoulder joints remain aligned with the palms as the pelvis goes up. Keep the knees bent till the toes are on the wall and the knees, hip joints, shoulder joints and palms are in vertical alignment. Then extend the legs up and proceed as in 1a.

1c. *Away from the wall*

When you have mastered jumping up with both feet, you can take the hands further away from the wall and jump up without allowing the feet to go on the wall. Keep the body just close enough to it to be able to put the feet on it in case you lose balance. Eventually, this pose has to be done in the middle of the room.

- In this free standing version, the head does not point straight down, but is flexed backwards and the eyes look at a point between the two hands. Fix the eyes on that point in order to keep the balance.
- Proceed with the rooting of the hands, the hasta bandha and the elongation of the whole body upwards from the middle bones of the hands to the middle bones of the feet, as described above.
- Hold for one minute.

2. Padma Adhomukha Vrksasana

padma=lotus; adho=downwards; mukha=face;
vrksa=tree

- Start with 1a, close to the wall.
- Cross the legs in padmasana (see page 72). Keep the knees on the wall, but bring the hips in alignment with the shoulder joints and the palms of the hands.
- For the rest follow the instructions given in adhomukha vrksasana (1).

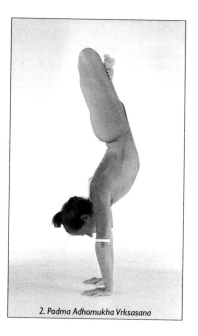

2. Padma Adhomukha Vrksasana

3. Pincha Mayurasana

pincha=chin,feather; mayura=peacock
(See also "Comparative Studies of Various Asanas", page 239)

3a. *Close to the wall*

- Kneel down on a 'sticky' yoga mat, close to a wall and facing it.
- Turn the arms as for savasana, so that the palms of the hands face upwards. Bend the arms and place the elbows on the mat, in alignment with the armpits. Then turn the palms of the hands down. The middle fingers are parallel to each other and the inner and outer wrists are equally long and parallel to each other. The tips of the middle fingers are on one line with the center of the palms and wrists, the center of the elbows and the center of the armpits. Make sure that the hands are even; do not keep one

hand further forward than the other. Spread the other fingers and extend them on the mat, rooting the knuckles of the fingers together with the ulnar wrist points. Perform hasta bandha to activate the shoulder joints and shoulder blades.

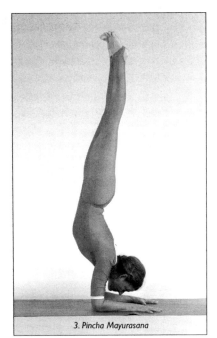

3. Pincha Mayurasana

- On an inhalation, raise the hips and knees and walk the feet in towards the arms, keeping the shoulders in vertical alignment with the elbows: the angle between the upper arms and the lower arms remains ninety degrees. Elongate the groins upwards and raise the pelvis and one leg, till the trunk and the leg are aligned almost vertically with the shoulder and elbow joints. Do not lose the height of the shoulders.
- In this pose it is even more important than in adhomukha vriksasana (1) not to jump up with the speed of the foot, dragging the pelvis and back up. The correct way of going into this pose is by using the abdominal and lower back muscles, so that you actually raise the body without jumping. Roll on the lower spring joint of the bottom foot and lift the trunk and bottom leg up into pincha mayurasana with the back muscles. Keep both legs straight, till the heels are on the wall (change legs each time you lift up, so as not to create an imbalance in the back muscles by always using the same leg).
- Keeping only the heels on the wall, bring the hip joints in alignment with the shoulder and elbow joints. Keep the arches of the feet strong (pada bandha) and the inner ankles together.
- Keep the top of the head first pointing straight downwards in between the inner arms. Keeping the head flexed backwards gives more curve in the upper thoracic spine, but makes it harder for the shoulders to elongate; on the other hand, keeping the head straight down in between the upper arms gives more freedom in the shoulder blades to slide the chest upwards, out of the shoulder joints.
- Root the hands, the ulnar wrist points, the lower arms and the elbows, performing hasta bandha. This creates the rebounce force in the upper arms and shoulder joints, so that they elongate automatically. Then flex the head backwards.
- On each mula bandha inhalation, elongate the body vertically upwards from the middle bones of the hands to the middle bones of the feet. Thus the whole body is connected into one unit through the five major bandhas: lifting the chest up from the shoulder heads, lifting the pelvis up from the lumbar spine and lifting the legs up from the hip joints.
- On each exhalation maintain that height.
- Hold for one minute.

3b. Away from the wall

- When you have gained confidence on the wall, you can start practicing further away from the wall, without allowing the feet to go to the wall. Keep the body just close enough to it to be able to put the feet on it in case you lose balance. Eventually, this pose has to be done in the middle of the room.
- In this free standing version, the head does not point straight down, but is flexed backwards and the eyes look at a point between the two hands. Fix the eyes on that point in order to keep the balance.
- Proceed with the rooting of the hands, the hasta bandha and the elongation of the whole body upwards from the middle bones of the hands to the middle bones of the feet, as described above.
- Hold for one minute.

4. Padma Pincha Mayurasana

padma=lotus; pincha=chin,feather; mayura=peacock

- Start with 3a close to the wall and cross the legs in padmasana (see page 72). Keep the hips in alignment with the shoulder and elbow joints.
- Hold for one minute; then change the crosslegs.

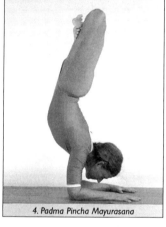

4. Padma Pincha Mayurasana

5. Vasisthasana I

Vasistha is the name of a sage

- Start with adhomukha svanasana (see page 210) on a 'sticky' yoga mat and then proceed:
- On an exhalation, roll over on the right hand and the right foot; the outer arch of the right foot is in line with the wrist and middle finger of the right hand.
- The right foot rests on the outer edge, more on the plantar than on the dorsal side of the foot. Place the left foot on the right one, so that the inner ankles touch and all the toes are in line as in paschimotta-nasana. Perform pada bandha to stabilize the trunk and to lighten the weight of the pelvis on the femur heads.
- The distance between the right hand and the right foot is such that the right arm forms an angle of ninety degrees with the chest. Thus the arm is not vertical, but slants forward from the shoulder joint.
- Rotate the right arm as in savasana: the biceps muscle rotates towards the right hand and the triceps muscle towards the ribs.

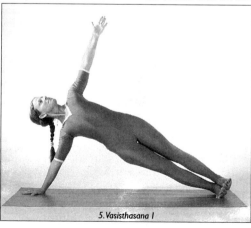

5. Vasisthasana I

- Seen from the side, the back of the head is in line with the sacrum and the back of the heels, and the ears, shoulder joints, hip joints, knees and ankles are in one line. Seen from the front, the bridge of the nose is in line with the sternum, the pubic bone and the inner ankles.

- Extend the left arm up towards the sky, in line with the right arm. This means that the arm does not point straight up, but is slanted, so that here too there is an angle of ninety degrees in the left arm pit. Turn the face to look up.
- Do not sink the chest into the right shoulder joint. Create space by rooting the right hand into the earth, performing hasta bandha, so that the arm is elongated and the chest is lifted up from the right shoulder head. Do not disturb the alignment of the body, however.
- Do not sink the pelvis into the right hip joint. Create space by rooting the outer edge of the right foot into the earth, performing pada bandha, so that the leg is elongated and the pelvis is lifted up from the right femur head.
- On each mula bandha inhalation, extend the coccyx towards the heels and elongate the lower abdomen and spine towards the back of the head. On each exhalation, turn the trunk and head further up towards the sky.
- Hold for three breaths. On the fourth exhalation, place the left hand on the mat, at shoulder width from and parallel to the right one, roll over on the right foot, place the left foot at hip width, parallel to the right one, on the mat and return to adhomukha svanasana.
- Hold adhomukha svanasana for three breaths.
- On the fourth exhalation, turn over on the left foot and repeat on the left side.

6. Vasisthasana II

Vasistha is the name of a sage

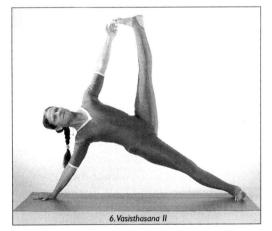

6. Vasisthasana II

- Start with adhomukha svanasana on a 'sticky' yoga mat and then proceed:
- On an exhalation, turn over on the right hand and the right foot and go into vasisthasana I (5).
- Bend the left leg, with the index and middle finger of the left hand hold the big toe (palm facing forward) and extend the leg up towards the sky.
- For the rest follow the instructions given in vasisthasana I (5).
- Keep the straight lines of the body, especially the line between the back of the head, the sacrum and the right heel. To stay in line, take the head and left leg backwards and the pelvis forwards, without turning it upwards. To avoid sagging the pelvis, you have to root the outer edge of the right foot, and elongate the left leg upwards, out of the left hip joint. That will automatically pull the pelvis upwards.
- Hold for three breaths. On the fourth exhalation, release the left foot, return to vasisthasana I (5), and then to adhomukha svanasana.
- Hold adhomukha svanasana for three breaths.
- On the fourth exhalation, turn over on the left foot and repeat on the left side.

7. Kasyapasana

Kasyapa is the son of Marichi and grandson of Brahman

- Start with adhomukha svanasana on a 'sticky' yoga mat and then proceed:
- On an exhalation, turn over on the right hand and the right foot and go into vasisthasana I (5). Cross the left foot as for padmasana (see page 72), swing the left arm around the back and hold the foot. If you cannot do this, you can start from the mat.
- Sit in siddhasana (see page 78), with the left foot in the groin of the right leg. Swing the left arm around the back in a circular motion and hold the metatarsal of the left big toe.
- Roll over onto the right hip and extend the right leg, but not fully; keep the knee slightly bent. Place the right hand on the mat in line

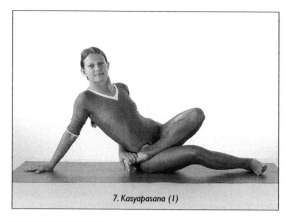

7. Kasyapasana (1)

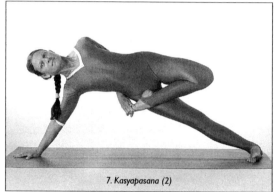

7. Kasyapasana (2)

with the right foot, with the fingers pointing in a straight line away from the right hip. The right arm makes an angle of ninety degrees with the chest, and thus is not perpendicular, but slants forward, away from the shoulder joint. The right foot rests on the outer edge, more on the plantar than on the dorsal side.
- On an exhalation, push up on the right hand and foot, till the right leg is straight and in alignment with the trunk. Extend the coccyx towards the right heel, and elongate the left thigh and knee out of the left hip joint. At the same time, elongate the lower abdomen and the two frontal hip bones up towards the ribs. Thus the left groin is opened.
- For the rest follow the instructions given in vasisthasana I (5).
- Keep the alignment of the body, especially between the back of the head, the sacrum and the right heel. To stay in line, bring the head and left knee back and the pelvis forwards, without turning it upwards. To avoid sagging the pelvis, you have to root the outer edge of the right foot and elongate the left thigh out of the left hip joint. That will automatically pull the pelvis upwards.
- Hold for three breaths. On the fourth exhalation, release the left foot, return to vasisthasana I (5), and then to adhomukha svanasana.
- Hold adhomukha svanasana for three breaths.
- On the fourth exhalation, turn over on the left foot and repeat on the left side.

8. Visvamitrasana

Visvamitra is the name of a sage

In the three previous positions the body balances on a unilateral line, that is, either on the right hand and right foot, or on the left hand and left foot. In visvamitrasana, the body balances on a diagonal line, that is, on the left hand and right foot, or on the right hand and left foot.

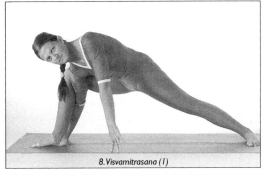

8. Visvamitrasana (1)

- Start with adhomukha svanasana (see page 210) on a 'sticky' yoga mat, but keep a shorter distance between the hands and feet. Then proceed:

- As the right hand has to end up in line with the left foot, you have to displace both hands slightly towards the left before swinging the right leg forward. On an exhalation, lean the body weight forward, bend the right arm and, lifting the right hip up, swing the right leg forward

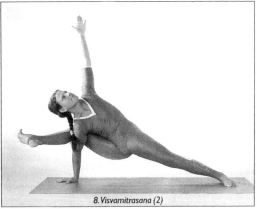

8. Visvamitrasana (2)

in a large, circular movement around the outer side of the right arm, so that the foot lands next to the inner border of the fingers of the right hand, with the knee bent at an angle of ninety degrees and the back of the thigh resting on the deltoid muscle of the right arm.

- Turn the left foot over, so that the sole of the foot rests on the mat, and the inner arch of the left foot is in line with the wrist and middle finger of the right hand.

- Turn over on the right arm and lift the right foot in the direction you are facing, perpendicular to the line between the right hand and the left foot. Then extend the right leg forward in a circular movement, till it is in line with the line between theright hand and the left foot, with the knee straight.

- Extend the left hand up to the sky at an angle of ninety degrees to the chest and look up at the sky.

- For the rest follow the instructions given in vasisthasana I (5). Keep the alignment of the body, especially the line between the back of the head, the sacrum and the left heel. To stay in line, bring the head back while extending the right leg, and bring the pelvis forwards.

- Hold for three breaths. On the fourth exhalation, place the left hand back on the mat, at shoulder width from and parallel to the right one. Lifting the heel of the left foot and rolling on the ball of the foot, swing the right leg back around the outer side of the right arm in a circular movement, lifting the right hip up, to return to adhomukha svanasana. Place the hands back again in their original position, in line with the feet.

- Hold adhomukha svanasana for three breaths.

- On the fourth exhalation repeat on the left side.

The next three positions are done in the *vinyasa* mode, that is, flowing directly from one into the next.

9. Dvihasta Bhujasana

dvi=two; hasta=hand; bhuja=arm

- Start with adhomukha svanasana (see page 210) on a 'sticky' yoga mat, but keep a shorter distance between the hands and feet. Then proceed:
- On an exhalation, jump the feet forward around the outer arms in a circular movement, till they land on the mat next to the outer borders of the hands. In this way the distance between the knees is shoulder width. Keep the hips high while jumping, so that you land with the knees just slightly bent.
- Widen the knees a little and, elongating the ribs forward from the groins, place the hands on the back of the calves, with the thumbs on the inner sides of the lower legs, pointing towards each other, and the fingers on the outer sides.
- Insert the shoulders underneath the knees, keeping the hips up and the knees slightly bent. Press the inner thighs against the ribs and the inner knees against the deltoid muscles, and elongate the buttock bones and the back of the thighs up towards the sky. This is kurmasana (see page 140) standing on the feet.
- Release the hands and place them behind the heels on the mat, with the fingers pointing forwards and the index fingers in line with the back of the heels. Extend the wrists down, lower the pelvis and sit down on the upper arms, near the deltoid muscles.
- Then bring the weight of the body slightly backwards, till the feet lift up from the mat. This is dvihasta bhujasana.
- Hold for a few seconds; then proceed to 10.

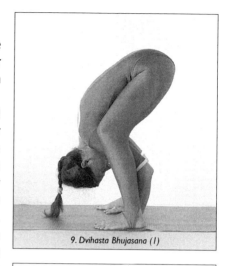

9. Dvihasta Bhujasana (1)

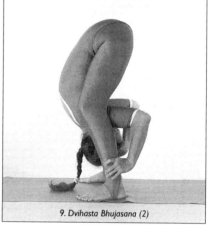

9. Dvihasta Bhujasana (2)

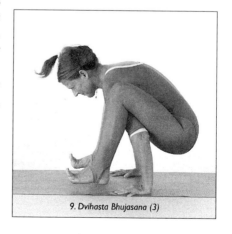

9. Dvihasta Bhujasana (3)

10. Titthibhasana

titthibha=firefly

- Elongate the legs forward, lifting the feet and the pelvis simultaneously: as the lower legs elongate forwards, the buttock bones and the back of the thighs elongate backwards, so that the backs of the legs are extended.
- Press the inner thighs against the ribs, and the inner knees against the deltoid muscles to avoid sliding off the arms.

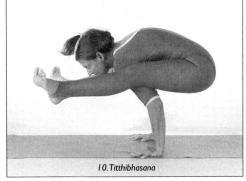

10. Titthibhasana

This is kurmasana (see page 140) standing on the hands: the trunk and the legs, from the buttock bones towards the heels, are parallel to the earth. Perform pada bandha to stabilize the legs and pelvis.
- Root the hands, performing hasta bandha, so that the arms elongate and the chest is lifted up from the shoulder heads. The back is not straight, but arches upwards: the more you elongate the arms, lifting the chest up from the shoulder heads, the more the back arches upwards (turtle back). Look straight forward.
- Hold for a few seconds; then proceed to 11.

11. Bhujapidasana

bhuja=arm; pida=pressure

- On the exhalation, bend the knees and cross the ankles in front of you. Do not lower the hips as you cross the ankles, but keep extending the buttock bones backwards while pressing the inner thighs against the upper arms.
- Root the hands, performing hasta bandha, so that the arms elongate and the chest is lifted up from the shoulder heads. The back is not

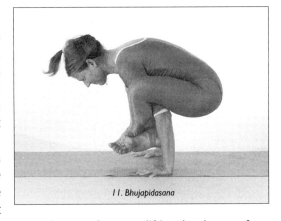

11. Bhujapidasana

straight, but arches upwards: the more you elongate the arms, lifting the chest up from the shoulder heads, the more the back arches upwards (turtle back). Look straight forward.
- Hold for a few seconds; then cross the ankles the other way.
- Return to dvihasta bhujasana (9). Turn the feet sideways on the upper arms, the right foot towards the right and the left foot towards the left, lift the hips and jump back into chaturanga dandasana (see page 52). Keep the head up and bend the arms as you jump, so that the shoulders end up above the hands. Always use the exhalation to jump, and the inhalation to stabilize your position.
- Proceed through urdhvamukha svanasana (see page 210) and adhomukha svanasana (see page 210).

The next two positions are done in the *vinyasa* mode, that is, flowing directly from one into the next.

12. Ekahasta Bhujasana

eka=one; hasta=hand; bhuja=arm

- Start with adhomukha svanasana (see page 210), but keep a shorter distance between the hands and feet. Then proceed:
- On an exhalation, jump the feet forward: the left foot ends up in between the two hands, and the right foot swings around the outer right arm in a circular movement to land next to the outer border of the right hand. Thus the hands and feet are on one line. Keep the hips high while jumping, so that you land with the knees just slightly bent.

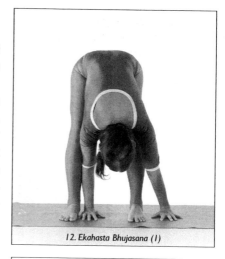

12. Ekahasta Bhujasana (1)

- Place the right hand on the back of the right calf muscle, with the thumb on the inner side of the lower leg, and the fingers on the outer side, and insert the right shoulder underneath the right knee. Then release the right hand and place both hands behind the feet on the mat, with the fingers pointing forwards.
- Extend the wrists down, lower the pelvis and sit down with the right thigh on the right upper arm, near the deltoid muscle. Bring the weight of the body slightly backwards till the right foot lifts up from the mat, keeping the leg bent as in dvihasta bhujasana (9).
- Then lift the left foot and extend the leg forward, parallel to the earth.

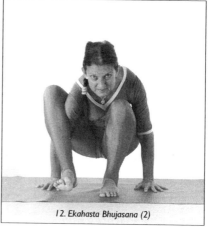

12. Ekahasta Bhujasana (2)

- Press the inner right thigh against the ribs, and the inner knee against the right deltoid muscle, to prevent the leg from sliding off the arm. Perform pada bandha with both feet to stabilize the legs and pelvis.
- Root the hands, performing hasta bandha, so that the arms elongate and the chest is lifted up from the shoulder heads. The back is not straight, but arches upwards: the more you elongate the arms, lifting the chest up from the shoulder

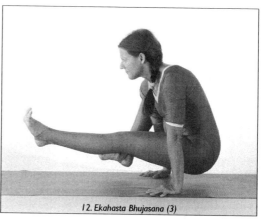

12. Ekahasta Bhujasana (3)

heads, the more the back arches upwards (turtle back). Look straight forward.
- Hold for a few seconds; then proceed to 13.

13. **Astavakrasana**

Astavakra is the teacher of King Janaka

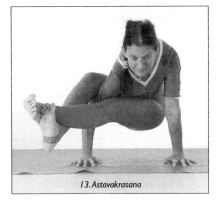

13. Astavakrasana

- Cross the left foot over the right, and extend both legs forwards and slightly sideways; the left foot crosses over the right one, so that the right leg supports the left one.
- Press the inner right thigh against the ribs, and the inner knee against the right deltoid muscle, to prevent the leg from sliding off the arm. Perform pada bandha with both feet to stabilize the legs and pelvis.
- Root the hands, performing hasta bandha, so that the arms elongate and the chest is lifted up from the shoulder heads. The back is not straight, but arches upwards: the more you elongate the arms, lifting the chest up from the shoulder heads, the more the back arches upwards (turtle back). Look straight forward.
- Hold for a few seconds.
- Release the crossing of the feet and bend the legs again, the left one in between the arms and the right one on the right arm, turning the foot sideways. Then lift the hips, bring the feet back, the left foot through the arms and the right one around the outer side of the right arm, and jump back into chaturanga dandasana (see page 52).
- Proceed through urdhvamukha svanasana (see page 210) and adhomukha svanasana (see page 210), and repeat 12 and 13 on the left side.

14. **Mayurasana**

mayura=peacock

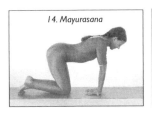

14. Mayurasana

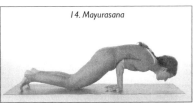

14. Mayurasana

- Kneel on the mat on hands and knees, with the knees slightly spread and the hands close together, fingers pointing backwards.
- Bend the elbows, keeping them close together, lift the knees and pelvis, and place the lower abdomen on the bent elbows: the elbows are in between the two frontal hip bones. Keep the head up.
- Bring the body weight slowly forward, supporting yourself on the toes and hands, till the feet lift off the mat by themselves. The whole body is now supported only on the hands, and makes one line, from the ankles through the knees to the shoulders and ears. The lower arms are not perpendicular to the earth, but slant forwards, with an angle of about a hundred degrees in the elbows.
- Hold for a couple of seconds. On an exhalation, bring the body weight back again, so that the feet go back onto the mat.

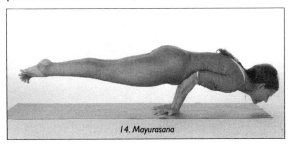

14. Mayurasana

15. Padma Mayurasana

padma=lotus;
mayura=peacock

- Thls is the same position as the previous one, performed with the legs in padmasana (see page 72).

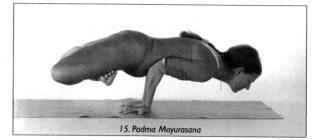

15. Padma Mayurasana

16. Hamsasana

hamsa=swan

- This is the same position as mayurasana (14), but here the fingers point forward. This produces a tighter angle in the wrist joints.

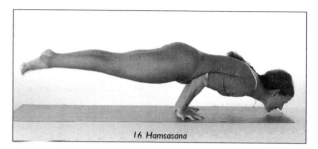

16. Hamsasana

17. Bakasana

baka=crane

- Start with salamba sirsasana II (see page 165) and then proceed:
- On an exhalation, lower the legs in between the arms, till the feet are about ten inches from the mat. Keep the knees straight and together.
- Bend the knees between the inner upper arms, keeping the elbows in line with the armpits and an angle of ninety degrees in the elbows.
- Spread the knees, keeping the feet together, and take the shins deep into the armpits. The tibial bones rest on the triceps muscles of the upper arms, and the inner thighs press against the sides of the rib cage. The weight of the body is on the center of the palms.
- Squeeze the knees inwards towards each other, so that the elbows stay in line with the armpits, and keep the inner ankles together, so that all the toes are in line. Perform pada bandha with both feet to maintain the compactness of the legs and hips. The upper and lower spring joints of the feet control the hip joints; they are of vital importance in all the bakasana poses, where you have to

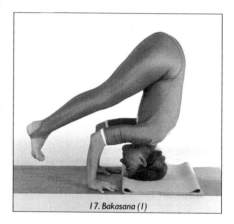

17. Bakasana (1)

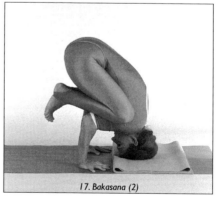

17. Bakasana (2)

maintain the compactness and coherence of the body. Keeping the feet and spring joints inactive would mean that the body would fall apart in the hip joints, and therefore it would be impossible to perform these poses.

- To lift the head up from the mat, bring the weight of the body back onto the wrists. As soon as the head is loose from the mat, however, you have to bring the weight of the body again forward onto the center of the palms. The central point of gravity is in the center of the palms. Thus, to maintain an even and effortless equilibrium, the weight of the body at the front of this central point and at the back of it should be even: the head, shoulders, upper chest and knees at the front of this central point should be in

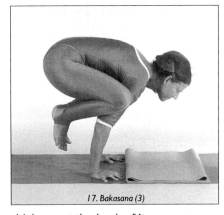

I7. Bakasana (3)

balance with the lower trunk, thighs and feet, which are at the back of it.
- As the head lifts, the feet will go down (see-saw action around the shoulder joints), but do not lower them too much, and do not lose the action in the spring joints (pada bandha).
- After reaching the balance, work on the lightness of the pose, the rooting and the elongation. Pressing the tibial bones against the triceps muscles to maintain the compactness of the body, root the hands and perform hasta bandha, so that the arms elongate and the chest is lifted up from the shoulder heads. The back is not straight but arches upwards; the more you elongate the arms, lifting the chest up from the shoulder heads, the more the back arches upwards (turtle back). Thus the pose is high and light.
- As bakasana is the true counterpose for back bendings, the back should not be concave but, on the contrary, should make a 'cat-back,' that is, the whole spine, from the base up to the neck, should push up towards the sky. The first thoracic vertebra and the coccyx are at the same height; they form the extreme ends of the bow, while the spine forms the drawn bow itself. This is the reversed bow: whereas in dhanurasana (see page 209) the bow of the spine is curved into the trunk, here it is curved backwards, out of the trunk. Therefore bakasanas are the counter poses for back bendings, and in both cases the coccyx and first thoracic vertebra form the extreme end points of the bow.
- The neck should be loose; do not try to lift the head up too much: the eyes look at an angle of forty-five degrees forward and downward.
- To come out of the pose, the movement of lowering the head onto the mat and bringing the weight of the body back onto the wrists should be synchronized, so that at all times the weight at the front and back of the central point of gravity is maintained.
- Once the head is on the mat, release the shins from the upper arms by lifting the pelvis and bringing the knees again in between the inner upper arms. Then extend the legs and return to salamba sirsasana II.

18. Parsva Bakasana

parsva=sideways; baka=crane

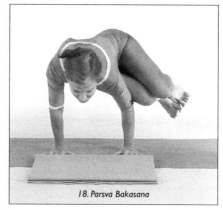

18. Parsva Bakasana

- Start with salamba sirsasana II (see page 165) and proceed:
- On an exhalation, lower the legs between the arms, till the feet are about ten inches from the mat. Keep the knees straight and together.
- Bend the knees between the inner upper arms, keeping the elbows in line with the armpits and an angle of ninety degrees in the elbows.
- Then lift the knees slightly above the level of the upper arms and, rotating the back, especially the lumbar spine, swing the legs over the left upper arm, till the outer side of the right thigh rests on the triceps muscle of the left arm. Turn the back enough so that you do not come to rest on the quadriceps muscle of the right thigh, but rather on the fascia lata.
- Keep the inner ankles together, so that all the toes are in line. Perform pada bandha with both feet to maintain the compactness of the legs and hips.
- The upper and lower spring joints of the feet control the hip joints; they are of vital importance in all the bakasana poses, where you have to maintain the compactness and coherence of the body. Keeping the feet and spring joints inactive would mean that the body would fall apart in the hip joints, and therefore it would be impossible to perform these poses.
- Even though the thighs rest only on the left upper arm, the weight of the body is still distributed evenly between both hands, on the center of the palms.
- To lift the head up from the mat, bring the weight of the body back onto the wrists. Keep lifting the feet, though. As soon as the head is loose from the mat, you have to bring the weight of the body again forward, onto the center of the palms. The central point of gravity is in the center of the palms. Thus, to maintain an even and effortless equilibrium, the weight of the body at the front and back of this central point should be even: the head, shoulders, upper chest and knees in front of this central point should be in balance with the lower trunk, thighs and feet, which are behind it.
- As the head lifts, the feet will go down (see-saw action around the shoulder joints), but do not lower them too much, and do not lose the action in the spring joints (pada bandha).
- After reaching the balance, work on the lightness of the pose, the rooting and the elongation. Pulling the heels close to the buttocks while keeping the inner ankles together, root the hands and perform hasta bandha, so that the arms elongate and the chest is lifted up from the shoulder heads. This rooting, elongation, lightness and lifting will be easier to feel on the right (free) side of the body, but try nevertheless to create some of it on the left side too.
- Here too the spine should push up to the sky, even though in this pose it is much less obvious than in the previous one, due to the turning of the spinal vertebrae. To give an extra accentuation to this turning of the spine, you have to synchronize the lifting of the feet with the lifting of the right shoulder blade, so that the first thoracic vertebra and

the coccyx have the same height from the earth. Keep the hips exactly in the middle, in between the two elbows, so that the spine from the coccyx to the back of the head remains perpendicular to the line between the hands.

- The neck should be loose; do not try to lift the head too much; the eyes look at an angle of forty-five degrees forward and downward.
- To come out of the pose, the movement of lowering the head onto the mat and bringing the weight of the body back onto the wrists should be synchronized, so that at all times the weight at the front and back of the central point of gravity is maintained.
- Once the head is on the mat, release the thighs from the left upper arm by lifting the pelvis and bringing the knees again in between the inner upper arms. Then extend the legs and return to salamba sirsasana II.
- Repeat on the other side.

19. Ekapada Bakasana I

eka=one; pada=leg,foot; baka=crane

This pose is a combination of bakasana (17) and titthibhasana (10).

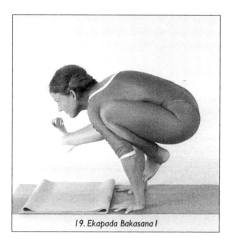

19. Ekapada Bakasana I

- Start with salamba sirsasana II (see page 165) and proceed:
- On an exhalation, lower the legs between the arms, till the feet are about ten inches from the mat. Keep the knees straight and together.
- Bend the knees between the inner upper arms, keeping the elbows in line with the armpits and an angle of ninety degrees in the elbows.
- Lift the left knee and bring the left shin into the left armpit as in bakasana (17).
- Press the left thigh against the left side of the rib cage, keeping the lower spring joint of the left foot active (pada bandha). The weight of the body is on the center of the palms.
- Lift the right knee and turn the right leg out, so that the toes of the right foot point away from the trunk, at an angle of ninety degrees to the right. Then swing the right leg forward in a circular movement, till the inner side of the thigh comes to rest on the deltoid muscle of the right arm. The right knee is still bent, and the right foot is still pointing away from the trunk.
- To lift the head up from the mat, bring the weight of the body back onto the wrists. Keep lifting the feet, though. As soon as the head is loose from the mat, bring the weight of the body again forwards, but not completely onto the center of the palms.
- While lifting the head, extend the right leg forward as in titthibhasana (10): keeping the toes pointing sideways extend the right foot forward in a circular movement, till the knee is straight and the sole of the right foot faces forward at an angle of forty-five degrees. Thus the left shin bone and the inner right thigh rest on the upper arms.
- After reaching the balance, work on the lightness of the pose, that is, on the rooting and the elongation. Pressing the left shin bone and the inner right thigh against the triceps muscles of the upper arms to maintain the compactness of the body, root the

hands and perform hasta bandha, so that the arms elongate and the chest is lifted up from the shoulder heads. The back is not straight, but arches upwards; the more you elongate the arms, lifting the chest up from the shoulder heads, the more the back arches upwards (turtle back). Thus the pose is high and light.

- To come out of the pose, the movement of lowering the head onto the mat and bringing the weight of the body back onto the wrists should be synchronized, so that at all times the weight at the front and back of the central point of gravity is maintained.
- Once the head is on the mat, release the left shin and right thigh from the upper arms by lifting the pelvis, and bring the knees again in between the inner upper arms. Then extend the legs and return to salamba sirsasana II.

20. Ekapada Bakasana II

eka=one; pada=leg, foot;
baka=crane

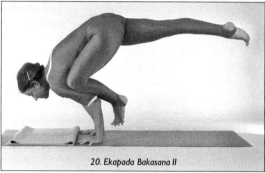

- Start with salamba sirsasana II (see page 165) and proceed:
- On an exhalation, lower the legs between the arms, till the feet are about ten inches from the mat. Keep the knees straight and together.
- On the next exhalation, bend the

20. Ekapada Bakasana II

left knee and bring the left shin into the left armpit as in bakasana (17). Lift the right leg high, keeping the knee straight. The weight of the body is on the center of the palms.
- To lift the head up from the mat, bring the weight of the body back onto the wrists. As soon as the head is loose from the mat, however, you have to bring the weight of the body again forwards, onto the center of the palms.
- This pose is the hardest of the bakasana poses, because the weight of the body back of the central point of gravity is greatly increased due to the backward extension of the right leg. Therefore it is imperative to keep the right leg raised high throughout the pose. Press the left shin down on the left arm, performing pada bandha to support the action in the pelvis and lower abdomen.
- To come out of the pose, the movement of lowering the head onto the mat and bringing the weight of the body back onto the wrists should be synchronized, so that at all times the weight at the front and back of the central point of gravity is maintained.
- Once the head is on the mat, release the left shin from the left upper arm, lift the pelvis and extend the left leg, joining it with the right one. Then return to salamba sirsasana II.

21. Dvipada Koundinyasana

*dvi=two; pada=leg, foot; Koundinya is
the name of a sage*

- Start with parsva bakasana (18) on the
  left arm and proceed:
- After reaching the balance, extend both
  legs so that they point forward at an
  angle of forty-five degrees.
- For the rest follow the instructions given
  in parsva bakasana (18).

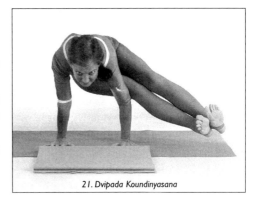

21. Dvipada Koundinyasana

22. Ekapada Koundinyasana

*eka=one; pada=leg, foot;
Koundinya is the name of a
sage*

- Start with parsva bakasana (18)
  on the left arm and proceed:
- Cross the left knee behind the
  right one, and extend the right
  leg forward. Keep the left knee
  bent. The right foot points
  forward in the direction you will

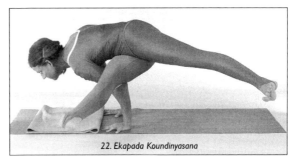

22. Ekapada Koundinyasana

  be facing, and the left foot points backwards.
- To lift the head, keep the left leg bent and proceed as usual.
- After reaching the balance, extend the left leg backwards. This means that the weight
  of the body is increased back of the central point of gravity. If this situation is not
  corrected, the weight of the left leg will inevitably drag you down. Thus, while
  extending the left leg backwards, you have to simultaneously bring the chest and
  shoulders slightly forwards, so that you maintain an even weight at the front and back
  of the central point of gravity.
- Before lowering the head again, bend the left leg, bringing the chest and shoulders
  slightly backwards (otherwise there will be too much weight on the front of the central
  point of gravity and you will fall on your head), and return to parsva bakasana.
- To come out of the pose, the movement of lowering the head onto the mat and bringing
  the weight of the body back onto the wrists should be synchronized, so that at all times
  the weight at the front and back of the central point of gravity is maintained.
- Once the head is on the mat, release the thighs from the left upper arm by lifting the
  pelvis and bringing the knees again in between the inner upper arms. Then extend the
  legs and return to salamba sirsasana II.
- Repeat on the other side.

23. Ekapada Galavasana

eka=one; pada=leg, foot;
Galava is the name of a sage

This pose is a preparation for urdhva kukkutasana (24).

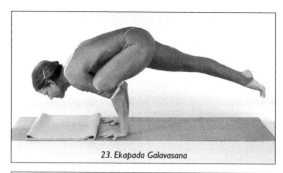

23. Ekapada Galavasana

- Start with salamba sirsasana II (see page 165) and proceed:
- Bend the left leg and place the left foot in the right groin as for padmasana (see page 72).
- Bend the right knee and bring the legs down to the arms. Place the left shin on the triceps muscle of the left arm and the left foot on the triceps muscle of the right arm, hooking the toes around the outer edge of the right upper arm and performing pada bandha to stabilize the hips. The right knee is still bent, with the right foot pointing backwards.

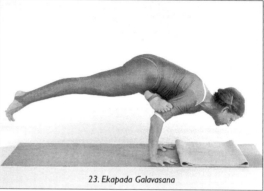

23. Ekapada Galavasana

- Lower the hips, so that the rib cage rests on the left lower leg, and then extend the right leg backwards.
- To lift the head, proceed as usual. Keep the right leg raised high with the help of the back muscles. The rib cage rests throughout on the lower left leg. Do not lose the grip of the left foot on the outer right arm.
- Before lowering the head onto the mat again, bend the right leg and then proceed as usual.

The last three positions of the bakasana series (24, 25 and 26) are done in padmasana (see page 72). In urdhva kukkutasana (24), both shins rest on the upper arms; therefore the padmasana should be fairly wide. In galavasana (25), the crossed shins rest on one arm, and thus the padmasana has to be tighter. In parsva kukkutasana (26) the padmasana should be very tight.

24. Urdhva Kukkutasana

urdhva=upwards; kukkuta=cock

If you can do padmasana in salamba sirsasana II, this pose is actually the easiest of all the bakasana poses.

- Start with salamba sirsasana II (see page 165), cross the legs in padmasana (see page 72) and, on an exhalation, lower the legs and place the shins on the triceps muscles of the upper arms, close to the armpits.

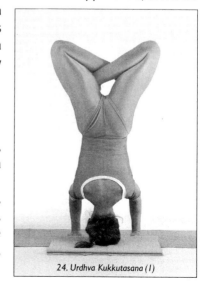

24. Urdhva Kukkutasana (1)

- To lift the head up from the mat, take the pelvis slightly back and down, and proceed as usual.
- Squeeze the thighs inward towards each other, and pull the knees up into the abdomen to maintain the compactness of the pose. Root the hands, performing hasta bandha, so that the arms elongate and the chest lifts up from the shoulder heads.
- This position is yoga mudrasana I (see page 81) while balancing on the hands, thus the body is

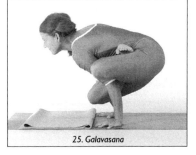

24. Urdhva Kukkutasana (2)

parallel to the earth. Like in bakasana (17), do not make the back concave but, on the contrary, make a 'cat-back', that is, the whole spine, from the base up to the neck, pushes up towards the sky. The first thoracic vertebra and the coccyx have the same height from the earth; they form the extreme ends of the bow, while the spine forms the drawn bow itself.
- The neck should be loose, do not try to lift the head up too much; the eyes look at an angle of forty-five degrees forward and downward.
- To come out of the pose, proceed as usual.

25. Galavasana
Galava is the name of a sage
As mentioned before, the padmasana here should be tighter than in the previous pose.
- Start with salamba sirsasana II (see page 165), cross the legs in padmasana (see page 72) and proceed:
- On an exhalation, lower the legs to the arms. Turn the hips to the left and place the point where the shins cross each other on the triceps of the left upper arm. The left knee is now on the left side of the left arm, and the right thigh is in between the two arms.
- Pull the right knee up towards the chest, almost as if you want to bite it. This involves strong action of the adductor muscles of the right thigh and of the oblique abdominal muscles.
- To lift the head, proceed as usual.
- This pose is like a twisted yoga mudrasana I (see page 81) performed while balancing on the hands. Thus the body is parallel to the earth as in urdhva kukkutasana (24).
- Pull the right knee up towards the chest, and keep pointing it straight forward in the direction you are facing, in the middle of the two elbows. Perform pada bandha to maintain the compactness of the thighs and hips.
- To come out of the pose, proceed as usual.

25. Galavasana

25. Galavasana

26. Parsva Kukkutasana

parsva=sideways; kukkuta=cock

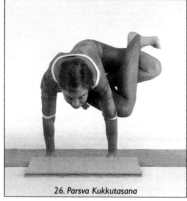

26. Parsva Kukkutasana

As mentioned before, in this position the Padmasana is tightest.

- Start with salamba sirsasana II (see page 165), cross the legs in padmasana (see page 73) and proceed:
- Hook the toes around the outer edges of the thighs, so that the arches and ankles are very strong (pada bandha).
- On an exhalation, lower the legs to just above the level of the upper arms. Inhale, and with a strong exhalation swing the legs to the left till the quadriceps muscle of the right thigh comes to rest on the triceps muscle of the left arm. The left knee points upwards.
- To lift the head, proceed as usual.
- To come out of the pose, proceed as usual.This pose is the most difficult of the Bakasana series, partly because of the extreme twisting of the trunk, and partly because of the balance.

Part 12 Back Bendings

Back Bendings

a. *Simple Back Bendings*
b. *Urdhva Dhanurasana*
c. *Back Bend Variations*

---

12 Simple Back Bendings

Simple Back Bendings

1. *Urdhvamukha Salabhasana*
   a. *Arms backwards*
   b. *Arms sideways*
   c. *Arms forwards*
   d. *Makarasana*
2. *Dvipada Adhomukha Salabhasana*
   a. *Arms backwards*
   b. *Arms sideways*
   c. *Arms forwards*
   d. *Makarasana*
3. *Ekapada Adhomukha Salabhasana*
   a. *Arms backwards*
   b. *Arms sideways*
   c. *Arms forwards*
   d. *Makarasana*

4. *Dvipada Salabhasana*
   a. *Arms backwards*
   b. *Arms sideways*
   c. *Arms forwards*
   d. *Makarasana*
5. *Ekapada Salabhasana*
   a. *Arms forwards, same side arm and leg up*
   b. *Arms forwards, opposite arm and leg up*
6. *Dhanurasana*
7. *Bhujangasana I*
8. *Urdhvamukha Svanasana*
9. *Adhomukha Svanasana*
10. *Purvottanasana*
11. *Ustrasana*

---

1. Urdhvamukha Salabhasana

urdhva=upwards; mukha=face; salabha=locust

1a. Arms backwards

- Lie on the stomach on a blanket with the legs extended straight backwards and the inner ankles together. Extend the arms backwards and clasp the hands on the back.

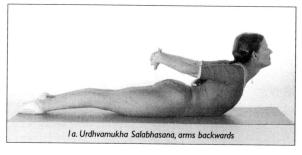

1a. Urdhvamukha Salabhasana, arms backwards

- On the inhalation, lift the head, chest and arms up, pulling the body up from the kidney region. Elongate the arms backwards out of the shoulder joints. Do not flex the head too far back, but keep the neck long and fairly relaxed.
- Keep the legs and feet on the blanket and the inner ankles together, rooting the top of the arches into the earth.
- Hold for a few seconds, retaining the breath. On the exhalation, lower the head, chest and arms. Repeat three times.

1b. Arms sideways

- Lie on the stomach on a blanket with the legs extended straight backwards and the inner ankles together. Extend the arms sideways on the blanket, at an angle of ninety degrees to the chest, with the palms of the hands turned down.

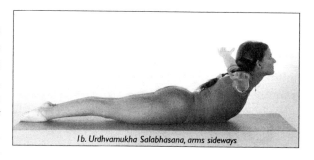

1b. Urdhvamukha Salabhasana, arms sideways

- On the inhalation, lift the head, chest and arms up, pulling the body up from the kidney region. Elongate the arms sideways out of the shoulder joints. To keep the arms at an angle of ninety degrees to the chest, elongate the ulnar side of the wrists more. Do not flex the head too far back, but keep the neck long and fairly relaxed.
- Keep the legs and feet on the blanket and the inner ankles together, rooting the top of the arches into the earth.
- Hold for a few seconds, retaining the breath. On the exhalation, lower the head, chest and arms. Repeat three times.

1c.   Arms forwards

- Lie on the stomach on a blanket with the legs extended straight backwards and the inner ankles together. Extend the arms forwards on the blanket, keeping them parallel to each other and the palms of the hands turned down.

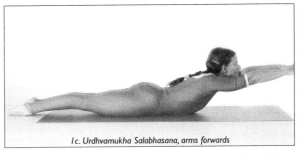

1c. Urdhvamukha Salabhasana, arms forwards

- On the inhalation, lift the head, chest and arms up, pulling the body up from the kidney region. Elongate the arms forwards out of the shoulder joints, keeping them parallel to each other. Do not flex the head too far back, but keep the neck long and fairly relaxed.
- Keep the legs and feet on the blanket and the inner ankles together, rooting the top of the arches into the earth.
- Hold for a few seconds, retaining the breath. On the exhalation, lower the head, chest and arms. Repeat three times.

1d.   Makarasana

makara=crocodile

- Lie on the stomach on a blanket with the legs extended straight backwards and the inner ankles together. Bend the arms and clasp the hands in the neck.
- On the inhalation, lift the head, chest and arms up, pulling the body up from the

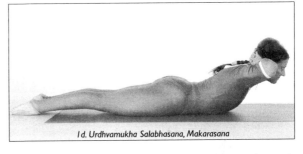

1d. Urdhvamukha Salabhasana, Makarasana

kidney region. Keep the elbows up. Do not flex the head too far back, but keep the neck long and fairly relaxed.
- Keep the legs and feet on the blanket and the inner ankles together, rooting the top of the arches into the earth.
- Hold for a few seconds, retaining the breath. On the exhalation, lower the head, chest and arms. Repeat three times.

2. Dvipada Adhomukha Salabhasana

dvi=two; pada=leg, foot; adho=downwards; mukha=face; salabha=locust

2a. Arms backwards

- Lie on the stomach on a blanket with the legs extended straight backwards and the inner ankles together. Extend the arms backwards on the blanket next to the trunk, with the palms of the hands turned up. Rest the forehead or chin on the blanket.

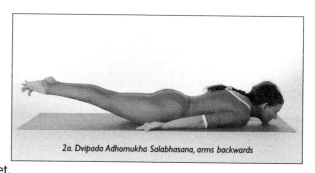

2a. Dvipada Adhomukha Salabhasana, arms backwards

- On the inhalation, lift the legs up, keeping the knees straight and elongating the legs backwards out of the lumbar spine. The inner ankles stay together and the head, trunk and arms stay on the blanket.
- Hold for a few seconds, retaining the breath. On the exhalation, lower the legs. Repeat three times.

2b. Arms sideways

- Lie on the stomach on a blanket with the legs extended straight backwards and the inner ankles together. Extend the arms sideways on the blanket, at an angle of ninety degrees to the chest, with the palms of the hands

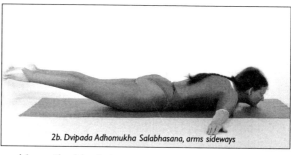

2b. Dvipada Adhomukha Salabhasana, arms sideways

turned down. Rest the forehead or chin on the blanket.
- On the inhalation, lift the legs up, keeping the knees straight and elongating the legs backwards out of the lumbar spine. The inner knees stay together and the head, trunk and arms stay on the blanket.
- Hold for a few seconds, retaining the breath. On the exhalation, lower the legs. Repeat three times.

2c.   *Arms forwards*

- Lie on the stomach on a blanket with the legs extended straight backwards and the inner ankles together. Extend the arms forwards on the blanket, keeping them parallel to each other and

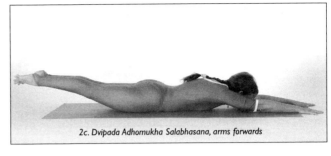

2c. Dvipada Adhomukha Salabhasana, arms forwards

the palms of the hands turned down. Rest the forehead or chin on the blanket.
- On the inhalation, lift the legs up, keeping the knees straight and elongating the legs backwards out of the lumbar spine. The inner ankles stay together and the head, trunk and arms stay on the blanket.
- Hold for a few seconds, retaining the breath. On the exhalation, lower the legs. Repeat three times.

2d.   *Makarasana*
makara=crocodile

- Lie on the stomach on a blanket with the legs extended straight backwards and the inner ankles together. Bend the arms and clasp the hands in the neck. Rest the forehead or chin on

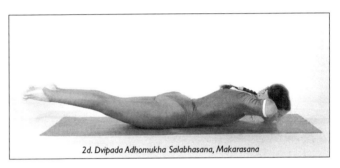

2d. Dvipada Adhomukha Salabhasana, Makarasana

the blanket, but keep the elbows up.
- On the inhalation, lift the legs up, keeping the knees straight and elongating the legs backwards out of the lumbar spine. The inner ankles stay together and the head and trunk stay on the blanket.
- Hold for a few seconds, retaining the breath. On the exhalation, lower the legs. Repeat three times.

3. Ekapada Adhomukha Salabhasana

eka=one; pada=leg, foot; adho=downwards; mukha=face; salabha=locust

3a. Arms backwards

- Lie on the stomach on a blanket with the legs extended straight backwards and the inner ankles together. Extend the arms backwards on the blanket next to the trunk, with the palms of the hands turned up. Rest the forehead or chin on the blanket.

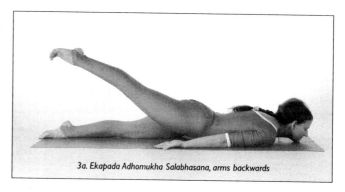

3a. Ekapada Adhomukha Salabhasana, arms backwards

- On the inhalation, lift the right leg up, keeping the knee straight and elongating the leg backwards out of the lumbar spine. Do not tilt the right side of the pelvis up to lift the leg, but use the biceps muscle at the back of the thigh to lift it. Both the frontal hip bones stay on the blanket.
- Hold for a few seconds, retaining the breath. On the exhalation, lower the leg and repeat with the other one. Repeat three times with each leg.

3b. Arms sideways

- Lie on the stomach on a blanket with the legs extended straight backwards and the inner ankles together. Extend the arms sideways on the blanket, at an angle of

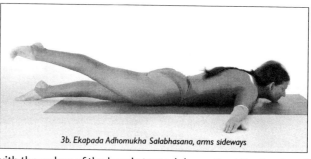

3b. Ekapada Adhomukha Salabhasana, arms sideways

ninety degrees to the chest, with the palms of the hands turned down. Rest the forehead or chin on the blanket.
- On the inhalation, lift the right leg up, keeping the knee straight and elongating the leg backwards out of the lumbar spine. Do not tilt the right side of the pelvis up to lift the leg, but use the biceps muscle at the back of the thigh to lift it. Both the frontal hip bones stay on the blanket.
- Hold for a few seconds, retaining the breath. On the exhalation, lower the leg and repeat with the other one. Repeat three times with each leg.

3c. *Arms forwards*

- Lie on the stomach on a blanket with the legs extended straight backwards and the inner ankles together. Extend the arms forwards on the blanket, keeping

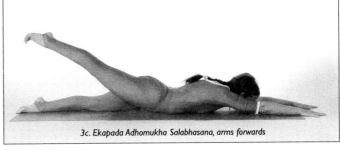

3c. Ekapada Adhomukha Salabhasana, arms forwards

them parallel to each other and the palms of the hands turned down. Rest the forehead or chin on the blanket.
- On the inhalation, lift the right leg up, keeping the knee straight and elongating the leg backwards out of the lumbar spine. Do not tilt the right side of the pelvis up to lift the leg, but use the biceps muscle at the back of the thigh to lift it. Both the frontal hip bones stay on the blanket.
- Hold for a few seconds, retaining the breath. On the exhalation, lower the leg and repeat with the other one. Repeat three times with each leg.

3d. *Makarasana*

makara=crocodile

- Lie on the stomach on a blanket with the legs extended straight backwards and the inner ankles together. Bend the arms and clasp the hands in the neck. Rest the

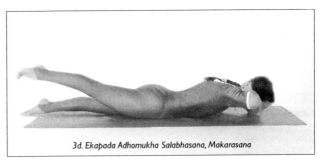

3d. Ekapada Adhomukha Salabhasana, Makarasana

forehead or chin on the blanket, but keep the elbows up.
- On the inhalation, lift the right leg up, keeping the knee straight and elongating the leg backwards out of the lumbar spine. Do not tilt the right side of the pelvis up to lift the leg, but use the biceps muscle at the back of the thigh to lift it. Both the frontal hip bones stay on the blanket.
- Hold for a few seconds, retaining the breath. On the exhalation, lower the leg and repeat with the other one. Repeat three times with each leg.

4. Dvipada Salabhasana

dvi=two; pada=leg, foot; salabha=locust

4a. Arms backwards

- Lie on the stomach on a blanket with the legs extended straight backwards and the inner ankles together. Extend the arms backwards and clasp the hands on the back.
- On the inhalation, lift the

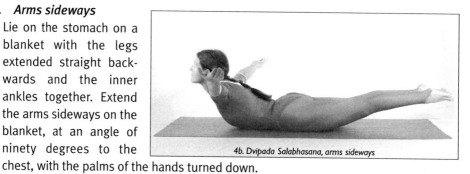

4a. Dvipada Salabhasana, arms backwards

  head, chest, arms and legs up, pulling the body up from the kidney region. Elongate the arms backwards out of the shoulder joints, and the legs backwards out of the lumbar spine.
- Keep the knees straight and the inner ankles together, and do not flex the head too far back, but keep the neck long and fairly relaxed.
- Hold for a few seconds, retaining the breath. On the exhalation, lower the head, chest, arms and legs. Repeat three times.

4b. Arms sideways

- Lie on the stomach on a blanket with the legs extended straight backwards and the inner ankles together. Extend the arms sideways on the blanket, at an angle of ninety degrees to the

4b. Dvipada Salabhasana, arms sideways

  chest, with the palms of the hands turned down.
- On the inhalation, lift the head, chest, arms and legs up, pulling the body up from the kidney region. Elongate the arms sideways out of the shoulder joints and the legs backwards out of the lumbar spine. To keep the arms at an angle of ninety degrees to the chest, elongate the ulnar side of the wrists more.
- Keep the knees straight and the inner ankles together, and do not flex the head too far back, but keep the neck long and fairly relaxed.
- Hold for a few seconds, retaining the breath. On the exhalation, lower the head, chest, arms and legs. Repeat three times.

4c. *Arms forwards*

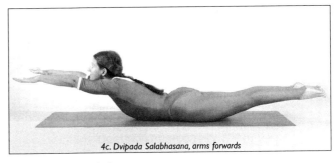

4c. Dvipada Salabhasana, arms forwards

- Lie on the stomach on a blanket with the legs extended straight backwards and the inner ankles together. Extend the arms forwards on the blanket, keeping them parallel to each other and the palms of the hands turned down.
- On the inhalation, lift the head, chest, arms and legs up, pulling the body up from the kidney region. Elongate the arms forwards out of the shoulder joints and the legs backwards out of the lumbar spine. Keep the arms parallel to each other.
- Keep the knees straight and the inner ankles together, and do not flex the head too far back, but keep the neck long and fairly relaxed.
- Hold for a few seconds, retaining the breath. On the exhalation, lower the head, chest, arms and legs. Repeat three times.

4d. *Makarasana*

makara=crocodile

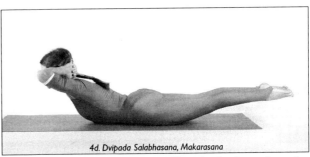

4d. Dvipada Salabhasana, Makarasana

- Lie on the stomach on a blanket with the legs extended straight backwards and the inner ankles together. Bend the arms and clasp the hands in the neck.
- On the inhalation, lift the head, chest, arms and legs up, pulling the body up from the kidney region. Keep the elbows up and elongate the legs backwards out of the lumbar spine.
- Keep the knees straight and the inner ankles together, and do not flex the head too far back, but keep the neck long and fairly relaxed.
- Hold for a few seconds, retaining the breath. On the exhalation, lower the head, chest, arms and legs. Repeat three times.

5.   Ekapada Salabhasana

eka=one; pada=leg, foot; salabha=locust

5a.   Arms forwards, same side arm and leg up

- Lie on the stomach on a blanket with the legs extended straight backwards and the inner ankles together. Extend the arms forwards on the blanket, keeping them

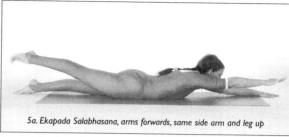

5a. Ekapada Salabhasana, arms forwards, same side arm and leg up

parallel to each other and the palms of the hands turned down.
- On the inhalation, lift the head, chest, right arm and right leg up. Do not flex the head too far backward, but keep the neck long and fairly relaxed.
- Do not tilt the right side of the chest and pelvis up to raise the right arm and leg, but use the back muscles and the biceps muscle of the right leg. Both frontal hip bones stay on the blanket and the shoulder blades stay parallel to the earth.
- Keep the knees straight, the right leg in line with the right hip and the right arm in line with the right shoulder. Elongate the right arm forward out of the right shoulder joint, and the right leg backward out of the lumbar spine.
- Hold for a few seconds, retaining the breath. On the exhalation, lower the head, chest, right arm and right leg, and repeat with the other leg and arm. Repeat each side three times.

5b.   Arms forwards, opposite arm and leg up

- Lie on the stomach on a blanket with the legs extended straight backwards and the inner ankles together. Extend the arms forwards on the blanket, keeping them parallel to

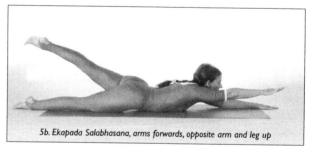

5b. Ekapada Salabhasana, arms forwards, opposite arm and leg up

each other and the palms of the hands turned down.
- On the inhalation, lift the head, chest, right arm and left leg up. Do not flex the head too far backward, but keep the neck long and fairly relaxed.
- Do not tilt the right side of the chest and the left side of the pelvis up to raise the right arm and left leg, but use the back muscles and the biceps muscle of the left leg. Both frontal hip bones stay on the blanket and the shoulder blades stay parallel to the earth.
- Keep the knees straight, the left leg in line with the left hip and the right arm in line with the right shoulder. Elongate the right arm forward out of the right shoulder joint, and the left leg backward out of the lumbar spine.
- Hold for a few seconds, retaining the breath. On the exhalation, lower the head, chest, right arm and left leg, and repeat with the other leg and arm. Repeat each side three times.

6. Dhanurasana

dhanu=bow

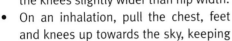

- Lie on the stomach on a blanket with the legs extended straight backwards and the inner ankles together. Bend the knees, and hold the arches of the feet with the hands, curling the toes around the fingers. Keep the feet together and the knees slightly wider than hip width.
- On an inhalation, pull the chest, feet and knees up towards the sky, keeping

6. Dhanurasana

the arches active against the fingers. The body arches like a bow (dhanu), till the trunk rests only on the abdomen.
- Do not flex the head too far backwards, but keep the neck fairly long and relaxed, and pull the trunk up from the kidney region.
- Hold for a few seconds, rocking the body gently on the mula bandha breathing; this gives the lower abdomen an excellent massage.
- On the exhalation, release the feet and lower the body onto the blanket.

7. Bhujangasana I

bhujanga=serpent

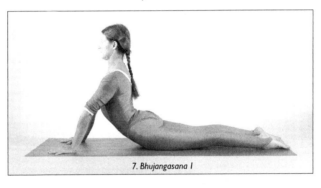

7. Bhujangasana I

- Lie on the stomach on a blanket with the legs extended straight backwards and the inner ankles together. Place the hands on the blanket next to the head, with the palms of the hands turned down and the fingers pointing forwards. The elbows point backwards.
- On a mula bandha inhalation, raise the head and chest and straighten the arms. Do not sink the chest into the shoulders, but lift it up against gravity. This is done by performing hasta bandha with the hands, so that the arms are elongated. Keep the lower abdomen on the earth and the knees straight.
- On the exhalation, curve the spine and head backwards, and roll the shoulders back by turning the pit of the elbows forwards: this lowers the shoulder blades.
- On each inhalation pull the two frontal hip bones forwards and up to elongate the spine upwards, and on each exhalation curve the spine backwards, creating a round movement which starts in the lower abdomen and ends in the back of the head.
- Hold for a few seconds, breathing normally. On the exhalation, bend the arms and lower the chest and head onto the blanket.

8. Urdhvamukha Svanasana

urdhva=upwards; mukha=face; svana=dog

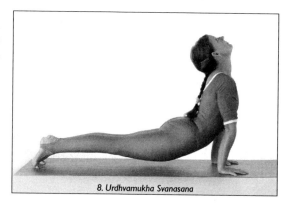

8. Urdhvamukha Svanasana

- Lie on the stomach on a mat with the legs extended straight backwards. Keep the feet at hip width so that the legs are parallel to each other.
- Place the hands on the blanket underneath the shoulders, with the palms of the hands turned down and the fingers pointing forwards. The elbows point backwards.
- Turn the toes under and straighten the knees, lifting them off the blanket.
- On a mula bandha inhalation, raise the head, chest and pelvis, straightening the arms till the whole body is supported only on the hands and the balls of the feet. The legs are parallel to the earth, and the knees are straight. Do not sink the chest into the shoulders, but lift it up against gravity. This is done by performing hasta bandha with the hands, so that the arms are elongated.
- On the exhalation, curve the spine and head backwards, and roll the shoulders back by turning the pit of the elbows forwards: this lowers the shoulder blades.
- On each inhalation pull the two frontal hip bones forwards and up to elongate the spine upward, and on each exhalation curve the spine backwards, creating a round movement which starts in the lower abdomen and ends in the back of the head.
- Hold for a few seconds, breathing normally. On the exhalation, bend the arms and lower the pelvis, chest and head onto the blanket.

9. Adhomukha Svanasana

adho=downwards; mukha=face; svana=dog

- Start with urdhvamukha svanasana (8) and proceed:
- On an exhalation, raise the pelvis and extend it backwards, keeping the arms and legs straight, till the body forms a unilateral triangle.
- The hands are at shoulder width, so that the arms are parallel to each other. The

9. Adhomukha Svanasana

fingers point straight forward, with the middle fingers parallel to each other.
- The feet are at hip width, so that the legs are parallel to each other. The inner borders of the feet are also parallel to each other.
- Make sure that your weight is evenly distributed between the two hands and between the two feet.
- Rotate the arms as in savasana, which means that the inner elbows rotate forwards:

the biceps muscles rotate outwards, and the triceps muscles rotate towards the ribs.

- Extend the fingers evenly on the earth, almost as if you are going to lift the wrists up. This is important for the shoulders; elongating the shoulders while carrying weight on the wrists will jam the shoulder joints. Pressing the metatarsals of the fingers down as if you want to lift the wrists up lifts the shoulder blades; then, when you elongate the shoulders, the movement is circular and there is no jamming in the shoulder joints.
- On a mula bandha inhalation, lift the heels up and extend the buttock bones upwards, spreading them at the same time. Then extend them backwards and elongate the back of the thighs from the knees to the buttock bones, so that the lumbar vertebrae move in.
- After reaching the maximum elongation, lower the heels and lower the head in between the arms.
- Root the hands and perform hasta bandha, so that the arms elongate and the chest and trunk are drawn up from the shoulder heads in the direction of the buttock bones. Thus the shoulders, the arm pits and the spinal column are elongated. At the same time, root the feet and perform pada bandha, so that the legs elongate and the pelvis is drawn up from the femur heads. Thus the whole spinal column is elongated harmoniously and the highest point in the body is in the buttock bones.
- On each mula bandha inhalation elongate the spine and shoulders further, and on each exhalation lower the head further to the mat. The groove of the spine is even, from the first cervical vertebra to the sacrum.
- Hold for one minute. Then lower the pelvis and return to urdhvamukha svanasana (8).

10. Purvottanasana

purva=East;
uttana=intense stretch

When the yogi performs the sun salutation (surya Nama-skar, see page 51), he faces the East. Therefore, the frontal side of the body is considered the East, the back side of the body the West, the right side

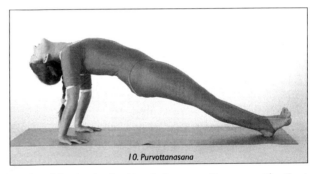

10. Purvottanasana

of the body the South and the left side of the body the North. In purvottanasana the East side of the body is extended, while in paschimottanasana (see page 121) the West side of the body is extended (*paschima=the West*).

- Sit on a mat with the legs extended straight in front of you. Lean the trunk backwards at an angle of forty-five degrees and place the hands on the mat, in line with the shoulders, so that the arms are perpendicular; the fingers point towards the heels.
- On an exhalation lift the pelvis up, till the whole trunk forms one line from the feet to the top of the sternum. The feet are resting on the heels, not on the soles.
- Root the hands and perform hasta bandha to elongate the arms and to lighten the chest on the shoulder heads. After elongating the cervical and thoracic spine with jalandhara bandha, curve the head backwards.
- On an exhalation, lower the pelvis again on the mat and turn the hands around, so that the fingers point away from the trunk, backwards. Then repeat purvottanasana. This position of the hands gives a more extreme rotation in the shoulder joints.

11. Ustrasana

ustra=camel

As ustrasana is an intermediate pose between the simple back bendings and the more advanced ones, it is described here in great detail to lay the foundation for the next series of poses.

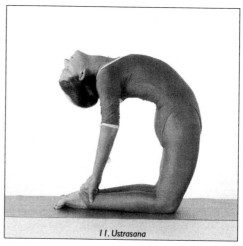

11. Ustrasana

- Kneel on a mat with the feet and heels together, and the knees slightly wider than hip width. The stable part of the body is the one which is in contact with the earth; this forms the basis for the mobile part to pull away from, upwards against gravity, or in any other direction.
- In ustrasana, the basis is formed by the entire lower leg, from the knees to the tips of the toes. On this basis the femur heads have to be fixed in such a way that they, in turn, provide the stable basis for the pelvis and the rest of the body to pull up from. This is done by constricting the outer hips and the inner thighs inwards towards each other while keeping the thighs perpendicular, at an angle of ninety degrees with the lower legs.
- The thighs are like a pillar, and on top of this vertical pillar the spine has to form a crescent moon shape, which has to retain its shape and coherence right from the beginning and throughout the pose.
- Lighten the weight of the body on the femur heads by lifting the pelvis and entire body up from the femur heads (rebounce action). This is done by elongating the inner arches of the feet backwards and rooting them into the earth while performing pada bandha, lengthening the thighs, and maintaining the constricting action of the outer hips and inner thighs.
- The act of lengthening the thighs and lifting the pelvis up from the femur heads on the mula bandha inhalation pulls the energy upwards along the interior spinal column. mula bandha is that lifting of the pelvis, but not only of the physical structure. It is the mula, the root of the body, which has to pressurize upwards, thus shooting the energy upwards. This upward movement of the energy travels along the line of gravity, and thus goes from the base of the pelvis straight up into the kidneys, lifting the kidneys (uddiyana bandha) up from the lumbar vertebrae. From the kidneys, still traveling in a straight line upwards, the energy goes up into the top of the sternum, lifting that up to the sky (the lower part of jalandhara bandha). This is the crescent moon shape: it has to retain its shape and integrity throughout.
- Keeping the thighs perpendicular, extend the arms horizontally sideways. Then elongate them out of the shoulder joints and bring the hands back in a circular movement to hold the heels, curving the spine backwards. Even though the hands hold the heels, there should be no weight on them.
- As the spine curves backwards, the thighs should remain perpendicular. Constrict the outer hips inwards with the support of the pada bandha, and pull the two frontal hip bones up towards the ribs, so that on each mula bandha inhalation the trunk lifts further up from the femur heads. Keeping the thighs perpendicular helps the body to

curve in the kidneys and the thoracic spine, instead of in the lumbar spine.

- The head is the last to curve backwards; this curving backwards of the head has to come out of the action of jalandhara bandha, so that the cervical spine retains its length.
- To come out of the pose, return to the original kneeling position: release the hands from the heels and, reversing the process, bring both the shoulder joints and the hip joints simultaneously back to the central line of gravity, keeping the sternum high and the head back: the head is the last to come up again.

12 Urdhva Dhanurasana

urdhva=upwards; dhanu=bow

Urdhva Dhanurasana is the basis for the more advanced back bending positions. We have therefore given quite an extensive description here, so that this will help you to understand the other back bendings better.

In no other pose is the interaction between the five bandhas more obvious than in this pose. Even though in the beginning you can practice pushing up from the earth, you can

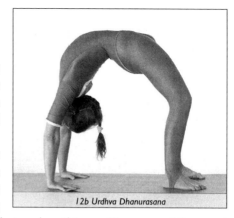

12b Urdhva Dhanurasana

never attain in that way the full elongation that makes this position one of the most beautiful and elegant of all the asanas. Therefore, once you have gained enough elasticity, start to practice dropping down from tadasana (see page 44), first onto the wall, and then onto the earth.

Thus, whereas in version 1 the body pushes up from the earth into urdhva dhanurasana (for beginners), those who are sufficiently acquainted with the pose and have acquired sufficient suppleness in the spine, hip and shoulder joints, can start practicing this pose going down from tadasana onto the wall (version 2).

The final stage is dropping from tadasana backwards into urdhva dhanurasana in the middle of the room (version 3), after having acquired sufficient understanding and suppleness on the wall.

1.　Pushing up from the earth

Lie on the back on a 'sticky' yoga mat and proceed:

- Pull the feet in towards the buttocks till the back of the heels are in contact with the buttocks. The width between the feet is slightly wider than the width of the hips. Keep the feet parallel to each other, do not turn them out, and do not keep one foot further forward than the other, but keep them even, rooting them like in tadasana. The feet are intimately connected with the spine, especially with the lower part of the spine; if they are weak and do not root, the spine will be weak and out of control, and you will damage the vertebrae by incorrect bending. Keep the knees at the same width as the feet, and rotate the thighs inwards as in virasana I (see page 96).
- Place the palms of the hands on the mat next to the ears with the fingers pointing towards the shoulders, so that the width between the hands is the same as the width of the shoulders. Keep the hands parallel to each other; do not turn the hands in or out and do not keep one hand further forward than the other, but keep them even. As the feet are rooting into the earth, so too the hands should be rooting. Keep the elbows close to the head, squeezing the ears in between the lower arms, and rotate the upper arms as in savasana, which means that the triceps muscles roll towards the face. The width between the elbows is the same as the width of the shoulders.
- On an exhalation lift the lower part of the pelvis (the coccyx) off the mat, keeping the upper rim of the pelvis and the lumbar area on the mat. The pelvis has to rotate

backwards around the femur heads, so that the lumbar spine elongates and the coccyx rolls towards the pubic bone. When you have reached maximum rotation, lift the pelvis and lower part of the trunk off the mat, supporting the body on the feet, shoulders, hands and the back of head. The pubic bone is now the highest point in the body, not the two frontal hip bones. If the two frontal hip bones are higher than the pubis the pelvis has not been rotated enough, and as a result the body bends in the lumbar spine and the groins do not open.

In this context it is important to note that in forward bendings the two frontal hip bones move towards the thighs, so that the biceps muscles at the back of the thighs are elongated and the buttock rims (which are at the back of the legs where the legs join the buttocks) are opened. Thus the body bends in the femo-iliac joints, closing with the thighs in the groins like a book. In back bendings, the opposite takes place. Here the two frontal hip bones move up in the direction of the ribs, so that the quadriceps muscles at the front of the thighs are elongated and the groins are opened. Thus the body bends in the buttock rims, and the femo-iliac joints are extended.

Do not attempt to go further as long as you cannot do this movement correctly. It is always better to go slowly and imprint the correct movement on the body than to go fast and move incorrectly. Once a wrong habit is created it is very difficult to undo it.

- Raise the body further, until it is only supported on the feet, hands and crown of the head (as in head balance). Work again on the backwards rotation of the pelvis: the pubic bone should be higher than the two frontal hip bones. Then push the body completely up till the arms (elbows) are straight.
- As the body goes up, the pubis remains the highest point in the body as long as possible. If the lower ribs are higher, the lumbar spine has lost control, bending is mainly done in the lumbar vertebrae and the shoulder and hip joints do not extend.
- Keep the heels down and the feet parallel to each other. Rotate the knees and thighs inwards, so that the width between the knees remains the same as at the start. Rooting the feet put more weight on the inner edges of the heels and on the big toe bones than on the outer edges of the heels and the little toe bones. If the outer edges of the heels and the little toe bones root more, the adductor muscles on the inside of the thighs become passive and the knees fall apart.
- As the arms are shorter than the legs the knees will not be completely straight. Nevertheless, try to straighten them as much as possible. Rooting the inner edges of the heels and the big toe bones, resist the knees towards the hands, and at the same time elongate the back of the thighs upwards, from the back of the knees towards the buttock bones. The pelvis, rotating backwards around the femur heads, and the back of the thighs, elongating upwards towards the buttock bones, meet in the buttock rims. The result is that the groins at the front of the body open. The lower legs are at right angles to the soles of the feet as in tadasana.
- Keeping the arms straight and the inner elbows facing each other, bring the shoulder joints in line with the wrist joints. The lower arms are at right angles to the palms of the hands. The shoulder blades are flat and the arms make a continuous line with the sides of the chest. This means that the shoulder joints are fully extended, the arm pits are opened and the sides of the arm pits are elongated; there should be no angle between

the upper arms and the chest in the arm pits. The action in the arms is the same as the action in the legs: as the knees rotate towards each other, the inner elbows too rotate towards each other, so that the width between the elbows remains the same as the width of the shoulders. Rooting the palms of the hands, put more weight on the inner edges of the palms and the knuckles of the index fingers than on the outer edges of the palms and the knuckles of the little fingers. If the outer edges of the palms and the little fingers root more, the muscles of the inner arms become passive and the elbows fall apart.

- The pelvis and chest rotate in opposite directions. The pelvis rotates backwards around the femur heads, so that the two frontal hip bones are drawn up towards the lower ribs and the coccyx rolls towards the pubic bone. The pubic bone moves up towards the sky, while the lower legs remain at right angles to the earth. The chest rotates around the shoulder joints in such a way that the lower ribs and the bottom point of the sternum are drawn towards the two frontal hip bones and the upper part of the thoracic spine rolls towards the upper point of the sternum. The upper point of the sternum moves forwards in the direction you are facing, while the arms remain at right angles to the earth.

- The action from the waist down is that the legs elongate and the knees resist backwards towards the hands; the backward rotating pelvis and the upward elongating thighs meet in the buttock rims. The result is that the femo-iliac joints are fully extended, the groins are opened and the sides of the hips are elongated. The action from the waist up is that the arms elongate and the elbows resist backwards towards the feet; the forward rotating upper chest and the upward elongating arms meet in the shoulder joints. The result is that the shoulder joints are fully extended, the arm pits are opened and the sides of the arm pits are elongated.

- Thus the pelvis and the chest rotate in opposite directions: the coccyx and first thoracic vertebra move away from each other, while the frontal hip bones and the lower ribs (+ bottom end of the sternum) move towards each other. The result is that the whole spinal column is elongated harmoniously and bends evenly in all its vertebrae. Dhanu means 'bow': the spine is drawn like a bow between the fulcrum points of the shoulder joints and hip joints.

- This whole movement is based on the rebounce force which comes from the rooting hands and feet: pada bandha elongates the legs and lifts the pelvis up from the femur heads, and hasta bandha elongates the arms and lifts the chest up from the shoulder heads.

- Keep the head and neck initially straight as in head balance; then, when you have reached the maximum height in the shoulder and hip joints, curve the head backwards to look at the heels.

2. Dropping down from Tadasana onto a wall

- Stand close to a wall with the back towards it and the heels about thirty centimeters distance from it. Keep the feet slightly wider than hip width, with the inner borders of the feet parallel to each other, and keep the feet even. On a mula bandha inhalation, raise the arms over the head till they point straight up towards the sky, parallel to each other.
- The most important thing is to create length in the hip joints and the lower abdomen before starting to curve the spine backwards. Thus it is important to start from the 'ski-jumping' stance described in tadasana (see page 44), in which the body slants slightly forward, so that the lower abdomen is directly above the lower spring joints. Performing pada bandha, lift the pelvis up on an inhalation, creating space and bounciness in the hip joints. As described in standing poses, elongation of the arms over the head starts in the lower spring joints and legs, with the first rebounce 'split' occurring in the ankles, and the second in the hip joints. From here the mula bandha inhalation picks up the elongation and carries it on through the whole spinal column, the shoulder blades, the shoulder joints and the arms: keeping the arms parallel to each other and rotating the triceps muscles forward, lift the lower abdomen (mula bandha) and kidney region (uddiyana bandha) on each inhalation.
- Elongate the upper thoracic spine and the cervical spine by performing jalandhara bandha at the end of the inhalation, and then curve the head back. Thus the shoulder blades elongate and move into the upper rib cage, and the curve starts in the upper thoracic spine and the cervical spine. Then, vertebra per vertebra, roll the curve down along the thoracic spine. In this way the sternum remains lifted and does not drop into the kidney region.
- As you curve the spine, the weight back of the central line of gravity is increased; therefore you have to simultaneously increase the body weight in front of the central line of gravity in an even measure. This means that the legs, from the slightly forward slanting position of tadasana, have to start slanting further forward, so that the hip joints are brought in front of the central line of gravity. Keep the legs completely straight, however, and keep the elongation of the legs through the action of the pada bandha.
- Up till now the groins are still in, and the trunk forms a crescent moon on top of the femur heads, with the spinal column drawn like a bow from the coccyx up to the first cervical vertebra. Do not pull the coccyx into the lumbar spine, but elongate it out of the lumbar spine as you lower the curve from the thoracic into the lumbar spine.
- Then drawing the frontal hip bones up in the direction of the lower ribs, continue curving the spine, till the groins are completely opened and the whole front of the body, from the front of the ankles to the pit of the throat, forms one even, round line.
- Finally place the hands on the wall with the fingers pointing downwards, but do not put any weight on them.
- To come up again you have to bring the whole body back to the central line of gravity. Thus you have to reverse the process, taking first the femur heads and groins back to the wall while pulling at the same time the frontal hip bones up, so as to maintain the integrity of the curve in the kidney region and in the upper chest.

When you feel comfortable doing this pose close to the wall, you can start walking the feet further away, till the heels are about fifty centimeters away from the wall. Then repeat all the steps described above. Again place the hands on the wall at the end, keeping the legs completely straight. Press the hands lightly against the wall, and on each mula bandha inhalation, which starts with the pada bandha and the elongation of the legs, lift the chest further up, out of the lumbar spine. Then slide the hands further down, without bending the knees and without collapsing the chest.

• To come back up follow the same steps as described above.

When you feel comfortable doing this pose at this distance from the wall and have gained enough control in the feet, the legs and the hip joints, you can move the feet still further away from the wall (one meter) and again follow the above described steps. Curve the body backwards with the legs straight, till the hands are on the wall.

• When you have reached the deepest point in the curve where you can still keep the knees straight, start walking the hands down on the wall. As the hands go down, the knees start to bend gradually, but only as much as necessary to facilitate going down. Keep the heels on the mat and keep the action in the lower spring joints (pada bandha) so as to maintain the rebounce effect in the ankles, knees and hip joints.
• Finally place the hands on the mat with the arms straight and the pits of the elbows facing each other. Keep the palms of the hands flat on the earth with the middle fingers pointing straight towards the heels, and keep the head straight in between the arms with the forehead touching the wall.
• By rooting the hands, performing hasta bandha, and applying a slight pressure with the forehead against the wall the arms elongate as in adhomukha vrksasana (see page 178). Thus the chest is lifted up from the shoulder heads by the rebounce action in the shoulder joints.
• By rooting the feet and performing pada bandha, the legs elongate as in tadasana. Thus the pelvis is lifted up from the femur heads by the rebounce action in the femur joints. The knees are bent just enough to accommodate for the difference in length between the legs and the arms.
• The name of this position is urdhva dhanurasana, which means the 'upward bow'. In this pose we can discern two bows, a short one and a long one. The short one is the bow or curve between the coccyx and the first cervical vertebra, in which the whole spine elongates and curves harmoniously. The long bow is the curve which starts on the front of the ankles and runs across the front of the knees, the frontal hip bones, the lower ribs and the elbows towards the wrists. Even though the knees are bent, this bow should also be as harmonious as possible, which means that the frontal hip bones are at the same height from the earth as the lower ribs. Therefore the knees should bend minimally, because it is the angle in the knees which determines the height of the frontal hip bones: the more the knees are bent, the lower the hip bones are.

3. Dropping down from Tadasana onto the earth

When you have reached sufficient control in this pose on the wall, you can learn to do it in the middle of the room. Follow the steps given under **2**.

- To take the hands down to the earth you have to keep lifting the pelvis up from the femur heads with the mula bandha breathing, while bending the knees. This means that the frontal hip bones keep contact with the lower ribs. Then drop the hands to the earth.

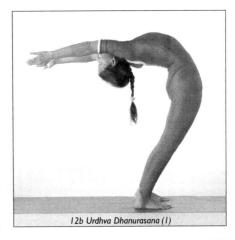
12b Urdhva Dhanurasana (1)

- Before curving the head backwards, lift the chest up from the shoulder heads by rooting the hands and performing hasta bandha, so that the arms elongate and the shoulder blades are lifted. Keep the head initially in between the upper arms. Once you have created the rebounce effect in the shoulder joints curve the head back and bring the shoulder joints vertically above the hands.

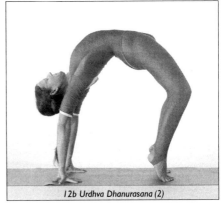
12b Urdhva Dhanurasana (2)

- Rooting the feet and performing pada bandha elongate the legs, keeping the chest stable. Thus the lumbar spine is elongated as the pelvis is lifted up from the femur heads.
- To come back up to tadasana, you have to reverse the process.

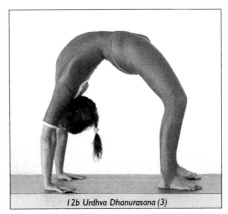
12b Urdhva Dhanurasana (3)

12c Back Bend Variations

These positions can be done in three different modes:

a. **Performing each position separately** and holding it for a few seconds.

b. **Vinyasa**
Connecting two or more positions by flowing from one into the other, using the breathing.

c. **Mala**
Connecting all the positions through surya namaskar, using the breathing and holding each of the back bend variations for the duration of three breaths.

Back Bendings Variations

1. Ekapada Urdhva Dhanurasana
2. Dvipada Viparita Dandasana
3. Ekapada Viparita Dandasana I
4. Mandalasana
5. Ekapada Viparita Dandasana II
6. Chakra Bandhasana
7. Vrschikasana I
8. Vrschikasana II
9. Kapotasana
10. Laghu Vajrasana
11. Padangustha Dhanurasana
    a. Padangustha Dhanurasana I
    b. Padangustha Dhanurasana II

12. Rajakapotasana
    a. Rajakapotasana I
    b. Rajakapotasana II
    c. Bhujangasana II
13. Gherandasana
14. Kapinjalasana
15. Ganda Bherundasana
16. Ekapada Rajakapotasana I
17. Ekapada Rajakapotasana II
18. Ekapada Rajakapotasana III
19. Ekapada Rajakapotasana IV
20. Natarajasana
    a. Natarajasana I
    b. Natarajasana II

---

1. Ekapada Urdhva Dhanurasana

eka=one; pada=leg, foot; urdhva=upwards; dhanu=bow

- Start with urdhva dhanurasana (see page 214) and then proceed:
- Root the left foot further into the earth, performing pada bandha, and raise the right leg with bent knee. Keep the weight even on both hands, and continue rooting them, performing hasta bandha to maintain the lightness and curve in the chest.
- Keep the two frontal hip bones parallel to each other, as well as parallel to the earth. Then elongate the right leg up towards the sky.
- For the rest follow the instructions given for urdhva dhanurasana.

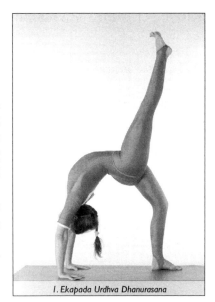

1. Ekapada Urdhva Dhanurasana

2. Dvipada Viparita Dandasana

dvi=two; pada=leg, foot; viparita=reverse; danda=staff

- Start with salamba sirsasana I (see page 157) on a 'sticky' yoga mat and then proceed:
- Bend the knees backwards, keeping the groins in: as in urdhva dhanurasana (see page 214), you have to bring the curve first into the upper back.
- Before curving a joint, however, you have to elongate it, creating the feeling of an 'airbag' inside it. In this pose, you have to pay special attention to rooting the head, together with the ulnar wrist points. Collect the upper arms inwards towards the center, so that the shoulder joints form the stable basis; then lift the chest up from the shoulder heads, rotating

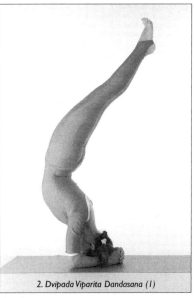

2. Dvipada Viparita Dandasana (1)

the triceps and latissimus dorsi muscles towards the front.
- Elongate the thoracic spine, and move the shoulder blades deep into the rib cage; then curve the upper thoracic spine. To bring the curve into the lumbar spine, you have to bring the chest forwards, retaining, however, the attraction between the frontal hip bones and the lower ribs.
- In all the back bendings, the two frontal hip bones and the lower ribs have to retain their magnetic attraction towards each other to keep the length in the lumbar spine. If they lose this attraction, the lumbar spine will be compressed in the curve. Thus, there is again a crescent moon shape, this time with the shoulder joints as the lower point (the base) and the hip joints as the top points.

- To drop backwards, constrict the outer hips inwards and elongate the upper thighs upwards out of the hip joints: then bend the knees, till the trunk forms one curve from the top of the knees to the arm pits. Thus the groins are completely open and form one continuous line between the upper thighs and the frontal hip bones. Then drop the feet onto the mat.

- Place the feet slightly wider than hip width, with the inner borders parallel to each other, and keep them in alignment; do not keep one foot further forward than the other.

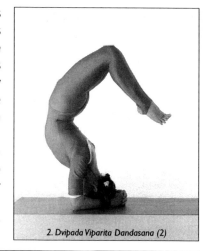

2. Dvipada Viparita Dandasana (2)

- To create one smooth curve at the front of the body, from the frontal hip bones to the arm pits, separate the pelvis from the femur heads by rooting the feet and elongating the legs; at the same time, extend the coccyx out of the lumbar spine towards the heels, so that the lumbar vertebrae do not become compressed.

- To lighten the chest up from the shoulder heads, root the top of the head and the ulnar wrist points as in salamba sirsasana I (see page 157), so that the thoracic spine in

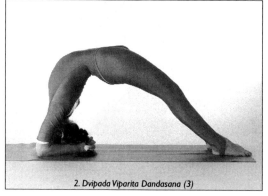

2. Dvipada Viparita Dandasana (3)

  between the shoulder blades elongates. Do not push the lower ribs forwards, but lift the chest up vertically.

- To get the even curve of the bow, the first thoracic vertebra has to move towards the sternum, while at the same time the coccyx moves out of the lumbar spine towards the heels; in this way the attraction between the frontal hip bones and the lower ribs, on the front of the body, is maintained.

- By resisting the knees slightly backwards towards the shoulders, and the shoulder blades towards the knees, the chest and pelvis have no other choice but to go up: this gives height and lightness to the body.

- Use the mula bandha breathing to attain further height: on each inhalation the body becomes lighter by connecting the pada bandha, the mula bandha, the uddiyana bandha and the jalandhara bandha, rooting the feet, the head and the ulnar wrist points.

- On an exhalation, walk the feet further out on the mat and extend the legs, till the knees are straight. Keep the feet at hip width, evenly forward with the inner borders of the feet parallel to each other. This pose is called dvipada viparita dandasana, which means the reversed walking stick.

- Hold for a few seconds, and then proceed to 3.

3. Ekapada Viparita Dandasana I

eka=one; pada=leg, foot; viparita=reversed; danda=staff

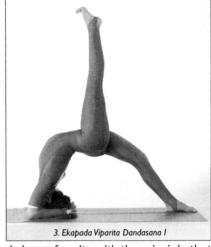

3. Ekapada Viparita Dandasana I

- When you have reached a stable position, lift the right leg up with bent knee and then extend it straight up towards the sky. Do not tilt the pelvis; the two frontal hip bones stay parallel to each other and to the earth.
- The right leg extends upwards in vertical alignment with the right groin, while the left foot and knee are extended in alignment with the left groin.
- To get height and lightness in the pelvis, root the left foot (pada bandha), elongating the left leg, and at the same time elongate the right leg upwards out of the right hip joint. This is in conformity with the principle that the part of the body which is below, forms the stable base for the part of the body, which is above, to elongate upwards against gravity.
- Hold for a few seconds. Place the foot back on the mat and repeat with the other leg. Return to dvipada viparita dandasana (2) and then proceed:
- Walk the feet in towards the head. On an exhalation, jump back up to salamba sirsasana I, keeping the head on the mat and the feet together. From salamba sirsasana I, come down in the usual way.

4. Mandalasana

mandala=circle

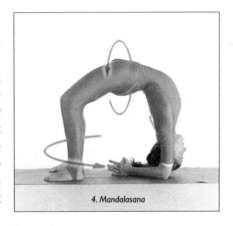

4. Mandalasana

- Start with dvipada viparita dandasana (2) and then proceed:
- Walk the feet towards the left. Turn the left foot ninety degrees outwards and place the right foot on the left ankle. Shift the body weight onto the left foot and, lifting the right hip up vertically, roll it over the left hip, till the right foot is again down on the mat, next to the left foot. Both legs are now straight again and at an angle of ninety degrees to the left side of the trunk.
- Walk the feet to the front, till they are in front of your face.
- Keeping the legs straight, walk the feet around to the right, till the legs are at a ninety degree angle to the right side of the trunk.
- Place the left foot on the right ankle. Shift the body weight onto the right foot, lift the left hip up vertically and roll it over the right one, till the left foot is down on the mat again, next to the right foot.
- Continue walking, till you are back again in dvipada viparita dandasana (2).
- Repeat the same procedure, walking the other way around.

- The front of the body is considered the East side of the body (purva), as it faces the rising sun in Hindu worship. Thus, when the feet are in front of the face, they are on the East side of the body. When the feet are behind the head (in dvipada viparita dandasana) they are at the West side of the body (paschima). When the feet are on the left side of the body they are in the South and when they are on the right side of the body they are in the North. Mandala means 'circle'. Thus the feet describe a complete circle around the head (the North pole).

5. Chakra Bandhasana
chakra=wheel; bandha=bound

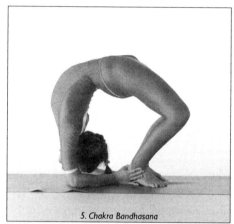

5. Chakra Bandhasana

- Start with dvipada viparita dandasana (2) and then proceed:
- Lift the head and hands up, bring the body weight forward onto the elbows, and walk the feet in towards the head. Keep the head between the arms initially, rooting the elbows to create the rebounce in the shoulder joints.
- On an inhalation, lift the chest up vertically from the shoulder heads, and on the exhalation, bring the upper chest, the arm pits and the shoulder blades forwards over the elbows. Resist the kidney region slightly backwards towards the heels to prevent the lower ribs from collapsing forwards, in which case they would lose the magnetic attraction to the frontal hip bones: the upper ribs and the upper part of the sternum should go faster and further forward than the lower ribs and the lower point of the sternum.
- Keeping the chest stable and the head lifted between the upper arms, raise the heels and walk the feet further in towards the hands, hold the ankles and then lower the heels again.
- To maintain the height and lightness of the body, especially of the pelvis, root the feet. By performing pada bandha, the legs elongate up towards the pelvis on the rebounce force. At the same time, the coccyx has to extend out of the lumbar spine towards the knees. Thus the pelvis rotates backwards around the femur heads, and the two frontal hip bones are drawn towards the lower ribs. The upwards elongating legs, and the backwards rotating pelvis, meet in the buttock rims (at the back of the upper thighs where the thighs and gluteus muscles meet). The result is that the groins are opened and the pelvis is lifted.
- To complete the pose, curve the head backwards and look at the heels.
- On an exhalation release the ankles, place the head back on the mat and return to dvipada viparita dandasana (2), and then proceed to 6.

6. Ekapada Viparita Dandasana II

eka=one; pada=leg, foot;
viparita=reversed; danda=staff

- Start with dvipada viparita dandasana (2) and then proceed:
- Lift the head and hands up, bring the body weight forward onto the elbows and walk the feet in towards the head. Keep the head between the arms initially, rooting the elbows to create the rebounce in the shoulder joints.
- On an inhalation, lift the chest up vertically from the shoulder heads, and on the exhalation, bring the upper chest, the arm pits and the shoulder blades forwards over the elbows. Resist the kidney region slightly backwards towards the heels to prevent the lower ribs from collapsing forwards, in which case they would lose the magnetic

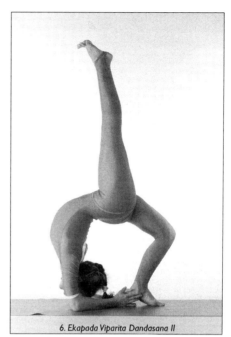

6. *Ekapada Viparita Dandasana II*

attraction to the frontal hip bones: the upper ribs and the upper part of the sternum should go faster and further forward than the lower ribs and the lower point of the sternum.
- Keeping the chest stable and the head lifted between the upper arms, raise the heels and walk the feet further in towards the hands. Hold the left ankle and lower the heel again.
- Lift the right leg up with bent knee and then extend it straight up towards the sky. Do not tilt the pelvis; the two frontal hip bones stay parallel to each other and to the earth.
- The right leg extends upwards in vertical alignment with the right groin, while the left foot and knee remain in alignment with the left groin.
- To get height and lightness in the pelvis, root the left foot (pada bandha), elongating the left leg, and at the same time elongate the right leg upwards out of the right hip joint. This is in conformity with the principle that the part of the body, which is below, forms the stable base for the part of the body, which is above, to elongate upwards against gravity.
- Hold for a few seconds. Place the foot back on the mat and repeat with the other leg. Return to dvipada viparita dandasana (2), and then proceed:
- Walk the feet in towards the head. On an exhalation, jump back up to salamba sirsasana I, keeping the head on the mat and the feet together. From salamba sirsasana I, come down in the usual way.

7. Vrschikasana I
vrschika=scorpion

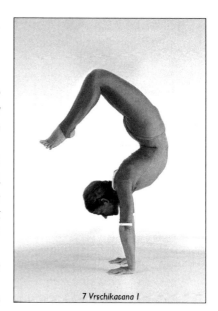

7 Vrschikasana I

7a. *Close to a wall*
- Start with adhomukha vrksasana (see page 178) close to a wall (between thirty and fifty centimeters distance from the wall) and then proceed:
- Bend the knees, place the toes on the wall and lift the head, curving the spine. Push the wall lightly with the toes as you lift the head, at the same time rooting the hands and performing hasta bandha, so that the chest is lifted up from the shoulder heads.
- Walk the feet down on the wall and raise the head further up towards the feet.
- Return to adhomukha vrksasana and come down again.

When you have gained enough confidence on the wall, and have mastered adhomukha vrksasana in the middle of the room, you can try this pose in the middle of the room.

7b. *In the middle of the room*
- Start with adhomukha vrksasana (see page 178) in the middle of the room and then proceed:
- Bend the knees and curve the spine. Raising the head further up, bring the feet down to the head. Root the hands and perform hasta bandha, so that the chest is lifted up from the shoulder heads.

This position resembles the scorpion as it stings its own head.

8. Vrschikasana II
vrschika=scorpion

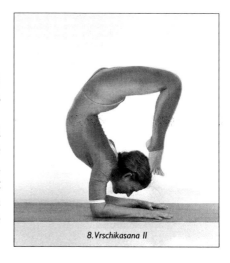

8. Vrschikasana II

8a. *Close to a wall*
- Start with pincha mayurasana (see page 180) close to a wall (about thirty centimeters distance from the wall) and then proceed:
- Bend the knees, place the toes on the wall and lift the head, curving the spine. Push the wall lightly with the toes as you lift the head, at the same time rooting the ulnar wrist points and the hands, performing hasta bandha, so that the chest is lifted up from the shoulder heads.

- Walk the feet down on the wall and raise the head further up towards the feet.
- Return to pincha mayurasana and come down again.

When you have gained enough confidence on the wall, and have mastered pincha mayurasana in the middle of the room, you can try this pose in the middle of the room.

8b. *In the middle of the room*
- Start with pincha mayurasana (see page 180) in the middle of the room and then proceed:
- Bend the knees and curve the spine. Raising the head further bring the feet down to the head. Root the ulnar wrist points and the hands, performing hasta bandha, so that the chest is lifted up from the shoulder heads.

This position resembles the scorpion as it stings its own head.

9. Kapotasana

kapota=pigeon

(For an additional, detailed description, see "Comparative Studies of Various Asanas", page 239)

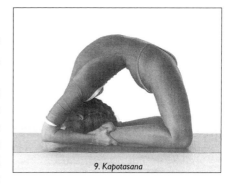

9. Kapotasana

- Kneel on a blanket with the feet and heels together and the knees slightly wider than hip width. The stable part of the body is the one which is in contact with the earth; this forms the basis for the mobile part to pull away from, upwards against gravity, or in any other direction. In kapotasana, the basis is formed by the entire lower leg, from the knees to the tips of the toes.
- On this base, the femur heads have to be fixed in such a way that they, in turn, form a stable basis for the pelvis and the rest of the body to lift up from. This is done by constricting the outer hips and the inner thighs slightly inwards towards each other, while keeping the thighs perpendicular, at an angle of ninety degrees to the lower legs.
- Thus the thighs are like a pillar, and on top of this vertical pillar the trunk has to create a crescent moon shape which has to retain its shape and coherence right from the beginning and throughout the pose.
- Lighten the weight of the body on the femur heads by lifting the pelvis and trunk up from the femur heads (rebounce action). To do this, you have to elongate the inner arches of the feet backwards and root them into the earth while performing pada bandha; at the same time elongate the thighs, maintaining the squeezing action at the outer hips and inner thighs.
- The act of elongating the thighs and lifting the pelvis up from the femur heads with the mula bandha inhalation, pulls the energy upwards along the interior spinal column. mula bandha is that lifting of the pelvis, but not only of the physical structure. It is the mula, the root of the body, which has to pressurize upwards, thus shooting the energy upwards. This upward movement of the energy travels along the line of gravity, and thus goes from the base of the pelvis straight up into the kidneys, lifting the kidneys

(uddiyana bandha) up from the lumbar vertebrae. From the kidneys, still traveling in a straight line upwards, it goes into the top of the sternum (jalandhara bandha), lifting that up to the sky. This is the crescent moon shape: this crescent moon has to retain its shape and integrity throughout. On a mula bandha inhalation, raise the arms over the head.

- To go down into kapotasana, the body has to balance around the central line of gravity: as the trunk and arms curve back and down, the upper thighs have to move forwards (maintaining the squeezing action of the outer thighs inwards) to balance the weight of the body, until the moment when the pelvis forms one continuous curve with the thighs through the groins. Whereas in the initial crescent moon shape the trunk formed one curve from the two frontal hip bones to the collar bones, and the groins were dipped inwards, this curve now starts at the knees, and continues through the groins up to the collar bones, forming one smooth and even line.

- Then, 'hanging' from the upper thighs, the groins and the iliopsoas muscles, bring the hands to the feet and hold the heels. Keep the upper arms parallel to each other, the elbows on the blanket and the top of the head in the arches of the feet. Do not put any weight either on the hands or on the elbows; the entire body weight should be suspended from the thighs, groins and iliopsoas muscles.

- On each mula bandha inhalation, root the top of the feet into the earth, thus elongating the thighs upwards, so that the angle in the back of the knees increases. This lifts the pelvis up from the femur heads, allowing the wave of the mula bandha breathing to create a deeper curve in the kidney region and the upper chest. The head too can, in its turn, move deeper into the arches.

- To come out of the pose, release the hands from the heels and, reversing the process, bring both the shoulder joints and the hip joints simultaneously back to the central line of gravity, by bringing the thighs back to the vertical line. Keep the head back and the sternum raised high to come back to the original kneeling position. In this way, the length in the lumbar spine and the curve in the kidney region and upper chest are maintained, and the trunk ends up in the same crescent moon shape as from where it started. The head and arms are the last to come back up again.

10. Laghu Vajrasana

laghu=small, beautiful;
vajra=thunderbolt, the weapon of Indra

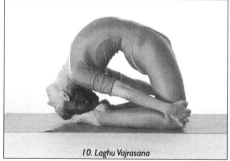

10. Laghu Vajrasana

- Kneel on a blanket with the feet and heels together and the knees slightly wider than hip width. Place the hands on the front of the thighs, close to the knees.
- Follow the instructions given in kapotasana (9) to create the curve in the spine. Then take the head down into the arches of the feet, crawling the fingers down on the front of the thighs towards the knees to maintain the curve. When the head rests in the arches, the fingers are holding the top front portion of the knees.

In this position one can clearly recognize the bow: the wooden part of the bow is the curving trunk, which starts between the knees and runs over the pubic bone, the lower point of the sternum, the upper point of the sternum and the forehead, and the string of the bow is formed by the extended arms, which pull the shoulder joints and knees towards each other: the closer these are pulled towards each other, the higher the curve of the wooden part of the bow.

11. Padangustha Dhanurasana

padangustha=big toe; dhanu=bow

11a. *Padangustha Dhanurasana I*

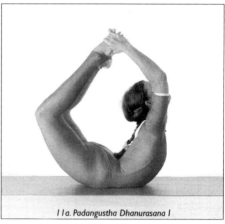

I Ia. Padangustha Dhanurasana I

- Start with bhujangasana I (see page 209) and then proceed:
- Bend the right knee and turn the right foot out so that it is at an angle of ninety degrees to the ankle, with the toes pointing sideways, away from the trunk.
- Support yourself on the left hand, turn the right arm as for savasana, and with the right hand hold the right foot: the palm of the hand covers the top of the foot, and the fingers curve around the inner arch.
- Rotate the arm in the shoulder joint, till the elbow points up towards the sky. In order to help this movement, and to take the load off the shoulder joint, pull the right leg up to the sky, so that the right foot pulls the right arm up, not vice versa. Both the right hand and the right foot now point up towards the sky.
- Keeping the upwards extension of the right leg, lift the left hand off the earth, bend the left leg and hold the left foot in the same way as described above; the trunk rolls from the bhujangasana I (see page 209) position forwards onto the stomach.
- Repeating the same procedure as above, rotate the left arm in the shoulder joint, till both hands and feet point up towards the sky: this is the bow when it is slack. To draw the bow (for shooting the arrow), both the hands and the feet have to elongate up towards the sky.
- The wooden part of the bow is formed by the entire spinal column, from the coccyx to the first cervical vertebra, while the arms and legs form the string of the bow. The juncture where the hands hold the arches of the feet forms the point where the arrow would be notched.
- On each mula bandha inhalation, draw the lower abdomen up into the kidney region (uddiyana bandha), and still further upwards into the upper thoracic spine and the cervical spine (jalandhara bandha): this allows the spine to curve deeper backwards. Then look up. In this final pose the trunk rests on the stomach, in between the two frontal hip bones and the lower ribs.
- Curl the toes around the fingers (pada bandha), so that the feet hold the hands as much as the hands hold the feet, and elongate the arches up towards the sky. As in kapotasana (9) and laghu vajrasana (10), the knees should be kept slightly wider than hip width.
- Hold for a few seconds, and then proceed to 11b.

11b. Padangustha Dhanurasana II

- Bend the elbows and knees and pull the feet to the head.
- Keep the upward extension of the thighs out of the hip joints, and of the upper arms out of the shoulder joints, so that the wooden part of the bow (the spinal column) stays tightly bent.
- Hold for a few seconds. Return to padangustha dhanurasana I.
- As the bow is tightly strung, do not release both hands at the same time to come out

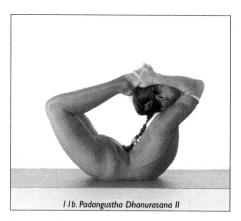

11b. Padangustha Dhanurasana II

of this pose, but release first one hand and place that hand and foot back on the earth to support the trunk. Then release the other hand and foot and return to bhujangasana I (see page 209).

12. Rajakapotasana

rajakapota=king of the pigeons

12a. Rajakapotasana I

- Start with bhujangasana I (see page 209) and then proceed:
- Bend the knees to an angle of about eighty degrees, supporting yourself on the hands. Keep the knees slightly wider than hip width, but the feet together.
- On a mula bandha inhalation, following the line through the spinal column and the bandhas as described in padangustha dhanurasana (11), curve the spine and the head back, till the head comes to rest in the arches of the feet.

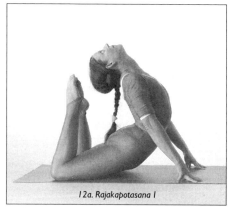

12a. Rajakapotasana I

- Here too, the pada bandha stabilizes the femur heads, so that you can draw the pelvis forwards and upwards on the inhalation, thus elongating and curving the spinal column into an even and harmonious bow.

Hold for a few seconds, and then proceed to 12b.

12b. Rajakapotasana II

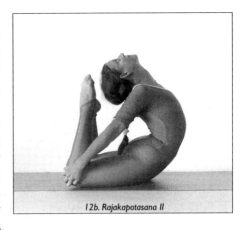

- Lift the right hand, supporting yourself on the left hand, and bring the right hand back in a circular movement to hold the right shin bone, close to the right knee (on the tuberositas of the knee).
- Resist the right shin bone against the hand to stabilize the right side of the body, lift the left hand and bring it back in a circular movement to hold the left shin, close to the left knee (on the tuberositas). At this point the body rests only on the lower abdomen, the groins and the upper thighs.

12b. Rajakapotasana II

- To prevent the body from rolling forwards onto the stomach, the shins have to continue resisting backwards against the hands, so that they pull the hands, the arms and the shoulders backwards: thus the body stays in balance. Keep the head in the arches of the feet.
- Hold for a few seconds, and then proceed to 12c.

12c. Bhujangasana II
bhujanga=serpent

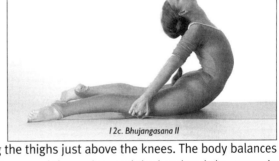

- Increase the resistance of the shins backwards against the hands and extend the legs, till the knees are straight and the feet are on the earth, with the toes pointing straight backwards.
- While extending the knees, you have to crawl the fingers from the tuberositas of the shins over

12c. Bhujangasana II

the knee caps, till you are holding the thighs just above the knees. The body balances on the lower abdomen, the pubic bone and the groins, and the head and chest remain curved backwards.
- Hold for a few seconds.
- To come out of this pose, release the knees one hand at a time to prevent the trunk from falling forwards (see padangustha dhanurasana (11)).

13. Gherandasana

*Gheranda is the name of a sage,
author of the Gheranda Samhita.*

This pose is a combination of bhekasana
(see page 102) and padangustha dhanurasana
I (11a).

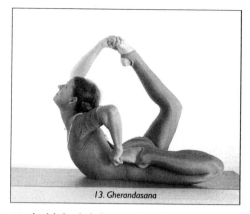

13. Gherandasana

- Start with padangustha dhanurasana I
  (11a) and then proceed:
- Keep the right hand and the right foot
  raised high to maintain the balance on
  the abdomen. Release the left hand,
  bend the left knee and bring the left arm
  down and backwards in a circular movement to hold the left foot again. The palm of the
  hand now covers the top portion of the foot and pushes it down to the earth, next to
  the left hip. The left elbow points upwards and slightly sideways, but keep the
  shoulders in line, the sternum central and the collar bones even; the left arm is now in
  the same position as in bhekasana (see page 102).
- At this point the right side of the body performs padangustha dhanurasana I (11a),
  and the left side bhekasana (see page 102).
- Release the left hand, and return to padangustha dhanurasana I (11a) with the left hand
  and foot.
- Release the right hand and foot, and repeat gherandasana on the other side.

14. Kapinjalasana

Kapinjala is a kind of partridge

This pose is a combination of
vasisthasana I (see page 182) and
padangustha dhanurasana I (11a). In this
position one leg is taken behind the
central line of gravity; therefore you have
to pay special attention to compensating
the body weight at the front of the central
line of gravity.

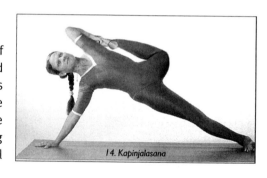

14. Kapinjalasana

- Start with vasisthasana I (see page 182) on the right hand and the right foot and then
  proceed:
- Bend the left knee, and with the left hand hold the left foot as described in
  padangustha dhanurasana I (11a) . Then rotate the upper arm in the shoulder joint, till
  it is next to the left ear, and the left hand holds the left foot behind the left shoulder.
- Rotate the left thigh inwards, so that the two frontal hip bones stay forward in an even
  line. This is padangustha dhanurasana I (11a). At this point the right side of the body
  performs vasisthasana I (see page 182) ,and the left side padangustha dhanurasana I
  (11a).
- In addition to the curve, the problem in this pose is the balance. If you do not bring
  the pelvis and chest forwards, while taking the left leg back into the padangustha
  dhanurasana I curve, the body weight behind the central line of gravity is not
  compensated and you will therefore lose your balance backwards.

15. Ganda Bherundasana
ganda=cheek; bherunda=terrible, formidable

15a. *Close to the wall*

- Kneel on a 'sticky' yoga mat close to the wall, facing it.
- Place the hands about thirty centimeters from the wall on the mat, keeping them at shoulder width, with the fingers pointing straight forward towards the wall.
- Bend forward like an animal drinking water, place the chin on the mat, and bend the elbows, till the shoulders are ten centimeters above the hands.
- Supporting the whole body weight on the chin and hands, jump the feet up on the wall. Then extend the knees so that the body forms one smooth curve from the shoulder blades to the back of the heels; the rib cage is wedged in between the inner upper arms.
- To get a deeper curve in the upper spine, bring the sternum gradually down towards the mat in between the hands, rooting the hands and performing hasta bandha to lighten the chest.
- The weight of the body has to be balanced evenly at the front and the back of the central line of gravity; thus, as the sternum sinks down, the pelvis has to lift up from the lumbar spine and move closer to the wall.

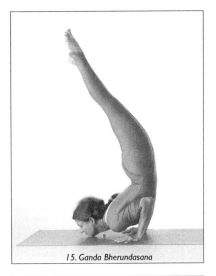

15. Ganda Bherundasana

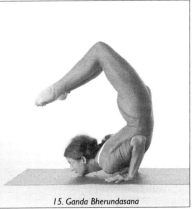

15. Ganda Bherundasana

15b. *Away from the wall*

- Perform ganda bherundasana further away from the wall and then proceed:
- Bend the knees and walk the feet down on the wall.
- When you have reached your deepest curve, take the feet one by one away from the wall, balancing only on the chin and hands.
- Pull the feet in towards the head and place the soles of the feet on the head.
- To come out of the pose, place the feet back on the wall again and come down, one foot at a time.

The next three positions are basically the same; the main difference is that in the first one (ekapada rajakapotasana I) the bent leg is bent as in janu sirsasana (see page 125), in the second (ekapada rajakapotasana II) it is bent as in marichyasana I (see page 132), and in the third (ekapada rajakapotasana III) it is bent as in triangmukhaikapada paschimottanasana I (see page 128). One could therefore consider these three positions the 'back-face' positions of those three forward bending positions.

16. Ekapada Rajakapotasana I

eka=one; pada=leg, foot;
rajakapota=the king of pigeons

In this pose the frontal leg is bent as in janu sirsasana (see page 125).

First part

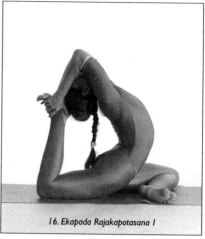

16. Ekapada Rajakapotasana I

- Sit on a mat and extend the right leg straight behind you, keeping the foot and knee in line with the back of the right groin (the buttock rim). The foot points straight backwards, the big and small toes rest evenly on the mat, and the back of the knee faces straight up to the sky.

- Bend the left leg at an angle of forty-five degrees to the trunk, and place the left foot in front of the right groin. Shift the weight of the trunk onto the right hip, and pull the left hip slightly backwards: thus the right hip joint and groin are elongated.

- At the same time, move the two frontal hip bones over towards the right, till the right frontal hip bone is in line with the outer edge of the right groin; both hip bones point forward evenly and have the same height from the earth.

- Extend the left thigh sideways out of the left hip joint and rotate it slightly inward. Thus the left knee is not only extended sideways, but is also rolled forwards on the tuberositas of the left tibia.

- The trunk, from the navel upwards, faces straight forward. Keep the weight of the trunk on the right hip, and rotate the right frontal hip bone, waist and rib cage forwards; thus the two sacro-iliac joints at the back of the pelvis are aligned.

- The pelvis should be almost vertical; if the right hip joint does not elongate sufficiently, the tendency is for the pelvis to fall forward, so that the two frontal hip bones collapse into the groins. To bring the pelvis close to a vertical position, pull the two frontal hip bones back and up in the direction of the ribs (the typical back bending movement). Be careful, however, not to twist the right side of the pelvis backwards.

- On a mula bandha inhalation, elongate the spinal column upwards out of the sacro-iliac joints. Root the buttock bones and the thighs into the earth, performing pada bandha with both feet, to get the rebounce action in the pelvis; thus the pelvis is lifted up from the femur heads, giving the thrust for the spinal column to elongate.

- On the exhalation, rotate the trunk and spinal column towards the left, until the right shoulder, the right side of the rib cage and the right waist are in alignment with the outer edge of the right groin, and the right frontal hip bone is above the right groin, one thirds distance from the right hip joint, and two thirds distance from the pubic bone.

- The spinal column forms a straight and even groove from the sacro-iliac joints to the cervical spine; it should not deviate to the left. To draw the groove up into the upper thoracic spine, elongate the ears out of the cervical spine. Elongate also the cervical vertebrae upwards and keep the head straight, in alignment with the chest. Keep the shoulders and shoulder blades down and relaxed.

Second part

- Place the right hand on the mat, next to the right thigh, to stabilize your position, and bend the right leg. On a mula bandha inhalation, raise the left arm over the head and elongate it out of the left sacro-iliac joint. Never make short movements in yoga: always first create length and lightness in the joints before bending them; this is especially important in the back bending positions.

- On the exhalation, bend the left arm and hold the right foot with the left hand. Even though the left hand holds the right foot, this is only meant to give you a frame within which to elongate and rotate; do not use the hand, the arm and the shoulder muscles to pull the spine and trunk upwards and to rotate them towards the left. That is only done on the breathing.

- On the next mula bandha inhalation, elongate the right arm upwards out of the right sacro-iliac joint and hold the right foot also with the right hand.

- When you have reached maximum elongation of the spinal column, start to curve the neck and chest backwards to take the head into the arch of the right foot. As usual, go in stages, using the mula bandha breathing: on each inhalation, elongate upwards, and on each exhalation, curve the head and chest further back and down. Curving the neck to take the head back into a back arch starts always with jalandhara bandha, so that the cervical and upper thoracic vertebrae are elongated before curving.

- In this whole process the movement is circular: on the inhalation, the lower abdomen moves forwards and up, and the chest moves up and curves back; on the exhalation, the head curves back and down. Thus, seen from the side, there is one smooth curve from the groins to the collar bones. In back bendings, one should always look at the front of the body: the line at the front of the body should be round and even. This is only the case if you use the wave of the mula bandha breathing correctly.

- Keep the neck, shoulders, shoulder blades and arms relaxed, and place the forehead in the arch of the right foot.

- Hold for a few seconds, and then repeat on the other side.

17. Ekapada Rajakapotasana II

eka=one; pada=leg, foot;
rajakapota=the king of pigeons

In this pose the frontal leg is bent as in marichyasana I (see page 132).

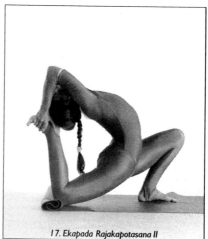

17. Ekapada Rajakapotasana II

- Kneel on a mat and bring the left foot forward, till there is an angle of ninety degrees in the left knee.
- Bend the left knee further, till the back of the left thigh is almost in touch with the calf muscle. As the pelvis is lowered, the right groin is completely opened.
- Keep the two frontal hip bones facing straight forward, and the pelvis and chest as vertical as possible. In all back bending positions, the two frontal hip bones move towards the lower ribs; this is to make sure that the extension is in the groins, not in the waist. Thus the lumbar spine is protected as the curve is brought into the hip joints.
- Place the hands next to you on the mat and, supporting yourself for balance on the fingers, curve the head and spine backwards as described in ekapada rajakapotasana I (16).
- Bend the right knee, so that the foot points up towards the sky. On a mula bandha inhalation, elongate the left arm up over the head, out of the left sacro-iliac joint. On the exhalation, hold the right foot with the left hand, curling the toes around the fingers, so that the foot holds the hand as much as the hand holds the foot. Perform pada bandha with both feet for the stability and rebounce of the body, and to lighten the pelvis on the femur heads.
- On an inhalation, elongate the right arm up, resisting the right leg backwards, and hold the right foot also with the right hand. The body now balances on the left foot and the right knee. Keep the left heel down, and the right frontal hip bone parallel to the left one. For the rotation of the right thigh and hip, follow the instructions given in ekapada rajakapotasana I (16).
- Using the mula bandha breathing and the action of the pada bandha in both feet, lift the pelvis up from the femur heads on each inhalation, rotating it backwards, so that the pubic bone moves forwards, and the two frontal hip bones move up towards the ribs: this brings the curve automatically into the upper back, and allows the head to curve deeper backwards. Rest the forehead into the arch of the right foot.
- Hold for a few seconds, and then repeat on the other side.

18. **Ekapada Rajakapotasana III**

eka=one; pada=leg, foot;
rajakapota=the king of pigeons

In this pose the frontal leg is bent as in triangmukhaikapada paschimottanasana I (see page
128).

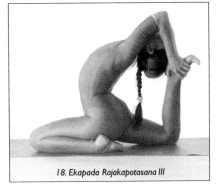

18. Ekapada Rajakapotasana III

- Sit in virasana (see page 96) and then
  proceed:
- Extend the right leg straight backwards. Due
  to the Virasana position of the left leg, the
  tendency to drop the upper part of the pelvis
  and the waist forward onto the left thigh is greater in this pose than in the two previous
  ones. Therefore you have to pay extra attention to the backward rotation of the pelvis,
  in which the pubic bone moves forwards and up towards the navel, and the two frontal
  hip bones move up towards the lower ribs: this brings the extension in the right groin,
  not in the waist.
- For the rotation in the right thigh and hip, follow the instructions given in ekapada
  rajakapotasana I (16).
- As all the back bending positions are bow positions, the accent is always on the
  extreme endpoints of the bow: these are the coccyx and the first cervical vertebra. To
  curve the whole spine evenly, the parts of the spine closest to those extreme points
  should be curved in the same measure as the middle part. This is done by drawing the
  two frontal hip bones up towards the ribs, at the same time drawing the ribs down
  towards the two frontal hip bones: thus the central parts of the bow (the lumbar spine
  and the lower thoracic spine) are lengthened, and the curve is brought into the sacro-
  iliac joints and into the upper thoracic spine.
- As said before, the tendency in this pose is to collapse the waist forward. By
  lengthening the spine as described above, the trunk retains its vertical position and its
  height.
- For the rest follow the instructions given in ekapada rajakapotasana I (16).
- Hold for a few seconds, and then repeat on the other side.

19. **Ekapada Rajakapotasana IV**

eka=one; pada=leg, foot; rajakapota=the king of pigeons

- Start with hanumanasana (see
  page 117) with the left leg
  extended forward and the right leg
  back and then proceed:
- Supporting yourself on the fingers,
  bend the right leg.
- For the rest follow the instructions
  given in ekapada rajakapotasana I
  (16).

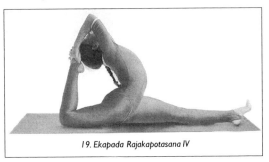

19. Ekapada Rajakapotasana IV

20. Natarajasana

nata=dance; raja=king; Nataraja is a name of Shiva, lord of dance and destruction (the Tandava is the dance of destruction)

Natarajasana is the last pose described in this book, and is also one of the most beautiful, elegant and symbolic poses in yoga: when performed correctly, the body takes on the shape of a tall wine glass. Yoga has always been considered a tool for reaching out to the universal force, in which the body becomes the recipient for that force. In many traditions, including the Christian and Sufi traditions, the universal force is compared to wine, which fills the human glass to produce divine ecstasy. Thus the ritual of drinking wine in the Catholic Church and in the famous Sufi poem, the Rubayat of Omar Khayyam.

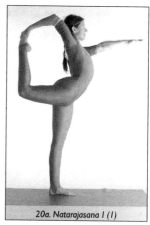

20a. Natarajasana I (1)

Natarajasana, as the last pose in this book, symbolizes the wine glass formed by the human body to be filled with the universal force. As the wine glass is completely transparent, the human body and mind too should be as transparent and empty as the crystal wine glass to receive the Divine ecstasy. This has been the aim of this book, to bring the attention of the student from the physical body to the transparent side of us, the one that we have called the Body of Light.

20a. Natarajasana I

- Stand in tadasana (which is the first asana described in this book) and proceed:
- Bend the right knee backwards and, holding with the right hand the right foot as described in padangustha dhanurasana I (11a), lift the foot up behind the trunk.
- For the rest follow the instructions given in ekapada rajakapotasana I (16).
- In this human wine glass, the foot of the glass is formed by the left, vertical leg. The glass itself is formed by the trunk and arms on the one side, and the right thigh and lower leg on the other side. To make this glass vertical and even, the upward elongation of the spinal column, from the coccyx to the back of the head, has to be equal to the upward elongation of the right leg, from the

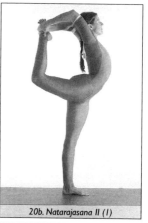

20b. Natarajasana II (1)

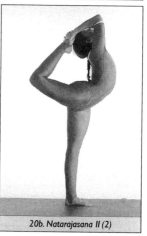

20b. Natarajasana II (2)

buttock rim to the arch of the right foot. Thus the top of the head, the hands and the right foot are equally high, and reach up to the sky in an even and harmonious way.

20b. Natarajasana II

- To close the wine glass at the top, curve the head backwards and place the arch of the foot on the top of the head. Thus the circle is closed.

Part 13 Comparative studies of various asanas

Let us now discuss a few asanas and compare them to each other in order to show that, in reality, the body knows only very few movements. These movements are: bending forward, bending backward, bending sideways and twisting around the vertical axis of the spine. One can add the movements of turning the body upside down, like in head balance, shoulder balance, full arm balance, elbow balance, etc.

Within these major groups of movements we can play around with an enormous amount of positions or asanas, using the Eight Vital Principles of Practice, in particular the force of gravity (rooting), to achieve slightly different effects on the body, even though the positions themselves are intrinsically the same or similar.

Comparitive studies of various asanas

1. *Playing with gravity*
   a. *Salamba Sirsasana and Pincha Mayurasana*
   b. *Halasana, Uttanasana, Urdhva Mukha Paschimottanasana II and Paschimottanasana*
   c. *Paschimottanasana and Upavistha Konasana*
   d. *Kapotasana and Urdhva Dhanurasana*

2. *Front face – Back Face*
   a. *Janu Sirsana and Ekapada Rajakapotasana*
   b. *Uttanasana and Urdhva Dhanurasana*

3. *Beauty and freedom in yoga*

---

1. Playing with gravity

1a. *Salamba Sirsasana and Pincha Mayurasana*

Salamba sirsasana is sometimes called the king of the asanas, as salamba sarvangasana is called the queen. One can also say that salamba sirsasana is a solar position (the *ha* part of hatha yoga) as it heats the body, while salamba sarvangasana is a lunar position (the *tha* part of hatha yoga) as it tends to cool the body. Salamba sirsasana in itself is not a complex pose, neither is it a very tiring one if one uses the external and internal forces intelligently. After all, it is tadasana upside down, and thus subject to the same forces as tadasana.

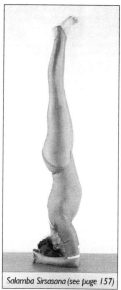
Salamba Sirsasana (see page 157)

The external force is the force of gravity. This force acts not only vertically downwards on the body but contains also a rebouncing aspect, as we have seen. Both the force of gravity and its rebouncing aspect can only function through those parts of the body which are exactly vertical, and this is where, in salamba sirsasana, many people get themselves into trouble. This is because they have the impression that, to stand on your head, you need to use the arm and shoulder muscles, which are exactly those muscles that you should not use.

Let us have a look at the arm and shoulder muscles. In salamba sirsasana I the arms are bent at the elbows at an angle less than ninety degrees, with the shoulders not vertically above the elbows, but a little backwards of them. This is very different from a pose like pincha mayurasana where the shoulders are directly above the elbows and the arms are bent at an angle of ninety degrees in the elbows. This means, on the one hand, that the head is lifted off the earth. On the other hand it means that the arms can use the gravity/rebounce action, as the upper arms, deltoid muscles and shoulder joints are in exact vertical alignment.

In salamba sirsasana this is not the case. As the shoulder joints are slightly backwards of the elbow joints the force of gravity exerts a tremendous pressure on those joints, a pressure that for most people is expressed in a sagging of the shoulders onto the neck. The reason for this is that muscles in general, and the big, peripheral muscles in particular, are not geared for static action, but only for dynamic action. In weight lifting the muscles of the arms and other parts of the body are used in a dynamic way, thus increasing their capacity of load carrying. Most asanas, on the other hand, are static poses, and thus need a different action.

In salamba sirsasana the deltoid muscles, which cover the shoulder joints, have no vertical rooting support like in pincha mayurasana, where the vertical rooting support is formed by the bones of the upper arms. The other muscle used by most people to hold the body up is the trapezius muscle. This muscle forms a kind of diamond shape at the back of the chest, running from the cervical and thoracic spinal column sideways towards the shoulders. This big, peripheral muscle is vital for many movements.

In salamba sirsasana, as it runs for the most part parallel to the earth, it forms however a kind of 'hanging bridge' between the spinal column and the shoulders. On this 'hanging bridge' the force of gravity exerts its pressure at an angle of ninety degrees to the fibers of the muscle. As these fibers are not geared for long term action, after a short while the trapezius will sag and the weight of the body will 'leak' into the cervical vertebrae.

Because the body has been counting on these big muscles to hold its weight up against gravity, it has not provided a 'back up' in case of failure. Thus, in order to be able to stay for some time in salamba sirsasana (ten minutes or more) without damaging the neck vertebrae, we have to approach it differently.

We have to go back to rooting, or the use of the gravity/rebounce force, and let that force do the work for us. Thus we have to find those muscles that are able to co-operate with that force, and not sag underneath it. Those muscles are the long muscles (the erector spinae) that run alongside the entire spinal column. In salamba sirsasana those muscles are aligned with the gravity/rebounce force and therefore can utilize that force through the action of rooting. These muscles, however, can only be reached if we move the outer, big muscles out of the way. Those outer, big muscles are the trapezius and the latissimus dorsi muscles that form the outer layer of the back. These muscles have to move sideways, away from the spinal column. This is done mainly by rolling the triceps muscles of the upper arms inwards towards the face (without displacing the elbows), and rolling the latissimus dorsi muscles forwards, which is experienced as a widening of the entire back. Once those muscles are out of the way, the interior muscle, the erector spinae, can go into action, elongating its fibers along the line of gravity.

Elongation can only take place, however, if you move a muscle in two opposite directions. Thus, in order to move the entire spinal column upwards along the line of gravity, something else has to move downwards along the line of gravity. That something is the head. Here we come to the crux of the matter. The more you root the head down into the earth, the more you save the neck in salamba sirsasana. The act of rooting the head enables the neck and upper thoracic spine to pick up the rebounce force so that they can elongate upwards, away from the earth towards the sky. Before doing this rooting movement into the earth, you can experiment standing in tadasana and placing a book on the top of your head. The book should be exactly on the middle of the head. You can feel with your fingers a kind of dip on the top of the head halfway between the forehead and the crown of the head. This is the fontanel, or the exact spot where the three joints of the skull meet at the top of the skull. Once you have placed the book on that spot, push it gently upwards towards the sky with the head without raising the shoulders, using only the spinal muscles. This movement starts with the rooting of the feet into the earth and the activating of the pada bandha. From there the rebounce force travels upwards through the legs, the lower abdomen and the chest towards the head (and the book).

To make sure that you do not tilt the head forwards or backwards, imagine that you have to elongate your ears upwards into the book. In this way both the back and the front of the neck extend upwards evenly. One can also feel the elongation in the upper back, on the spinal column in between the shoulder blades, as well as a lateral stretch between the shoulder blades themselves. Thus, not only are the ears, shoulder joints, hip joints and ankle joints all in a vertical alignment in salamba sirsasana, but the body is very light due to the fact that it is not holding itself up with the gross peripheral muscles, but only with the gravity/rebounce force. It is precisely the spinal column which, elongating upwards away from the downward rooting head, pulls the peripheral muscles, like the trapezius and deltoid muscles, with it upwards. Thus the shoulders are lifted and the angle in the elbows is increased, but not by the action of those same muscles, but by the action of the erector spinae.

The next step is to make sure that the back plate and the front plate of the body are parallel to each other. The back of the pelvis should not collapse into the lumbar spine, thus pushing the lumbar vertebrae into the body. Curving the lumbar spine too much forward results in an over-extension at the front of the body, especially in the region between the lower ribs and the navel. This eventually weakens the abdominal muscles as well as the lumbar spine itself.

The neck and thoracic vertebrae pick up the rebounce force of the rooting head in the first joint, the one between the skull and the atlas (the first cervical vertebra). This rebounce force, as it travels upwards, tends to slow down somewhere in the lower thoracic/upper lumbar region. Thus the internal spinal muscles in that region have to be on the alert to pick up the thread from there and continue up towards the sky, not letting that rebounce force collapse in the lumbar, thus dragging the lumbar vertebrae forward into the abdomen. In other words, the pelvis should sit lightly on the lumbar vertebrae, and the bowl of the pelvis, as in tadasana, should be vertical, not slanted.

At the lower end of the spinal column we have the coccyx. One of the main issues in yoga is that the coccyx should never collapse into the fifth lumbar vertebra. Many people interpret this as meaning that you have to 'tuck the coccyx under'. This, however, drags the lumbar vertebrae too far back, eventually resulting in a loss of the lumbar curve. The curves of the spinal column have to be respected at all cost. Though they should not be too deep, they should not be eliminated either. Thus the correct interpretation is that the coccyx should move away from the lumbar vertebrae through internal (ex)tension, not through flexion. This is facilitated by the action of the legs. If the legs are passive in salamba sirsasana their weight will sink heavily into the femur-iliac joints, thus compressing those joints and collapsing the pelvis into the lumbar vertebrae.

The legs, with the ankles in a vertical alignment with the hip joints, should be elongated upwards, out of the femur-iliac joints, so that space is created in those joints and the heads of the femurs sit lightly in the femur-iliac joints, not sink into them. To get the feeling in the legs and consequently in the lower back, you have to constrict the upper thighs slightly inwards so that, at the back, the gluteus muscles are widened across the sacro-iliac joints, thus pulling the big diamond-shaped ligamental plate that crosses over the lumbar spine (the lumbar aponeurosis) backwards. This action, in its turn, pulls the lumbar spine backwards and thus saves it from collapsing forward into the front of the body. By then elongating the inner thighs upwards you can feel the extension on the hip joints and the lumbar spine.

The breathing is vital in all the asanas. In general, the rule is that you use the inhalation to open the body, while you close the body on the exhalation. But when there is more force needed for a certain action, it is better to exhale, using the exhalation as a kind of jet to propel you through the movement. In using the mula bandha breathing in salamba sirsasana the wave action of the inhalation facilitates the elongation upwards of the spinal column towards the sky, while the exhalation consolidates your position.

Pincha mayurasana is also a vertically upside down position, but with a different action from salamba sirsasana. In the first place, due to the fact that in this position one stands on the lower arms and not on the head, it is not possible to hold this pose for as long as salamba sirsasana. Usually one holds it for about one minute. Where in salamba sirsasana I the hands are clasped, here the lower arms run parallel to each other and the hands rest straight on the earth with the palms facing downwards and the middle fingers parallel to each other. This means that the outer and the inner edges of the wrists are even.

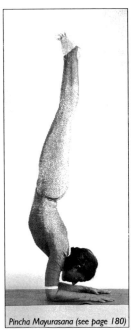

Pincha Mayurasana (see page 180)

Here we run into the first problem. If the shoulders are stiff it is hard to maintain this once the body is raised to a vertical position. The hands tend to move towards each other, so that the lower arms are no longer parallel to each other. For the hands to remain in their original position the shoulders need to be able to form a straight line through the upper arms and rib cage, with the shoulder joints vertically above the elbow joints and an angle of ninety degrees in those joints. Thus it is advisable to work first on loosening and lengthening the shoulder joints before attempting pincha mayurasana.

To go up into pincha mayurasana you have to keep the hands extended firmly on the earth and the head lifted. The rooting action of the ulnar wrist points and of the hands (hasta bandha) here is vital, as it will support the shoulders (rebounce) and will prevent the hands from slipping towards each other. Then raise the body up into pincha mayurasana.

Here we run into the second problem. Most people jump up. This means that the speed of the leg which jumps pulls the trunk up into the vertical position. The pelvis, being the heaviest part to pull up, though, tends to sag in the process and thus collides with the lumbar spine and the sacro-iliac joints. Moreover, because most people do not change legs each time they jump up, one side of the lumbar spine becomes stronger over time while the other side becomes weaker and compressed. You can easily verify this for yourself by jumping up next time with the leg that you never use. Thus, unwittingly, one can even create conditions of scoliosis through thoughtless practice.

Instead of jumping up with speed, there is a different way. Keeping the arms firmly planted on the earth with the ulnar wrist points and hands rooted and the shoulders in a vertical alignment with the elbows, raise the trunk and one leg as high as you can. You have to aim at being as close to the vertical as possible. Then, using the flexibility of the lower spring joint of the bottom foot rather than the force of the leg muscles, lift yourself up into pincha mayurasana.

With a little bit of practice you can raise the body up without jumping, by just continuing the lengthening upwards of the spinal column and the lower abdomen. Change leg every time you go up. In this way it is the spinal column and the pelvis which pull the bottom leg up, not the bottom leg jumping up which pulls the trunk and pelvis. Thus the pelvis does not collide with the lumbar, and the lumbar vertebrae and sacro-iliac joint are safe.

Once you are in the vertical position, you have to find again, like in salamba sirsasana, the central line of gravity, so that you can lift the chest up from the shoulder heads (the upper arms now being the base from which to pick up the rebounce action) and continue that action through the spinal column and legs. The part of the body which now has to cooperate with gravity is, of course, the lower arms.

It is advisable, if the shoulders are really stiff, to practice this pose by keeping the head forward in between the arms, in the direction you are facing. In this way you free the shoulder blades so that you can pull the chest up from the shoulder heads. Keeping the head flexed backwards blocks the shoulder blades and shoulders and thus makes it harder to pull the chest up. While going up, the shoulders should remain vertically above the elbow joints. Many people collapse in the shoulders while going up and thus end up on their foreheads or face as the ninety degree angle in the elbows collapses.

1b. Halasana, Uttanasana, Urdhva Mukha Paschimottanasana II and Paschimottanasana

Looking at these poses superficially one would consider them four different poses. Looking at them in a more holistic way, however, one can easily see that they are one and the same pose, subjected to the force of gravity in different ways.

In halasana gravity pushes the pelvis and spine down into the neck and shoulders, in uttanasana it pulls the spine out of the pelvis, liberating the lumbar and shoulders, in urdhva mukha paschimottanasana II it pushes the legs into the pelvic joints and in paschimottanasana it pulls the body down onto the legs. Even though the shape of the body in all these poses is more or less the same, the effect of gravity is different.

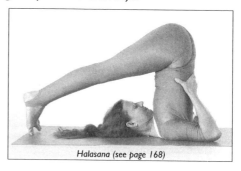
Halasana (see page 168)

To liberate the energy body we have to elongate the physical body always in opposite directions, not just in one direction. This involves a stable part and a mobile part which elongates out of the stable part. The stable part of the body is always that one which is in contact with the earth, from which it derives its stability, so that the mobile part can move away from it.

Thus, in halasana, the stable part is formed by the neck, shoulders, upper arms and feet, which rest on the earth, while the mobile part is formed by the spine and pelvis. As gravity pulls down in a straight line through the pelvis and the spine, which are vertically above the shoulders, they have to move upwards in a straight line, away from the shoulders. This is only possible if those stable parts co-operate fully with gravity, that is, if they root into the earth. The more those stable parts root into the earth, the more the mobile parts can elongate upwards along the line of gravity towards the sky.

In uttanasana the stable part is formed by the soles of the feet. Thus, like in tadasana, we have to root the soles of the feet into the earth, so that the ankles can lift. This lift is carried upwards through the legs and femur heads towards the lower abdomen. By then lifting the pelvis up

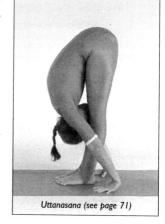
Uttanasana (see page 71)

from the femur heads on a mula bandha inhalation a wave is created for the spine to elongate forwards and downwards.

In urdhvamukha paschimottanasana II the stable part is formed by the back and the head, which rest on the earth. The mobile part is formed by the legs. In this pose one is tempted to pull the feet straight down to the earth along the line of gravity. In this way, however, we do not create any space in the lumbar vertebrae. So here too the spinal column and the legs should meet exactly in the femur-iliac joints. This happens by elongating the lumbar spine, or more precisely the groins and the

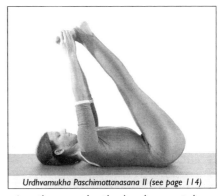
Urdhvamukha Paschimottanasana II (see page 114)

pubic bone, backwards as you pull the legs down. In other words, the lumbar vertebrae should not press onto the earth in this pose, but there should still be the slight natural curve of the lumbar spine, just above the pelvic rim at the back.

In paschimottanasana the stable part is, of course, the back of the legs and the buttock bones. So here too, the more those buttock bones and the back of the legs root into the earth, the more the rest of the pelvis and the trunk can lift, as it were, up from the femur heads and buttock bones, creating again a wave action which carries the whole spinal

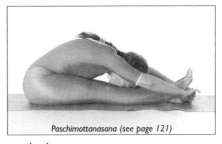
Paschimottanasana (see page 121)

column forward before gravity drops the trunk onto the legs.

These are simple physical adjustments in these poses, in which you have applied the principle of rooting. This rooting has to be guided by the breathing. Doing the asanas without the breath is like doing wind surfing without wind: you go nowhere.

Inhalation is that part of the breathing which helps the spine to elongate, to lift up from the stable underground. It is that part of the breathing which elongates the body in the opposite direction of the rooting action, so all the elongating and upward movements are done on the inhalation. Thus, in halasana you elongate the spine upwards on the inhalation, in uttanasana you elongate it forward, in urdhva mukha paschimottanasana II you elongate the lumbar and thoracic spine on the earth and in paschimottanasana you elongate it forward.

Exhalation is that part of the breathing which by nature follows gravity, in which the ribs drop with gravity, thus emptying the lungs. In halasana this means moving the spine forwards from the back to the front to bring the sternum closer to the chin, without pushing the chin down, however, which is a common mistake. The chin should always lift up on the sternum towards the sky in the jalandhara bandha movement, so that here too you maintain the slight natural curve of the neck vertebrae just underneath the skull. In uttanasana the exhalation helps to drop the whole trunk down to the earth, after you have elongated it forward on the inhalation. In urdhva mukha paschimottanasana II the legs come down, and in paschimottanasana the trunk drops onto the legs.

Thus, on each inhalation and exhalation you create a wave, which ripples throughout the whole trunk. This wave-like action of the inhalation starts always in the lower abdomen, and is carried upwards along the interior length of the spinal column to the top of the head, after which it is attenuated during the exhalation along the line of gravity.

Using rooting and breathing in this way is the first step on the road to an awareness and usage of the energy body or body of light.

1c.   *Paschimottanasana and Upavistha Konasana*

The word *paschima* means 'the back of the body' or 'the west'. The back of the body is considered in India the west side as one faces the east for sun worship and thus the front of the body represents the east.

Paschimottanasana is the basic pose from which is derived a whole series of variations. Most of these variations are one-legged variations, in which the hip joint of the bent leg is either rotated inward or outward. In paschimottanasana both legs are extended straight forward with the inner ankles touching each other and the feet placed in such a way that all the toes are in one line, as in tadasana. And as in tadasana, the heels and balls of the feet are in line, in this case in a vertical alignment. You can pull the gluteus muscles backwards and sideways with your hands, so that you feel that you are sitting on the bones rather than on the flesh. In this way you can understand better whether the body weight is divided equally over the two buttock bones. Due to certain habitual patterns you may feel that you have more weight on one buttock bone than on the other. You can correct this by shifting the weight of the trunk over the legs to the bone which has less weight. The center line of the quadriceps muscles, the central eye of the knee caps, and the central line of the tibia bones have to face straight upwards towards the ceiling.

Paschimottanasana is a forward bending movement. This means that the trunk has to hinge forward in the hip joints. Due to either shortness at the back of the hamstrings or to a certain configuration of the pelvis, this is sometimes not possible. Thus the trunk is bent forward from the lumbar vertebrae, leaving the pelvis in a rigid, upright position. This is the classical humpback position that especially beginner students show.

Therefore, as the root of forward bending is in the back of the legs, the most direct approach is to start by softening and lengthening the back of the legs. The biceps muscles at the back of the thighs are attached to the upper rim of the pelvis and so pull the rim of the pelvis backward if they are tight. This tightness of the biceps muscles is for the largest part caused by civilized living, which means the use of chairs as well as by certain sports, like bicycling, jogging, canoeing, etc.

There are several positions that can help to lengthen those muscles, like adho mukha svanasana, uttanasana, and prasarita padottanasana. In these positions the gravity helps to pull the weight of the trunk forward and thus the back of the legs can elongate more easily, whereas in paschimottanasana one has to work against gravity to do this.

As the body has to hinge forward in the hip joints and not in the waist area, you have to bring the movement first down into the lower abdomen. Holding the feet firmly without pulling them perform the mula bandha breathing. In this breathing the inhalation starts in the lower abdomen with the pulling up of the pelvic floor in general and for women the uterus in particular. This means that the pressure in the lower abdomen is brought slightly backwards towards the sacro-iliac joints. Thus these joints are widened slightly and do not collapse. From there the air moves upwards along the inner lumber spine into the kidney region, widening the lumbar region and the kidneys.

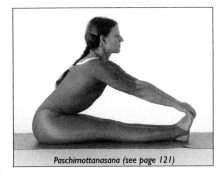

Paschimottanasana (see page 121)

The air then moves upwards along the inner thoracic spine into the upper chest, thus widening and lifting the upper chest. It finally moves up into the back of the head. In this way the body is elongated on each inhalation from the base of the pelvis to the head in a forty-five degree angle, like a jet plane taking off. In this movement the two frontal hip bones are brought forward and lifted towards the rib cage. Note that the pubic bone too is brought slightly forward and up. If the pubic bone is brought forward and down the sacro-iliac joints collapse and the lower abdomen loses its power.

With the exhalation the body goes down towards the legs with gravity, while maintaining the length on the front from pubic bone to throat. In other words, the trunk should not curl back into itself while going down into the final pose. When finally the face comes to rest on the shin bones this has to be well beyond the knees. The more the length at the front is maintained the closer the face will come to the feet.

Even in the final pose you should maintain the soft, even breathing. Each inhalation creates a gently rippling movement from the base of the pelvis along the inner line of the spine towards the head, while on each exhalation the weight of the trunk is abandoned to gravity. Using the breathing in this way you will find that the body can elongate further and further forward without using the arm muscles or the shoulders to pull. The arms should not pull, but you can include the shoulders and arms in the rippling motion of the breathing, elongating the hands further and further forward beyond the feet. When you do eventually clasp the hands beyond the feet you should turn the palm of one hand facing forward and with the thumb and fingers form a ring in which you insert the fingers of the opposite hand. In this way there is no limit to the elongation as the hand can slide further and further forward through the ring of the other hand. Keep the palm of the sliding hand straight, facing the earth, with the fingers pointing straight forward. Here too, however, you should not create one-sided habits. Change hands at regular intervals so as to get an even movement on both sides of the trunk.

The body is a finely tuned network of information. The minute you put your hands on something the body automatically transfers part of its weight to the hands and through the hands to the support on which the hands are resting.

There are three places where you can clasp the hands around the feet. You can rest them on top of the balls of the feet, clasp them in the arches or rest them on the earth. Many people prefer the first. This is because, by resting the hands on the balls of the feet, part of the weight of the trunk is transferred through the hands to the feet. This softens the lower back, which makes it easier to elongate it, and can be helpful for those students who need to soften the lower back in order to make it move forward. It is counter-productive, however, for those students who are already very flexible in paschimottanasana, in which case keeping the hands on top of the feet weakens the lower back even further and therefore creates an even more unstable situation in the lumbar spine and sacro-iliac joints. For those people it is advisable to clasp the hands in the arches so that, as there is no support for the hands, the weight of the trunk, arms and hands is sustained by the lower back. Thus the lower back is strengthened.

Even though there are many similarities between upavistha konasana and paschimottanasana, the difference is great.

In upavistha konasana there is an angle of ninety degrees or more between the legs so that the femur heads fit differently into the hip joints and the sacro-iliac joints have a greater tendency to collapse, due to the fact that the lower abdomen can go down to the earth in between the legs, unlike in paschimottanasana. Therefore it is easier to let the pubic bone roll too far forward and down. Thus it is even more necessary to keep elongating the coccyx backwards away from the lumbar spine in order to maintain the length at the front of the lower abdomen.

Many people experience discomfort in this position along the inner thighs as the adductor muscles and the gracilis muscles are greatly stretched. So here the softening and lengthening has to take place mainly along the inner line of the thighs and knees. One has to pay extra attention to elongating the inner ankles and the metatarsals of the big toes away from the groins, keeping the feet in a vertical position and the toes well spread. The elongation of the metatarsals of the big toes is connected to the inner groins, while the spreading of the other toes and especially of the little toes brings a greater awareness to the muscles around the outer hip joints.

This pose is slightly dangerous for the inner knees and the back of the thighs. To make it safer you have to pull the knee caps strongly up so that you maintain the control over the muscles of the legs. In this way you may go less forward but there is also less chance of hurting a leg muscle. For those students who are flexible and go easily forward it is advisable to keep the legs very strong and the arms spread sideways, resting the palms or wrists just lightly on the tips of the toes so that all the body weight is supported by the lower back.

Using the mula bandha breathing and at the same time slightly elongating the legs out of the hip joints elongate the whole trunk upwards and forward before going down on an exhalation to the earth in between the legs. Like in paschimottanasana the trunk should not curl into itself while going down but should maintain the length at the front so that eventually with a bit of practice you can rest the chest on the earth.

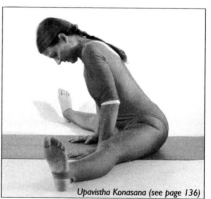
Upavistha Konasana (see page 136)

1d. Kapotasana and Urdhva Dhanurasana

As the technique for urdhva dhanurasana is basically the same as for kapotasana, which is a complex position, it is useful to have a look at kapotasana first. The main difference between the two is that kapotasana starts from a kneeling position, while urdhva dhanurasana starts from tadasana.

The art of the asanas is to liberate the energy trapped within the body by elongating all the joints of the physical body. To do this, we have to differentiate between the stable part(s) of the body and the mobile part(s). The stable part of the body is the one which is in contact with the earth. This forms the basis for the mobile part to pull away from, upwards against gravity, or in any other direction.

In kapotasana (as well as in ustrasana, which is the same position, but with the arms down), the basis is formed by the entire lower leg, from the knees to the tips of the toes, with the knees slightly wider than the hip joints. This is very important. Many people suffer in kapotasana and urdhva dhanurasana from a sharp pain at the outside of the knees. This is because, when the hips are stiff, the ligaments at the outside of the knees are overstretched. Moreover, keeping the

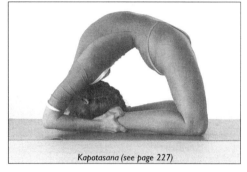

Kapotasana (see page 227)

knees in line with the hips or even more narrow than the hips eventually will put a load on the femur-iliac joints, producing stress there. Keeping the knees slightly wider than the hip joints gives a better, more natural, angle to the femur heads, and thus takes the stress off from those joints and from the knees. The feet and heels are kept together, however, with the toes pointing backwards.

This forms the basis. From here on we have to fix the femur heads in such a way that they, in their turn, form the stable basis for the pelvis and the rest of the body to pull up from. This is done by constricting the outer hips and the inner thighs slightly inwards, from the inner knees up to the inner groins, keeping the thighs perpendicular at an angle of ninety degrees with the lower legs.

To understand this movement better, imagine that you have a block in between the knees and squeeze it, at the same time lifting the arms up over the head. Hold the wrist of one arm and pull it upwards out of that same side femur head, so that you feel the elongation from the outer knee throughout the whole side of the body up to the wrist. Then do the same thing with the other arm and repeat this several times until you feel that you have reached maximum elongation.

This is very important. Many people make the mistake of straight away pushing the groins forward by putting their hands on the hips or at the back of the thighs, thus increasing the angle at the back of the knees. The thighs are like a pillar, and on top of this vertical pillar we have to create a crescent moon shape. This crescent moon shape has to retain its shape and coherence right from the beginning and throughout the pose. Lighten the weight of the body on the femur heads by lifting the pelvis and entire body up from the femur heads (rebounce action). This is done by elongating the inner arches of the feet backwards and rooting them into the earth while performing pada bandha, lengthening the thighs and maintaining the squeezing action at the outer hips and inner thighs.

The act of lengthening the thighs by lifting the pelvis up from the femur heads with the mula bandha inhalation pulls the energy upwards along the interior spinal column. mula bandha is that lifting of the pelvis, but not only of the physical structure. It is the mula, the root of the body, which has to pressurize upwards, thus shooting the energy upwards. This upward movement of the energy travels along the line of gravity, and thus goes from the base of the pelvis straight up into the kidneys, lifting the kidneys up from the lumbar vertebrae.

From the kidneys, still traveling in a straight line upwards, it goes up into the top of the sternum, lifting that up to the sky. This is the crescent moon shape. This crescent moon has to retain its shape and integrity throughout.

To go into kapotasana from here we have to balance the body around the central line of gravity. As the trunk goes back and down, the upper thighs have to move forward (maintaining the squeezing action at the inner sides of the thighs) to balance the weight of the body, until the moment when the pelvis 'clicks' with the femur heads.

Where in the initial crescent moon shape the trunk showed one round line from the pubic bone to the top of the sternum, and the groins were dipped inwards, this round line now starts at the knees and continues through the groins up to the top of the sternum, making one smooth and even curve.

This is in strong opposition to the way many people start, putting the hands on the hips or the back of the thighs and then pushing the trunk/groins forward. The result of this pushing forward is the immediate collapse of the crescent moon shape as the chest sinks down onto the kidney and lumbar area, while the head comes up to balance the uneven distribution of the body weight around the central line of the gravity. In this way the lumbar vertebrae and sacro-iliac joints are completely compressed and there is no smooth curve at the front of the body, but a jarred line of angles and bones (iliac crests and lower frontal ribs). With a little bit of practice (relaxed and with the breathing) one can take the hands all the way down to the earth.

In urdhva dhanurasana the start is the same. Stand with the feet at hip width or even slightly wider (again to protect the fitting of the femur heads in the femur-iliac joints). Fix the femur heads so that they in their turn can function as a stable underground for the pelvis to lift up from. Using a mula bandha inhalation lift the arms straight up over the head, hold the wrist of one arm with the hand of the other, and pull that arm out of the same side femur-iliac joint. Repeat this action several times, until you feel that you have reached maximum elongation. Keeping the legs

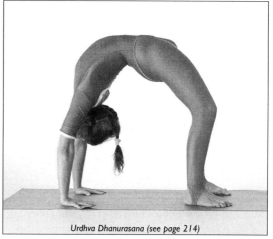

Urdhva Dhanurasana (see page 214)

straight, vertical, create that crescent moon shape by lifting the pelvis up from the femur heads. There should be one smooth curve from the pubic bone up to the top of the sternum. (There is again a dip in the groins). Then go back and down in the same way as for kapotasana till the hands reach the earth. At this point the smooth and even curve starts at the feet and continues through the knees, groins, and lower ribs up to the throat. For a more detailed description of this pose see urdhva dhanurasana (page 214).

2. Front face – Back face

2a. *Janu Sirsasana and Ekapada Rajakapotasana*

It is interesting to note that many asanas have a 'front face' and a 'back face'. That is, that the same pose has a forward form and a backward form.

Let us start with two positions which are fairly complicated, but at the same time very interesting. These positions, when performed wrongly, can easily harm the body, but, when performed correctly, can be of immense help in cases of scoliosis. Both in janu sirsasana and ekapada rajakapotasana I, two positions which at first sight seem very different, the emphasis is on correct alignment of the hip joints, the sacro-iliac joints and the lumbar vertebrae. If there is no proper alignment of these joints, these positions can lead to problems, especially in the sacro-iliac joints, but also in minor degree in the lumbar vertebrae.

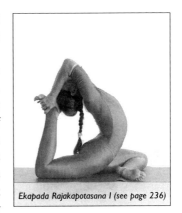

Ekapada Rajakapotasana I (see page 236)

Let us look at janu sirsasana first. Sit on a blanket and extend the right leg straight in front of you with the foot and knee in line with the right groin. The right foot should be vertical and the big and small toes (the inner

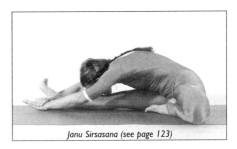

Janu Sirsasana (see page 123)

and outer borders of the foot) should be at equal distance from the trunk. The right knee should face straight up to the sky so that the inner and outer knee at the back rest evenly on the blanket. Bend the left leg and place the left foot against the inner side of the right thigh. There should be an angle of ninety degrees between the left and right thigh, and the sole of the left foot also makes an angle of ninety degrees with the left shin. Do not let the left foot slip underneath the right thigh.

In this position we have already a distortion of the pelvis, as the left hip joint is further back than the right. Proceeding with janu sirsasana without to a certain degree correcting this situation is precisely what would put a great strain on the left sacro-iliac joint and on the left side of the lumbar vertebrae, over-stretching them disproportionately to the right side. Thus, we cannot maintain the weight of the body equal on both buttock bones, but have to shift it onto the right one, even to the point of slightly lifting the left buttock bone off from the blanket. The left knee, however, has to stay on the blanket. In this way we get an opening or an elongation in the left groin and hip joint. As the weight of the body is shifted onto the right buttock bone, the left frontal hip bone also moves closer to the right thigh, while the right frontal hip bone moves over to the right, to come into alignment with the outer edge of the right thigh. Thus both the frontal hip bones will point evenly forward and have the same height from the earth.

Simultaneously with moving the left frontal hip bone over to the right, the left femur has to be elongated out of the left hip socket. This includes a forward rotation of the left thigh, which means that the left knee is not only extended sideways, but is also rolled forwards on the tuberositas of the left tibia. As the trunk, from the navel upwards, has to face straight forwards in the direction of the right foot, the left frontal hip bone, waist and rib cage should be rotated forwards at the same time as the weight of the body is shifted onto the right buttock bone. Only in this way does the left sacro-iliac joint come into a better alignment with the right one, and is thus less hyper-extended, as this extension is shifted to the left hip joint instead.

In this respect it is interesting to note that, if there is a problem in performing this preliminary movement, that is, elongating and rotating in the left hip joint, experience has shown that this is almost a sure indication of an already existing arthritis of the left hip joint, or a tendency to such.

Once the left sacro-iliac joint is eased, the whole spinal column has to elongate upwards. This movement has to start precisely from those sacro-iliac joints, thus the urgent necessity to first bring those into alignment. Not only does the whole spinal column have to elongate upwards out of the pelvis but, as mentioned previously, it also has to rotate towards the right. To get a better feeling of this hold the outer edge of the right foot with the fingers of the left hand, and keep the right hand loosely on the earth next to the right thigh.

Then, using the mula bandha breathing, start elongating the spinal column and turning. On the inhalation, which starts always in the lower abdomen, the pelvis is, as it were, lifted up from the femur heads, while at the same time the buttock bones are slightly extended backwards and downwards (with only the right one in touch with the blanket). On the exhalation the whole spinal column (and consequently the whole trunk), from the sacro-iliac joints upwards, is turned towards the right, until the right arm pit, the right side of the rib cage, and the right waist are in alignment with the outer edge of the right thigh. Thus the right frontal hip bone is above the right groin close to the right hip joints, one third distance from that joint and two thirds distance from the pubic bone.

At this point, seen from the back, the spinal column should form an even groove from the sacro-iliac joints to the cervical spine, and should run straight without any sign of deviation to the left. In order to create the groove also in the upper thoracic spine, the ears have to be elongated out of the cervical spine, leaving, of course, the shoulders and shoulder blades down and relaxed. Needless to say that the drive for this elongation and rotation comes entirely from the breathing, which creates the wave of the movement from the base upwards. Even though the left hand holds the outer edge of the right foot, this is only meant to give you a frame within which to elongate and rotate. Do not use the hand, the arm and the shoulder muscles to pull the spine and trunk upwards and to rotate them.

In this initial upward elongation the head has to stay in alignment with the chest, and the cervical spine has to stay natural. Do not push the cervical vertebrae backwards but, keeping the head in alignment with the chest, elongate them upwards. After reaching maximum elongation and rotation take the trunk down to the right leg. However, as usual, go in stages, using the mula bandha breathing. On each inhalation elongate forward, and on each exhalation take the trunk further down. With the right foot still vertical turn the palm of the right hand forward and with the thumb and the four fingers form a ring. Place the dorsal side of the wrist in the outer arch of the right foot, turn the palm of the left hand also forward and insert the fingers of the left hand in the ring formed by the right hand. In this way there is the possibility of future elongation. Many people just clasp the fingers beyond the sole of the foot like in head balance, which means that there is no room for future elongation. In the way described the left hand can keep on sliding forward within the ring formed by the right hand, till the fingers of the right hand hold the left wrist or even further.

It is important to note that, with the right leg elongated forward, it is the right hand which forms the ring for the left hand to slide through. This is because, by placing the back side of the right wrist in the small arch, that pressure stabilizes the right foot in its vertical position.

When going down onto the right leg, the lower abdomen has to arrive first on the right thigh, then the navel. The navel has to come to rest exactly on the midline of the right thigh. If this is not the case, but the navel stays on the inner side of the thigh, it means that you have not pursued the first part of this pose sufficiently.

After the navel, the sternum has to come to rest on the thigh, close to the knee. Here too, the sternum should be on the midline of the thigh, not on the inner side. The head is the last one to come and rest on the shin. You can either place the forehead on the shin, or, if you are more supple, the chin, so that the eyes look at the right foot. In both cases the neck, shoulders, shoulder blades and arms should remain relaxed and the head (and of course the whole trunk) should, with each mula bandha inhalation, move closer to the right foot.

Let us now look at ekapada rajakapotasana I. Sit on a blanket and extend the right leg straight back of you, with the foot and knee in line with the right groin. The right foot should be straight and the big and small toes should rest equally on the earth. The center of the right knee should rest on the earth so that the inner and outer knee at the back face straight up to the sky. Bend the left leg and place the left foot in front of the right groin. The left thigh comes out of the left groin at an angle of forty-five to the left, and the left foot should not be underneath the right groin, but in front of it.

In this position we have already a distortion of the pelvis, as the right hip is further back than the left. This is even aggravated if you do not keep the right leg back in a straight line, and if you do not rest it exactly on the center of the knee, but on the inside of the knee, shin and thigh (which many people tend to do). Proceeding with ekapada rajakapotasana I without correcting this situation puts great pressure on the right sacro-iliac joint and gives a wrong twist to the lumbar vertebrae.

In this wrong, twisted position, many people keep the weight of the body on the left hip, while the right hip is lifted up and twisted backwards. Thus, to correct this, you have to bring the weight of the body also onto the right hip, by shifting it to the right and at the same time taking the left hip slightly backwards. In this way we get an opening or an elongation in the right groin and hip joint. As the weight of the body is shifted onto the right hip, the left frontal hip bone also moves over to the right, while the right frontal hip bone moves over to the right to come into alignment with the outer edge of the right groin. Thus both the frontal hip bones will point evenly forward and have the same height from the earth. Simultaneously with moving the left frontal hip bone over to the right, the left femur has to be elongated out of the left hip socket. This includes a forward rotation of the left thigh, which means that the left knee is not only extended sideways, but is also rolled forwards on the tuberositas of the left tibia. As the trunk, from the navel upwards, has to face straight forwards, the right frontal hip bone, waist and rib cage should be rotated forwards at the same time as the weight of the body is shifted onto the right hip. Only in this way does the right sacro-iliac joint come into a better alignment with the left one, and is thus less compressed.

In this respect it is interesting to note that, if there is a problem in performing this preliminary movement, that is, elongating and rotating in the right hip joint, experience has shown that this is sure indication that the back bending is done from the lumbar vertebrae, not from the hip joints, and thus those vertebrae are placed under great stress and will sooner or later be weakened and give problems.

Once the right sacro-iliac joint is eased, the whole spinal column has to elongate upwards. This movement has to start precisely from those sacro-iliac joints, thus the urgent necessity to first bring those into alignment. Not only should those joints be in alignment, but the pelvis itself has to be brought as close as possible to a vertical position. As said just now, if there is no sufficient elongation in the right hip joint, the tendency is to let the pelvis fall forward so that the two frontal hip bones collapse into the groins. You can compare this to virabhadrasana I, where many people tend to do exactly that, that is, collapse the pelvis forward into the groins, thus having to pull the body back up to a more or less vertical position out of the lumbar vertebrae instead of out of those same hip joints.

To bring the pelvis up to as close a vertical position as possible, you have to pull the two frontal hip bones back and upwards in the direction of the ribs (of course without twisting the right side of the pelvis backwards). Not only does the whole spinal column have to elongate upwards out of the pelvis but, as mentioned previously, as the tendency is to twist it towards the right, you have to pay attention to keep it centered. Then, using the mula bandha breathing, start elongating the spinal column upwards. On the inhalation, which starts always in the lower abdomen, the pelvis is, as it were, lifted up from the femur heads, while at the same time the buttock bones and the two thighs are rooted into the earth. On the exhalation the whole spinal column (and consequently the whole trunk), from the sacro-iliac joints upwards, is slightly turned towards the left, until the right shoulder, the right side of the rib cage, and the right waist are in alignment with the outer edge of the right groin. Thus the right frontal hip bone is above the groin close to the right hip joint, one third distance from that joint and two thirds distance from the pubic bone.

At this point, seen from the back, the spinal column should form an even groove from the sacro-iliac joints to the cervical spine, and should run straight without any sign of deviation to the left. In order to create the groove also in the upper thoracic spine, the ears have to be elongated out of the cervical spine, leaving, of course, the shoulders and shoulder blades down and relaxed.

In this initial upward elongation the head has to stay in alignment with the chest, and the cervical spine has to stay natural. Do not push the cervical vertebrae forwards or backwards but, keeping the head in alignment with the chest, elongate them upwards. Then bend the right leg and take the left arm up over the head to hold the right foot, keeping the right hand loosely on the blanket next to the right thigh. To do this, you have to first elongate the left arm out of the left groin/sacro-iliac joint, up to the sky. Never make short movements in yoga, so do not just take the arm over the head to hold the right foot, but first create that length and lightness in the left shoulder joint by elongating the left arm out of this joint. Needless to say that the drive for this elongation comes entirely from the breathing, which creates the wave of the movement from the base (the left groin and sacro-iliac joint) upwards. Then, on an exhalation, hold the right foot with the fingers of the left hand. Even though the left hand holds the right foot, this is only meant to give you a frame within which to elongate and rotate. Do not use the hand, the arm and the shoulder muscles to pull the spine and trunk upwards and to rotate them (towards the left).

Then, on a mula bandha inhalation, take the right arm up over the head, elongating it upwards from the right groin/sacro-iliac joint, and hold the right foot also with the right hand, keeping the pelvis straight and vertical. After reaching maximum elongation of the spinal column, start to bend the head and chest backwards in order to take the head towards the arch of the right foot. As usual, go in stages, using the mula bandha breathing. On each inhalation elongate upwards, and on each exhalation take the head and chest further back and down. Thus the movement is circular: the lower abdomen up, the chest up and back, the head back and down, so that at the front of the trunk there is one round line from the groins towards the collar bones. The line of the back bendings should always be seen at the front, and should be round and even. This will only be the case if you use correctly the wave of the mula bandha breathing. Keep the neck, shoulders, shoulder blades and arms relaxed and the forehead in the arch of the right foot.

2b. Uttanasana and Urdhva Dhanurasana

Uttanasana and *urdhva dhanurasana* are both positions which start from tadasana, and thus, if we prepare ourselves really well in tadasana, those two positions should come accurately.

Standing in tadasana and, rooting the soles of the feet, rebouncing the body weight back upwards within the joints (lower and upper spring joints, knees and hip joints) against the pull of the gravity, we have to then rotate the pelvis forwards (uttanasana) or backwards (urdhva dhanurasana). One of the most important things to understand in yoga is that, to go down, one has to go up.

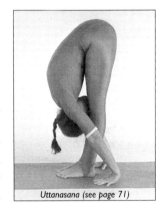

Uttanasana (see page 71)

Most people do not act with this understanding and thus, both in uttanasana and in urdhva dhanurasana, one sees that the body just collapses under the pull of gravity, without creating any resistance or inner space, inner elongation. Before rotating the pelvis forwards (to go into uttanasana) or backwards (to go into urdhva dhanurasana) one has to see if one can lift the pelvis up from the femur heads, creating that inner space or bounce within the femur-iliac joints before rotating those joints. Thus, when rotating,

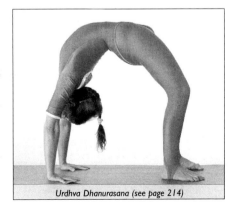

Urdhva Dhanurasana (see page 214)

elongation is brought in the case of uttanasana, in the upper part of the back of the thighs (the biceps muscle), and in the case of urdhva dhanurasana, in the upper part of the front of the thighs (the quadriceps and the iliopsoas muscles). Thus, in uttanasasa, the buttock creases in between the femur and the ischias bones are elongated, while in urdhva dhanurasana the groins are elongated.

At this point it is relatively easy to elongate the spinal column away from the pelvis against the gravitational pull (forward in uttanasana, upward in urdhva dhanurasana) to go into the final pose. Thus, one has to maintain throughout this inner elongation, this space within the vertebral and pelvic joints, and not collapse them, thus losing the height and beauty of the pose.

An asana, or any other pose, is only beautiful if it is powerful, but this power is not in relation to somebody else or something else. Power, beauty, is where there is space in the body, in the mind. It is only there where the power of the muscle, the power of ambition, the power of thought, is absent. It is only there where mind and body do not look ahead to a future, to the fruit of its present actions, but when both mind and body are fused in the moment, in the pose, without ambition, without fear, with interest and joy. When that happens, even for a split second, there is an inner explosion of energy which transforms that pose into a thing of beauty, into a thing spiritual, in which the position 'does itself', in which there is no warfare between wanting to do it and resisting doing it.

Thus asana and pranayama have to mingle, and our attitude in asana has to be the same as in pranayama. In pranayama one of the keys to a free and profound breathing is the release of the skin. If the skin on the chest and the rest of the body is hard, brittle, the body, the energy, is literally imprisoned within the skin.

Tension, under whichever form, is always from the periphery of the body towards the center. Clasping the arms as protection against cold (or as protection of the ego), frowning, the hunched-over position of a depressed mind, the so-called goose pimples on the skin itself, are all contractions of the body inward, an attempt, as it were, to make the body as small as possible within the surrounding space.

On the other hand, we 'heave a sigh of relieve', we feel as if a 'burden has been lifted from our shoulders', we yawn, stretch and smile in moments of relaxation, contentment, happiness, opening our body in all directions within the surrounding space, fusing, as it were, our inner energy with the surrounding energy. Thus, to elongate the body in the asanas, the first thing to do is to soften the skin, so that the underlying muscle and bone can expand. This is a mental process. We have to carefully and deliberately release the skin and the underlying tissues, moving the body from the bones and joints more than from the actual muscles, making, as it were, the muscles and the skin transparent, like an X-ray photograph.

In this process, the breathing is extremely important. If one can use the image of a surf board, the breathing is the wave which carries the surfboard a long distance. Without the underlying wave, the surf board and its rider would just be sitting in stagnant water.

Inhalation is an opening movement, a liberating movement, an expansion of the chest, of the body, in space. On the other hand, exhalation is an abandoning movement, a giving in to gravity, a controlled collapsing of the body. Thus, inhalation is that wave which carries the opening of the body, the elongation upwards (urdhva dhanurasana) or forwards (uttanasana) before the act of going down, which, in its turn, is smoothed out by the exhalation.

For this, one should never be in a hurry. In each pose, take a couple of breaths to prepare for the elongation, opening the body on each inhalation and maintaining and consolidating that new position on each exhalation. Then, when the body has reached its maximum elongation, move with a smooth and controlled exhalation into the final pose. Doing things in this way, riding on the waves of the inhalation and exhalation, you will find that there is very little fatigue in performing the asanas and the body does not fight the pose. Then there is beauty, and power, and joy, and out of that flows the pose.

3.   Beauty and freedom in yoga

In these two paragraphs, 'Playing with Gravity' and 'Front face – Back face', only a few asanas have been discussed. For fun's sake, find out for yourself all the different asanas that you can play these 'gravity games' with, or all the asanas that show a 'front face' and a 'back face'. Also, some asanas have a 'grounded' version as well as an 'elevated' version, like for instance anantasana and vasisthasana II, which are the same positions, the only difference being that in anantasana the body rests on the earth, while in vasisthasana II the body is elevated on one hand. Another such pose is titthibhasana, which is the 'elevated' form of kurmasana, or urdhva kukkutasana, which is the 'elevated' form of yoga mudrasana.

Looking at the asanas in such a way stimulates the creative vision and helps you to understand the poses better. As mentioned before, even though asanas are countless, the basic principles are few and simple. The important thing in all this is to look at yoga holistically, and not fragment either the asanas or yoga itself too much in a frantic search for more and more information. Information, beyond a certain point, beyond the 'point of no return', becomes a ballast, killing the very thing that you try to create, which is beauty and freedom in the asanas, in yoga.

part three
breathing

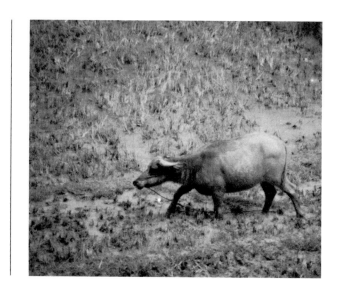

The soft awareness breathing

Normally we are not aware of our breathing, as it is supposed to be an automatic process of the body. Awareness, however, is always associated with chi energy, and so breathing with awareness, in addition to bringing a greater amount of oxygen to the body, also brings a greater amount of chi energy. Moreover, with the awareness one can direct the breathing to go wherever oxygen or chi energy is lacking, thus filling in the gaps in energy

The soft awareness breathing does not have a specific trajectory, but takes place as it were everywhere at the same time. It is very helpful to practice and integrate this type of breathing in your daily life to keep the body and mind in a mindfully relaxed and integrated way. In this way the breathing will support the first two principles, the not-doing of the mind and the not-doing of the body. While going about our daily chores, a small part of our awareness is employed to watch our breathing. Using the imagination or intent as well as the peripheral eyes we can feel that the breath is going down through our body into our center of gravity, and from there out into the rest of the body. Visualizing that we are breathing into our center of gravity helps to make the diaphragm descend.

Centering the breath

It is important to balance the breathing laterally and also between the front and the back. Most people are used to breathe more on the front of the body, which has to do with the fact that we have more awareness of the front of the body than of the back. To center the breathing we need to be able to breathe equally on the front and on the back. Even though on the back the ribs are attached to the spinal column, the ribs and the spine are two different systems. Therefore, breathing into the back does not mean that the spinal column should be pushed backwards. We just need to fill out the ribs at the back in the same way that we fill out the ribs at the front, while keeping the spine erect and firm. The amount of breathing on the front should be matched by the amount of breathing on the back.

In the same way we need to center the breathing laterally. The lateral balance is usually compromised by crooked habits, like carrying the shoulder bag always on the same shoulder, or using predominantly one hand to do things. To center the breathing laterally we therefore need to look at these habits, and try to even the left and right side out so that the breathing too will center in the middle. The back and the front of the body should always be balanced and the two sides also. You should always come in the middle of the body.

The accentuated awareness breathing or the mula bandha breathing

The trajectory of this type of breathing is through the bandhas. Though it actually starts in the feet, with pada bandha, I have called it the mula bandha breathing because its central collecting point is the hara in the lower abdomen. Pada bandha gives the tone to the lower abdomen, and as such it is indispensable, but the center of the radiation of the breathing is in the hara.

This breathing is done in all the postures to enhance the elongation of the body, but can also be applied in daily life when needed. Usually, when it is practiced independently as a breathing exercise, it is done sitting in siddhasana or padmasana.

Mula bandha breathing takes place in the lower throat. In order to understand exactly where in the throat, you can pretend that you want to yawn. Initiate the yawn, keeping your mouth closed, though, and then change it into an inhalation. Thus you can feel the opening or widening in the lower throat, close towards the back of the throat, the spinal column. That means that the air goes straight down into the lower abdomen, because the widening of the lower throat results in a widening of the lower thoracic diaphragm and therefore the movement of the breathing can go through it. Breathing in the lower throat also means that the breathing is soundless.

The diaphragm has fibers going down along the frontal line of the lumbar spine. As the center of the diaphragm goes down on the inhalation and 'collides' with the intestines, the abdominal muscles refuse to yield, and move even slightly backwards. At the same time the buttock bones root and thus do not receive the movement, and the sacrum is held firm and vertical. Between the three – the abdomen going backward, the sacrum holding or containing that energy and the buttock bones rooting – the movement of the inhalation, the wave action, has no other option but to loop back up again and go back up along the spinal column, on the frontal or interior side of the lumbar spine.

As it moves up along the spinal column, it has to pass through the spinal curves. The lumbar spine has the curve going forward (the lordosis), but at the height of the lower thoracic spine the lordosis turns into a kyphosis (the spinal curve going backwards). Thus the wave, moving up along the spine, does not end up in the front of the body at the height of the lower thoracic spine, but in the back, in the kidney area. It is interesting to note that in oriental arts both the lower abdomen and the kidneys were considered power spots in the body.

In the region of the lower thoracic spine the movement widens the lower ribs, which is their anatomical function, and thus it draws the diaphragm up into the chest into a kind of mild uddiyana bandha. Even though the center of the diaphragm goes down on the inhalation, the diaphragm on the whole goes up into the rib cage, leaving the upper abdomen slightly hollow as the kidney region widens and lengthens upwards. In the upper thoracic spine the kyphosis turns again into the cervical lordosis, and thus the wave of the inhalation comes back to the front of the body and ends up in the upper thoracic diaphragm, the manubrium, the upper part of the sternum, which is lifted as a result.

In the classical yoga texts there is a breathing technique called ujjayi. In this breathing technique the air is drawn into the lungs by slightly constricting the upper throat, thus producing a wind-like sound. As all techniques, this type of breathing forms part of a pranayama session, in which are included several types of breathing techniques. There are many excellent books that describe these techniques, amongst others Light on Pranayama, by BKS Iyengar.

The scope of this book (apart from the chapter on the asanas) is to provide the reader with clues on how to do things naturally, at any time and wherever one wants to, without being tied down to a particular place, time or posture. For this I devised mula bandha breathing.

We can do a very interesting experiment to see the effect of the use of the eyes on our breathing.

Do concentric vision, and watch internally where the air enters, where it goes, and how it goes where it goes. Then do the same thing with peripheral vision. We can clearly see that concentric vision produces automatically ujjayi breathing, that is, the air goes through the upper throat into the lungs, and as it enters, it opens the chest from inside. It does not go deeper than that, but stays confined in the chest above the diaphragm.

On the other hand, peripheral vision produces automatically mula bandha breathing. In peripheral vision the air enters through the lower throat, and goes straight away down into the pelvis, where the movement starts with the lifting of the pelvic floor. The whole body, chest and pelvis, through peripheral vision and the lower throat widening, is opened and widened, and this creates a kind of vacuum in which the air is drawn into the body.

The only problem one could say in the mula bandha breathing is that there is no control over the speed of the breathing, so the tendency for the breathing would be to go fast. Where in ujjayi breathing the control is in the upper throat, in mula bandha breathing the control of the speed and depth of the breathing is in the lowest part of the trunk, in the lower abdomen. The abdominal muscles control the speed and the depth of the breathing. They function like the reins on the horse – they give the exact amount of freedom to the breathing to go in the speed that you want. The more you tone those muscles the slower the breathing goes. Thus the breathing and its control are done from the hara.

The following essays are taken from tape recordings of courses that I conducted in the United States over a period of twenty years. As each class had its own mood, I thought it would be interesting to maintain that mood by not editing too much, so as to keep certain continuity.

Class I

Sitting

Sitting is something we do all day long, whether on a chair, on a bicycle or on the saddle. Let us see how we can make this simple activity as efficient as possible.

Sit on the floor in siddhasana or padmasana with the back straight and the hands on the knees, the palms facing upwards.

In this posture, the back of the thighs and the buttock bones form that part of the body which is in contact with the ground, and thus these parts have to utilize the force of gravity. Establish that link, feel the contact of the back of the thighs and the buttock bones with the ground, and then yield them to the force of gravity, following the line of gravity down into the ground. The buttock bones and the thighs should gradually, as it were, sink into the ground.

The bowl of the pelvis should be held completely vertical, neither tilted backwards nor forwards. This means that the two frontal hipbones are in a vertical alignment with the groins, at an angle of ninety degrees with the femurs. As you keep the pelvis firmly vertical, without collapsing, you have to 'grow' the buttock bones downwards. The body is like a tree. If one considers the hip joints, the groins and the sacro-iliac joints as 'ground level,' then the part which is below this 'ground level' has to 'grow' downwards, just like the roots of a tree, while the part which is above it has to 'grow' upwards, like the trunk of the tree.

This 'growing upwards' is done when the body picks up the rebounding force from the downward 'growing' *roots* (buttock bones). The exchange of the downward and upward forces takes place in the sacro-iliac joints, the hip joints and the groins.

One can divide the body roughly into three compartments: the pelvis, the chest and the head. Most people hold the body up from the chest or from the head, shoulders and neck. This means that the support for the weight of the body comes from the diaphragm or even from the shoulders.

In the first place, the body has to counteract that tendency by dropping the point of support into the third, the basic, compartment, the lower abdomen. Draw a line from hip joint to hip joint, and another one, a front-back line, from the mid point between the navel and pubis to the sacrum: where those two lines cross is the center of gravity. It is from here that the body should be upheld. Thus the energy in the neck and the shoulders, which is often used to hold the body up, has to be brought down into the lower abdomen. This is a question of internal weight; it is not a question of dropping the spinal column. It is the force with which the body is upheld which is lowered.

In the second place, the body has to shift the internal weight backwards as well, into the backside of the body. The frontal side of the body is in contact with the frontal brain and the eyes; it is that part of the body that we can see with our concentric vision and think about. The backside of the body, on the other hand, is that part which we cannot see, with which we don't have a relationship, and which is in contact with the back brain. We can only contact that part through peripheral vision.

Our actions are always focused on the front of the body, on the front of the face. If one says: 'Let me think,' one points to the forehead. If one says: '**I feel**,' one points to the chest. If one says: 'I am afraid,' one points to the diaphragm. This shows that we feel or experience our emotions on the front of the body. On the backside of the body we do not feel anything. Thus, after having lowered the internal weight of the awareness into the lower abdomen, you have to bring it also from the frontal side of the body into the backside, towards the sacrum, the 'sacred' bone.

It is easy to feel how the awareness is lodged on the frontal side of the diaphragm. The diaphragm, which is a negative emotional center, is hot. It is here that we find the solar plexus, the 'sun knot,' where we experience fear and anxiety, which, when excessive, the body expresses as 'ulcers.' On the backside of the body, we find the kidneys, which, in most Oriental disciplines, are associated with water, with the moon, with coolness.

One of the most important things is to bring the hot, solar energy of the frontal diaphragm, and the cool, lunar energy of the kidneys, into balance. The internal weight of awareness, which is lodged against the frontal wall of the abdomen, has to be brought backwards towards the kidneys, without disturbing the physical body, and without bending the spine.

In the chest, too, the awareness has to be moved backwards. The sternum is the center of positive emotions (love, affection) as the diaphragm is the center of negative emotions (fear, anger). From the sternum, the internal weight, the internal awareness, has to be brought backwards into the shoulder blades, without bending the chest or the thoracic spine. In this way the whole back of the chest, the shoulder blades, and even the kidneys, widen. The shoulder blades are the wings of the body. Use them!

These are the first two acts the body has to perform: after rooting the buttock bones, the upholding force of the body is lowered into the lower abdomen, and then shifted backward into the backside of the body, the part of the body that is unknown, mysterious.

The third act of the body is to become aware of the surrounding space, especially the space above the head. The body is a conduit for electrical energy, which passes between the ground and the sky, like lightning that goes from the ground to the clouds and back down again. Starting with the vertical space above the head, you can actually feel the weight of the sky on your head, pressing down on you. Part of this weight is gravity pulling the body down, and part is the actual weight of the air molecules pressing down on the head. Instead of struggling to elongate the body upwards against this weight, there is a much simpler way. This is by visualization.

In your imagination, 'take the sky away', the air above the head, as if you create a vacuum above the head. In this vacuum the spinal column will unfurl itself upwards, without any muscular effort. It is just the image of having 'taken the weight of the sky away' that makes the spine go up like a cork surfacing above water level after having been pressed underneath it and then released. Thus, you have to bring the inner awareness not only into the back of the body, but also deep within, into the skeletal structure, from where it can then expand outwards again.

With the buttock bones growing downwards like the roots of a tree, the spinal column growing upwards like the trunk of a tree, and the branches growing sideways - that is, the rib cage, the shoulder blades, the shoulders, and the kidney region widening – the picture of the human tree is complete. All the energies are in balance, the inner awareness moves freely in all directions, and the body is light, held up by its own inner expansion.

The last act of the body is to 'take the skin away' all over the body, this barrier between the inner energy and the outer space or energy. The skin is the 'bag' in which we live, like a leather bag, and basically what is inside the skin is the same 'substance' as what is outside, but it is contained. Due to our lifelong thoughts and emotions, the skin becomes tough to the point of brittleness, a barrier to hold the outer energies at bay, and to 'protect' the inner being from these outer energies. Thus the inner energy is trapped within this hard skin, and cannot mix with the energy that is outside, the sun and air that nourish it. Therefore, through visualization, the skin has to be 'taken away.'

To practice this, start with the hands. With the palms facing upwards, relax the hands and carefully 'take away' the skin. In doing this, you feel as if the hands swell and become big.

One can compare this sensation to a sponge. When the sponge is squeezed, it is small and tight, but when it is released, it immediately swells up, filling itself with air. As the hands become big, they also become warm and begin to tingle, as the energy within the hand spills out and mixes with the energy outside, till there comes a moment in which you no longer clearly feel where the hands end and the space around the hands begins. No longer feeling the boundaries of the hands, you do not feel whether they are resting on your knees, on the ground, or on nothing at all.

After the hands, you can do the same thing with the arms, 'taking the skin away,' feeling the swelling, the warmth, the tingling, and the melting of boundaries. Then move up to the shoulders, the shoulder blades, the neck and the chest. You can clearly feel how the skin holds the inner energy, the inner body, tight, so that when you 'take the skin away' from the shoulders, the shoulder blades, the sternum, and the rib cage, they become big, wide, open, vulnerable. Watch carefully that the skin dissolves everywhere evenly, that there are no hidden parts where it refuses to melt. Those are the places where the body has collected tensions, so you have to spend a little extra time undoing the skin in those parts.

Then move to the pelvis, the legs, the feet. Keeping the skeletal frame straight, upright, 'take the skin away' everywhere. It is like making an X-ray picture of your body, where the skeleton is outlined clearly, but the muscles and the skin are only vague shadows, transparent. The most difficult area to make transparent is the head, the face. Carefully dissolve the skin on the face till it is transparent, like a clear piece of quartz crystal, through which the inner light can shine out.

Class II

Part one: sitting

Sit in padmasana or half padmasana. Padmasana is not an ideal position in the sense that the pelvis in this position is always slightly uneven. Therefore you have to change legs at regular intervals so as not to permanently make the pelvis uneven. The line of the spine should end up exactly in the middle between the two buttock bones.

The first thing is to balance properly on the triangle of the legs. Close the eyes and keep the head up. Keep the hands loosely on the knees with the palms facing upwards. This helps to keep the shoulder blades down.

We have to find the balance on the gravitational line. The body should not come too far forward or too far backward. If the body is too far backward, you can feel that you are hanging from your frontal muscles in order not to fall over backwards. If the body is too far forward, the muscles in the back have to be tense in order to keep the body from falling forwards. So find the balance of the body on the thighs and the legs.

The spine, the body, should not collapse, it should be completely straight, but do not depend on the muscles for this. If the body is on the gravitational line, you don't need much effort to keep the body straight. The front and the back of the body should be parallel to each other and vertical, not leaning.

It is the same with the sideways balance. You should also feel that you are balancing evenly on both the buttock bones, the weight on both those bones should be even.

The head should balance evenly on the spinal column. If the head is too far forward, the muscles at the back of the upper trunk and neck are tense to prevent the head from falling forwards. The head should be on the gravitational line, straight above the rib cage and the pelvis, and all the vertebrae of the spinal column should be in alignment.

Find out where the central gravitational line of the body is, so that you relax most of the muscular system, resting almost entirely on the skeleton. The muscles relax; the skeleton remains firm. The body should not yield its weight to gravity; on the contrary, it should resist gravity, lifting itself up, through the act of rooting the buttock bones into the ground.

Feel whether the pelvis is sitting heavily and broadly on the buttock bones, of whether you are pricking the buttock bones into the ground, so that the pelvis is lifted up. Do not lift the pelvis up by lifting the rib cage; the movement has to come from the pelvis itself, not by pushing the solar plexus forward.

The beauty of the body is when it is light. Everybody knows how to be heavy, but find out how light the body can become. This lightness of the body comes when the whole skeletal frame of the body lifts up, and the muscles hang loose from the frame of the skeleton. Draw the spine upwards out of the muscular periphery of the body, like you draw a sword out of a scabbard. To do that you have to shift the weight of your awareness onto the back of the body; not the physical weight of your body, but the internal weight of your awareness.

People do not realize that awareness, consciousness, has bulk and weight, it can move around and throw light on different areas of the body. Usually the internal weight of the awareness is on the front of the body, the face, the throat, the sternum, the solar plexus, creating a lot of tensions there. This is where we feel most at home, and thus the neck and shoulders are pulled forward chronically and the back stoops. Moving the internal weight backwards automatically straightens the body and releases the tensions at the front of the body.

Moving the internal weight of the body backwards does not mean that the spine should bend backwards, rather the spine should be firm like a rod and the internal weight has to 'lean' against the spine. This automatically broadens the whole back, and this broadening of the back then allows the body to lengthen upwards. In this action there is no muscular effort involved.

The same thing applies in the region of the head and the neck. With eyes closed feel inside your body: You can feel that you are on the front of the face and the chest, and this drags the head and the neck forward. The usual remedy is to pull the chin in, which is again an action on the front. So instead of correcting one wrong action on the front by another, see if you can withdraw the internal weight backwards from the face, the throat and the chest into the back of the head.

If you manage to do this you can easily feel how the neck broadens and lengthens without any muscular effort; the whole head comes as it were out of the trunk, like a turtle drawing its head out of the shell. When the turtle pulls its head out, the shell stays where it is, so here too, he chest stays where it is and the head just comes out; the neck is lengthened not by pulling the chin in, but by internal weight shifting.

Part two: Breathing

Take the head down, but do not drag it down; never make heavy movements. Keep the head light, just tip it down lightly; the axis is in the ear holes, not in the shoulders.

Keep the hands loosely on the knees, palms facing upward.

When you breathe let the action be on the back, because this is where you get the depth of the breathing. If you breathe from the frontal ribs, you never obtain the same depth. Without bending the spine, breathe into the back.

In inhalation the diaphragm moves downwards and backwards, not forwards. And when you exhale, draw the air up out of the back. When you inhale, push the coccyx and the buttock bones down, and at the same time extend the lumbar and the thoracic vertebrae. Then, when you exhale, keep the coccyx down and maintain the length between the vertebrae that you got from the inhalation.

If you confine the breathing only to the chest, if you think that only the lungs are involved in the breathing, you automatically block the inhalation, you restrict the expansion of the lungs and chest. To get the depth of the inhalation, you have to think more comprehensively.

Start the inhalation by almost bypassing the lungs, and inhale way down, into the pelvis. Of course, this is by way of speaking, but the feeling is actually there. Bypassing the lungs in this way you automatically release the diaphragm, so that it is free to go down and back. The spinal column remains straight. Then the breathing becomes deep and wide.

The spine, the skeleton, should be completely straight and still, not shaking. The inhalation and the exhalation should also not shake or change the position of the spine and skeleton.

Anything you do, bringing the head down, sitting, breathing, can be done in two ways. You can put the energy of the movement in the muscles, which creates tensions so that that energy is lost, tied down in these tensions. The other way is not to tie the energy down in the muscles, but let it remain free and fluid. It is only this energy that can bring joy to the pose.

When you sit, the more you sit and breathe from the skeletal frame, the more you can release the grip of the muscles on the bones, and the more you release that energy which is locked up in the muscles as useless tension.

That does not mean that you have to be weak and floppy. On the contrary, withdrawing the energy from the muscles and investing it in the bones will make you stronger and give you more endurance than before. It will give you more power, but a different kind of power, a different kind of energy.

To bring the head down, lift the back of the head up. The neck should not move backward, but upward. Release the grip of the muscles on the bones, and release the grip of the skin on the muscles. How much is the skin of the hands holding onto the muscles of the hands? The maturity, energy wise, of the body comes when the skin, muscle and bone separate, then the body will be light.

The whole point is whether to do psychological warfare or not. If the muscles grip the bones unnecessarily, if there is unnecessary tension, then there is internal warfare. But one should not indulge the body either. We should find a state of peace in the body that is neither indulgence nor warfare. And that is only possible when you balance the body on the bones and use the muscles minimally, mainly for movement. Just use the muscles lightly to keep the body erect.

Thus, when you inhale, bypass the chest, as it were, so that the inhalation widens the back and elongates the spine. During exhalation that length has to be maintained, even though the back looses its width.

Fill the rib cage evenly in all directions, the ribs and the shoulder blades should widen, and the chest and shoulder blades should hang passively from the spinal column. Often we pull the body up from the rib cage, from the shoulders, from the shoulder blades, and the spine is dull.

Bring the dynamism of the periphery into the spinal column, pulling the spinal column out of the rib cage like a sword out of its scabbard. The brain, reason, is connected with the skeleton, while the emotions are connected with the muscles. If you lift the rib cage and the shoulders, that is an emotional and egoistic action, not a cool action. We have to learn to separate the muscles and the bones. If the whole body, muscles and bones, are 'soft', the body sags; there is no firmness. On the other hand, if the whole body (muscles and bones) are aggressive, there is a lot of stiffness and tension. One is indulgence and the other is warfare.

One has to strike a balance: the bones have to be firm while the muscles have to release: yin and yang. Get that balance between the masculine and feminine energy within the body, not overdoing either. The awareness should be absolutely clear and piercing; it should pierce the body. Then the breathing becomes slow and controlled.

When you inhale and exhale, the air should not disturb the skeleton. The lumbar vertebrae should elongate, but the skeleton should not oscillate. At the same time, the inhalation and the exhalation should not meet with any obstacles anywhere in the muscles. The muscles of the chest should be completely receptive to the breathing, but not the skeleton. If you can find that balance, then you have done ninety percent of the work.

Find out in the body where the muscle is obstructing the breathing. In the solar plexus, in the shoulders, in the chest, find out where the muscles are obstructing, and then gently, internally, remove that obstruction.

CLASS III

Part one: sitting

Sit in padmasana.

In any given position you have the base, (or basis), and an upper part. The basis, which is that part of the body that is on the ground, should move down with gravity so that the upper part of the body can move up and become light. There is always a division, or dual movement, in the body. You cannot only be light, but must also be grounded, or rooted. Nor can you only be heavy, as then the body and mind are depressed. One part of the body must be stable, in order that other parts of the body can be light. For instance, in head balance the head has to move downward with gravity for the rest of the body to be light, to go up. On the other hand, in tadasana, the feet are on the ground; thus the feet must move downward with gravity while the rest of the body becomes light in order to move upward.

In padmasana the two buttock bones, the coccyx and the pubic bone form a triangle with the legs. This whole triangle should move downward. You actually push it into the ground by using two pairs of muscles. The outside of the thighs and hips has to squeeze slightly inward as well as the inside of the thighs, so that the knees move slightly closer toward each other. With that slight muscular action you can then 'prick' the buttock bones down, so that the rest of the body rests or 'floats' on this stable basis.

The pelvis is kind of a bowl shape, and this bowl should rest vertically on the ground. Many people, however, slump, which means that the pelvis is in a backward rotated position.

By putting the fingers on the two frontal hipbones (the iliac crests), you can see which position the pelvis is in. If these bones are further backward than the groins, it means that the pelvis is sitting on the back of the buttock bones, and the coccyx is lower than the public bone. Therefore, the whole body is already slumped at the basis as the bowl of the pelvis is tilted backward, with the base of the pelvis moving forward and the top of the pelvis backward.

Most people try to correct this position by another wrong position, i.e. by rotating the pelvis too far forward, and pulling the coccyx up into the lumber spine. Thus, the top of the pelvis is further forward than the base, and the coccyx is back and up, while in the slumping position, the coccyx is forward and the top is back. In either case the position is wrong.

We have to find that position in which the pelvis is straight and vertical, which means that when you put you fingers on the two frontal hipbones, these should neither move backward, nor should they move forward in a downward direction, but rather, move forward in an upward direction. Lift the pelvis form the femur heads and then bring it slightly forward without capsizing it backward or forward.

Returning to the concept of the pelvis as a bowl, this bowl should be vertical and lifted. This means that the two frontal hipbones are high and aligned above the groins, not low in the groins. Thus, the buttock bones, coccyx and pubis press downward equally, and the two frontal hipbones move forward and up. As the two frontal hipbones move forward and up, the pelvis widens. Thus, the distance between the two frontal hipbones also widens and the abdomen becomes flat and firm. The firmness of the position is in the pelvis and in the hip joints.

Once the basis is firm, it is like a pillar. A pillar needs a base at its bottom, a round or a square base stone. Once you have built that base stone out of the pelvis, the spinal column is the pillar. Each vertebra then moves vertically upward from the one below, not by pushing it upward, but rather by removing the pressure at the top of the spine it is allowed to 'float' upward.

The pressure at the top of the spine is gravity, of which we are not usually aware. It 'presses' down on us and the body slumps underneath this pressure. Try to take this pressure mentally away. Then from the basis, the spine moves upward by itself because the head no longer presses on the shoulders, and because the shoulders no longer press on the lumbar spine. Taking the pressure away at the top allows the body to 'breathe'. Having taken away the outer constricting pressure, a space is created inside the body, and this, in itself, allows the body to breathe.

Returning to the widening movement of the pelvis, grip the muscles around the hips as the coccyx, pubis and buttock bones are anchored down, and as the rest of the pelvis is pulled up. Thus, the sacrum moves into the pelvis, pushing the sacro-iliac joints sideways.

In pregnancy there is a movement called counter-nutation. As the baby comes out, the joints have to widen, otherwise there in not enough space. To widen and narrow the hipbones at the same time is anatomically impossible, but energetically it is. It feels as if the body is widening and narrowing at the same time. However, this is because it is the muscles which squeeze inward that form the support for the pelvis to widen.

We are familiar with the above two movements: tilting the pelvis backward, or forward. When you tilt it forward, it means you rotate the whole pelvis, including the sacrum, and thus the coccyx moves backward and upward. When the pelvis tilts backward, the coccyx moves down and forward.

The sacrum and the coccyx are part of the spine. However, in the above example I am not using them as part of the spine, but as part of the pelvis. Thus, I am moving only in the lumber-sacrum joint and not in the sacro-iliac joints. To move in the sacro-iliac joints you have to do both nutation and counter-nutation. You have to rotate the pelvis forward and at the same time, you have to rotate the sacrum backward, anchoring the coccyx. Thus, the pelvis rotates forward, but without the sacrum and the coccyx.

If I only rotate forward, nothing happens. If I only rotate backward, nothing happens. Now if I push the coccyx and buttock bones down and lift the pelvis up, the pelvis neither tilts backward nor forward. The pelvis remains vertical and straight. Lifting it vertically up and bringing it forward creates the movement in the sacro-iliac joints.

Normally, when you rotate the pelvis forward, the buttock bones widen (as in forward bends). When you turn the pelvis backward, the two frontal hipbones widen (as in back bends). By moving the pelvis forward and up, and keeping the sacrum vertical, we are able to widen the pelvis at the front and back at the same time.

There are three joints around the pelvis: the hip joints, where the legs join the pelvis; the sacro-iliac joints, where the sacrum (the fused spinal vertebrae) joins the ilium part of the pelvis; and the lumbo-sacral joint (the joint between the last lumbar vertebra and the sacrum).

Because it is easy, we usually bend in this last joint. Again, as I said before, we incorrectly consider the sacrum and the coccyx as part of the pelvis. However, I want you to do something different. I want you to keep the sacrum exactly where it is and to move only the two frontal hipbones forward, together with the coccyx. This will allow you to move in the sacro-iliac joints.

What we usually do is to keep the pelvis, sacrum and coccyx as one whole unit, and then we rotate it forward or backward around the lumbo-sacral joint. This is because most people do not realize that the spinal column is actually one unit. Instead most people assume that the spine finishes in the lumbo-sacral joint, and the sacrum and coccyx form part of the pelvis, so that we only move in the lumbo-sacral joint.

I want to separate the spine from the actual pelvis. Instead of dividing yourself in the sacro-lumbar joint and putting the sacrum and coccyx in the unit of the pelvis, I want you to divide yourself in the sacro-iliac joint and put the sacrum and coccyx back in the unit of the spine. As I said, when you rotate the pelvis forward, including the sacrum, you tip the coccyx up and thus you bend in the lumbar spine. On the other hand, when you slump backward, rotating the pelvis, including the sacrum, backward, the coccyx rolls too far under, and the lumbar vertebrae come out backward. Therefore, keeping the firmness in the muscles, anchor the coccyx, and then move the pelvis horizontally forward by drawing the two frontal hipbones forward and up, without displacing the chest.

The story

I am watching the dressage champion and I do not like what I see: though her legs adhere fairly stable on the horse's rib cage, her pelvis moves forward on each canter stride, while her chest hits violently back. The whole thing gives a feeling of great un-restfulness, of untidiness. In classical riding the legs and the chest are held absolutely still. They form the framework for body and horse. The pelvis, which is in the middle, is the body part that drives the horse forward: on each stride, in rhythm with the horse, the pelvis is brought forward underneath the still chest, in a beautiful, round movement. This produces the still, meditative picture we can admire in classical schools like the school in Vienna, or in Spanish riding.

In many traditions, the lower part of the body is considered the ground and the chest air. Most people are very airy, which means that they pull the body up from the chest, so that air is pulling up ground, leaving ground hanging and not grounded. The ground part must descend in order for the air part, the honeycomb of the rib cage, to be light.

Usually, when we think of opening the chest, we divide the body in the middle, displacing the chest forward. The back is pushed forward into the front of the chest, making it narrow in order to make the front wide. However, this accomplishes nothing, as our actual goal is to open *both* back and front simultaneously.

Most of us have a lot of awareness in the chest, and very little in the pelvis. Thus, we usually tilt the chest forward in relation to the pelvis. Keeping the fingers on the lower frontal ribs, if you slump the body, those ribs go backward. Then, when you try to open the chest, you push those ribs forward by caving the lumbar inward.

What you want to do, instead, is to put the ground part of the body straight underneath the air part, creating one line between pelvis and chest, and not displacing one at the cost of the other. Keeping the chest where it is, bring the pelvis underneath and in line with the chest. As you will see, once they are in line, the body can then go straight up.

This means that as the pelvis moves forward, and as the body goes up, the chest automatically opens, not only forward, but in all directions. Therefore you have to leave the chest entirely alone and work on the pelvis to get it in line with the chest, allowing the spine to go up and the chest to open. We have to be very innocent in the chest, to keep it light. But we have to be grounded in the pelvis. To be innocent in the chest is a different way of life, it is a psychological state of mind.

As I said before, people think of the pelvis and the sacrum as one unit, dividing the body from the lumbo-sacral joint, instead of from the sacro-iliac joint. Now, exactly the same thing happens in the chest region. People think of the chest as consisting of the rib cage and the spine, all fused together.

When you slump in the chest, the spine also moves backward. When you push the chest forward, the spine moves forward. Pushing the ribs with the spine forward, or slumping the ribs with the spine backwards are both incorrect. The thoracic vertebral joints are not being used at all. Again, you must separate the spinal column from the rib cage. You must use the vertebral joints, which are the joints between the ribs and the vertebrae, and the joints between the vertebrae themselves.

Thus, the spine should move into the body, but not the ribs. However, the spine should never move horizontally into the body. The spine has curves, which exist for a reason, and must be respected. Usually, we either let the spine collapse backward, or we push it too far forward, always in a horizontal movement.

The thoracic spine has a backward curve by structure. What happens when you push that part of the spine horizontally forward? You compress the inter-vertebral spaces, so that the vertebrae are bumping into each other like the wagons of a train; they do not create space between themselves.

This is why I say, and it sounds funny: 'Grow your ears long'. If you *root* the buttock bones, sitting in the cross leg position, and then you elongate the holes of the ears upward, the spot where the cervical spines enters the skull, then the whole spine elongates without losing spaces. On the contrary, it gains space in between the vertebrae. Elongating the ears upward, so that the spine moves upward, brings us back to the psychological aspect of taking away the weight of gravity upon the head.

The reason why the curves are often too pronounced in both the thoracic and in the lumbar region is because the body is pressed down by the weight of gravity. That is why we become 'shorter' as we grow older. How can bones become shorter? The bones do not become shorter, but the space between the vertebrae diminishes. The skeletal structure collapses underneath the weight of gravity.

Root the pelvis, so that it cooperates with gravity, so that the spine and the rest of the body can rise above the level of gravity, floating, light and free. As if there were a string attached to the top of the head, pulling the body upward, without displacing the chest forward or backward.

Part two: Savasana

In this part I would like to show how the body functions. Many people do a lot of poses, and often they damage the body in the process. If you understand, however, how the body functions, you can do all the poses without damaging the body. It is an education to understand as clearly as possible how to do them.

When we work using the muscles, putting too much tension in them, we strain the joints, the body. Tense muscles 'break' the joints. So we have to learn to relax the muscles, we have to learn to release the muscles and to go deep inside the body, into the joints, not to remain in the muscular periphery of the body.

For instance, when you stand in tadasana with the lumbar spine (the lower ribs and the upper abdomen) pushed forward, you 'break' the trunk in the middle, and thus you have to use a lot of muscular tension to stay upright.

The trunk consists of two main parts, the lower part and the upper part.

In the lower part of the trunk we produce the energy (from the food we eat), which keeps the body going. The pelvis has to uphold all the weight of the trunk, and therefore the bone structure here is rather heavy, and the spinal vertebrae (the sacral and coccygeal vertebrae) are fused together to lend more strength to them.

The rib cage, on the other hand, is a light structure, containing the lungs (air) and heart. Technically speaking, the weight of the body should rest on and be upheld by the pelvis (the heavy structure), but many people hold the weight of the body higher up, in the rib cage and shoulders, and thus they create a lot of tension in those areas. We have to learn to lower the center of gravity, to uphold the weight of the body in the pelvis.

As the spinal vertebrae of the sacrum and coccyx are fused together, many people think that they form part of the pelvic (iliac) structure, and so they bend forward and backward from the joints in the lumbar spine, completely ignoring the sacro-iliac joints where the spinal column (the sacrum) connects with the pelvis. This puts a great strain on the lumbar vertebrae, especially on the joint between the fifth lumbar vertebra and the sacrum, the so-called lumbo-sacral joint.

We should always remember that the spinal column ends in the tip of the coccyx, and not in the fifth lumbar vertebrae. We have to learn to do the positions using all of the body and the spinal column, not forgetting any part of it.

Lie down in savasana

When the lower ribs go down to the ground, the shoulders lift up. When the shoulders go down to the ground, the lower ribs lift up. To open the rib cage harmoniously both the lower ribs and the shoulders have to go down to the ground simultaneously, then the sternum will lift, the upper part of the chest will open, and the thoracic spine will move into the body, elongating.

Do not shorten the back of the neck by lifting the chin up to the sky, but elongate the back of the neck so that the forehead and chin are parallel to the ground. This is very important, especially in poses like head balance. You have to make sure that the forehead and the chin are on the same level, parallel to the ground. If the chin is too much in, the neck is overstretched. That is also wrong.

The ribs and shoulders should widen, so that the sternum lifts up. The body is very tricky; you have to waken the intelligence of the body. We have many habits, and one is that we use the body mainly on the front, we are not conscious on the back of the body. If I say; 'elongate the neck', you pull the chin in. We think of the front of the body, not on the back.

Classical Savasana

Lie down in savasana.

Let the back of the neck lengthen, so that the chin comes down. Do not keep the legs too far spread apart, as that caves in the lumbar too much. Keep the heels together, and then let the feet drop sideways.

The pelvis should rotate slightly backwards, so that the lumbar spine is elongated and the coccyx moves down towards the heels. Then concentrate your attention on sinking the complete weight of your body to the ground; do not withhold any of this weight.

When we stand, sit or walk there is always the risk of falling, so the muscles are always in a state of alertness in order to prevent this. In savasana this risk is absent, the body has already completely fallen, there is no way it can fall further. Thus the muscles have no reason to grip or hold on to the bones. You have to gently convince the muscles to let go of their grip on the bones, and to relinquish the entire weight of the body to the gravity of the ground.

To do this the brain has to be very alert; it should not go to sleep. The brain should be the protector of the body, helping the body to release its weight to the ground. For most of us the brain is the attacker of the body, and this attacking manifests itself in physical tensions, the tensions of the muscles gripping the bones. In yoga the brain should become the protector of the body, it should neither attack nor indulge the body, but it should help the body to regain its own inner level of peace.

If you go to sleep in savasana, it means the brain is not interested in doing this, but is only interested in indulging in its own dull state of being. The brain should not be dull, and should not indulge itself, but it should be crystal clear, piercing the body with clarity and attention, helping it to release the parts where it has stored its anxieties. The brain should help the body to release those tensions, those anxieties, to undo them.

Watch inside; watch the upper chest between the shoulders, from one end to the other. Tension is always from the periphery of the body towards the center. Watch how tension pulls the shoulders nearer to the sternum, reducing the width across the upper chest. This is the psychological defense mechanism of the body.

See if gently, internally, you can convince the muscles of the upper chest to let go of the shoulders, to undo that tension that pulls them in towards the sternum. If you do that, you feel how the shoulders automatically, by themselves, move away from the sternum, away from the thoracic spine, sideways, thus widening the upper chest across the front and the back.

You can do the same thing in the solar plexus. Most people have a certain tension underneath the lower ribs, a tightness in the solar plexus, a squeezing inwards from the periphery towards the center. Here also, watch that unnecessary tension, and gently, internally, see if you can release that grip from the periphery to the center. Again you can feel how the solar plexus widens as it releases.

In the same way watch the skin, everywhere in the body. See how the skin is hard;

see how it forms a hard barrier between you and the external space around the body. There is a barrier between the inner body and the external space, and that barrier is the skin.

The relaxation of the body is when you manage to separate the muscle, the bone and the skin. Release the skin from the body; mentally take the skin away between you and the external space. If you can do that you will feel how the body kind of swells up. That swelling is the relaxation of the muscles that let go of their grip on the bones and flow out through the skin into the space around the body. It is like a sponge. If you squeeze the sponge, it becomes smaller, harder, but when you let go of it, it swells up to its natural size. The same thing with the body. If you take the skin away, the muscles swell up like the sponge.

Tension is from the periphery to the center, relaxation is from the center to the periphery, from the bones towards the skin. By separating the bones, the flesh and the skin one from the other tension is released.

In sitting the same process has to take place, but the skeleton should remain firm. In savasana everything should fall apart, the bones, the muscles, the skin, but not the brain. The brain has to be very clear, not sleeping. If the brain sleeps, there is no intelligence in the body to undo its tensions. The brain should be firm and non-oscillating, penetrating all the parts of the body.

CLASS IV

Part one: sitting against the wall

Use the blindfold, so that you screen out the rest of the universe. You are going to sit for ten minutes and I want you to keep the body still for ten minutes, because we do not want an interruption. If you do need to stretch your legs and change, do so without disturbing your body, and then bring your body back on the wall again, the head on the wall.

Sit with your back towards the wall and wedge the sacrum against the wall, but let the rest of the trunk lean forward at an angle of eighty degrees away from the wall. Between the shoulder blades and the wall there should be a couple of inches space. Do not keep the elbows on the wall; I want you to be fairly comfortable and relaxed. The head stays in line with the trunk; do not bring the head forward or down.

This is an exploration of your own inner universe. Each one of us is a grain of sand in the outer universe, but within the grain of sand there is also an inner universe. Originally I think that yoga was meant to get you in touch with that inner world; not with your inner head, but with the inner being, with the inner 'you'.

What happens nowadays is that people, through obeying, through getting the rules and obeying them, create an outer posture, which is like a shadow posture on the outside of the body, but within the body, within the skin, within the inner universe, there is no posture. The important thing is to not create an outer shadow play, but to create something real on the inside. To do that you have to take complete control.

That means that you are the only one who can deal with your own body, nobody else can do that for you. You alone can take your exploration, can take your expedition inside your body and inside the connection between your body and your mind. Nobody can tell you how to do it; this is not a how-to situation. This is a situation where you are the explorer, and you are the Amazon river or forest that you are exploring.

The body, this organ, which is inside the skin, in reality extends far beyond the skin. But for the moment we will just deal with the skin as a dividing line between the inner and the outer world. Later on we will change that. In this inner body we need to find out where the collisions are.

Most of us, through improper exercise, through stress, etc., create an enormous amount of collision areas inside the body. A collision area means that muscles and bones collide instead of co-operate. We need to find those places, and then we need to get rid of those collision areas. We need to re-structure the body in such a way that the body is again floating on the gravitational line, instead of sinking underneath it.

To do that, certain parts of the body need to be activated, and other parts of the body need to be softened or neutralized. The collision happens when we are using ineffective muscles to do certain things. The human body is a vertical body, which means that the spinal column is aligned vertically on the gravitational field. If you try to keep the body on the gravitational field with the wrong muscles, this is where you create collision areas.

The vertical body, the vertical spine has advantages and disadvantages. The disadvantage is that it is very unstable. As long as it is on the gravitational line it is ok, but the moment it goes off from it, it creates havoc because instability sets in. This is what you see in almost every human body. So the disadvantage is the instability. On the other hand, the instability is also an advantage, as it makes the body very mobile. If we manage to bring the body back on the gravitational line, the more you can do so, the more the body can let go of those collision areas, because it does not need all those muscles to keep from falling.

In all the poses, whatever you do, standing, walking, riding your horse, yoga postures, etc., there is always a chance of falling, because the whole structure of the human body balances on two small feet, or on the two sitting bones, or on two small hands, like in full arm balance. This is very precarious. The only posture that is totally safe, let us say, is savasana, because in savasana there is no way you can fall further. The whole body has completely fallen. Savasana is a horizontal posture where every single part of the body has fallen to the floor. Therefore it is a real good 'lie detector' to find collision areas.

Today we do padmasana against the wall, so we need to deal with the gravitational force. Place the shoulder blades flat against the wall and also the back of the head. This is your vertical alignment on the gravitation field, because the wall is completely vertical. In that way, your spine being aligned on the wall, it is vertical.

As I was saying before, the vertical body is always in a state of alarm, because anything can throw it for a loop, any movement you make can throw this whole body out of alignment and bring it crashing down to the floor. Anybody who has small children knows this. Therefore the body has an incredible amount of co-ordination and muscle activity - of which you are completely unaware - to prevent this structure from falling. The more you allow the structure to go out of the proper alignment, the more frantic this inner activity becomes in order to prevent it from falling. Thus that becomes a collision area.

The first thing to do is to come back to the gravitational alignment, and then we have to find those areas where there is a chronic alarm situation going on. Almost everybody has those, because almost everybody is out of alignment. We have to find out where those chronic alarm situations are, and then see if we can undo them and bring the relaxed tone of the body back into that area.

Most people are unaware of their spine, so I want to start right there. Keeping your body on the wall, focus your attention on your spinal column. When teaching we use the eyes, because you have to see the other person, but when we deal with our own body, we go through the ears, or something that you might call ears. It is not really ears, it is not hearing, but it is an inner ear, an inner awareness. It has something vaguely to do with the balance point inside the ears, that is why I like to call it the ears. Through that inner balance point in the ears the body always knows what is the upright position, otherwise we would all be dumplings.

That is why I make you practice blindfolded, so that you can listen inside your body and then zoom your attention in on the spinal column. Now, when you want to work on the body, and especially on the alignment and on the gravitational force, you start from the point of the body where you are in touch with the ground. Like when you build a house, you start with the first bricks on the floor, you do not start with the roof.

At the base of the spine are the sacroiliac joints, the sacrum and the coccyx. Just above the sacrum there is the sacral-lumbar joint, which is one of the most stressed joints in the body, because the spine makes a very sharp angle here to connect with the sacrum. By lifting heavy objects, by wrong posture etc. that angle, that pressure, is increased.

Bring your attention to that triangle of the two sacroiliac joints and the sacral-lumbar joint. Feel, in the first place, whether that triangle is pressing equally on the wall. If the pelvis is not completely straight, but tilted, then one sacroiliac joint may be more pressing into the wall than the other. In that case you have to slightly fidget to bring both sacroiliac joints equally onto the wall. Do so silently, though.

The first thing you need to learn in yoga in order to make the body a healthy instrument is to create space inside the body. The body needs very little. The body is made of zillions of atoms; it is for the largest part energy, and we constrict that energy, we tighten that energy. Energy, in nature, wants to take more space, it wants to move. When you look at clouds, which are a form of energy, or when you look at a steaming kettle, there is an expansion going on, a movement. That is the nature of energy. You can feel how this triangle is very small; the joints are all pulling into each other, and there is no expansion.

To undo tension, there is nothing you can do. Anything you do to undo tension is to create more tension. The only way to undo tension and to create space is by paying attention, by placing your attention in that area. Attention is the key that unlocks the energy; there is no other key. Just watch that triangle, watch it very friendly, and do not try to do anything about it. Just watch it like you would watch an animal. Then you can see how that triangle begins to expand, the sacroiliac joints start moving away from each other, and the sacrum begins to gently drop down to the floor. The breathing very soft and relaxed, do not make a noise with your breathing.

Then shift your awareness higher up, into the lumbar spine. You can feel that the more you place your attention on the lumbar spine, the more the vertebrae will stop colliding into each other, and will create space to go up.

Then move up into the thoracic spine. The thoracic spine especially is a very fertile area to feel the unfolding. The weight of the head is always pressing down on the vertebrae, so make the head light. Ideally, in order to elongate the spinal column, we need to bring the ears back in line with the shoulder joints, but there are two ways of doing it. Usually people use the muscles to do that. That is not what I want you to do. I want you to use your imagination. With your imagination move the head very slowly backwards. Imagination, or visualization, is a force. Not a muscle force; a different type of force.

Visualization or intent is a force that acts on the energy in the body, while thinking is a force that acts on the muscle. In visualization or intent there is no thought energy and no muscle energy involved. You simply kind of feel your way backwards with the back of the head. Feeling your way backwards will then pull your head back. Then feel your way upwards with the back of the head and the top of the head. Feel how gradually your head wants to go up. It is not that you want it to go up, but it is the head itself that wants to go up. That will then lighten the load on the thoracic spine.

Once the thoracic spine elongates upwards like this, bring your awareness to the sides of the body, the left and the right side of the spinal column. Again this is only a question of the imagination. Feel that the whole left and right side of your body, and the back, want to move sideways, away from the spinal column. It is not a question of you pulling it sideways. It is a question of your imagination giving the green light, as it were, to that squeezed up energy to expand.

Certain areas are heavy-duty collision areas, for instance the shoulders, the trapezius muscles. Keeping the head light and high watch your trapezius muscles, watch the shoulders; do not try to do anything. Trying to do something is the worst you can do. Just watch it, watch how the tension pulls the shoulders in towards the sternum, and up towards the ears. Keep the head high and backwards and do not allow it to drop. You can start first of all imagining that you have an iron hook on top of your head with a cord hanging from the ceiling, and this cord is attached to the iron hook, pulling you up.

Then go back to the trapezius muscles and the shoulders and just work your attention inside there. Do not do anything. Attention is the key that unlocks the tension. Just by watching the shoulders, by watching the trapezius, by watching the shoulder blades, you feel how gradually the tissues around those areas kind of swell up, like the steam, like the cloud. When you are heating water, it becomes steam, which then expands. Your attention is like the heating process that makes the energy inside those collision areas expand, and that is relaxation, that is real relaxation. Not just going dumb and limp, and falling asleep. The attention has to be very sharp, that is why nobody can do this for you, you are the savior of your body, and nobody else. To save your body, you need to train your attention to unlock the collision areas in your body.

Tomorrow we will add breathing, but now, without opening your eyes, just slide away from the wall, lie on your back and do savasana, without disturbing the body or the mind. Keep the eyes covered with the blindfold. Do not wriggle; do not do anything, just lie on your back. Let the energy continue expanding, let your body continue expanding in all directions, not because you use the muscle force, but because you look at your energy with your attention, and therefore you are giving it the green light.

Part two: sitting and breathing

Place the blindfold over your eyes and do not disturb. First find your sitting position. Take one or two minutes to find your balance.

Yesterday we brought the attention to the spinal column. The center of your body, in this position, starts in the pelvis. In circus language, there is a certain act, which is called the Russian bar. In this, there are two men holding a bamboo bar in between them, and there is a girl who stands on top of the bar. The men flip this girl up, and then she does all kinds of things, like hanumanasana, or full arm balance. The men are called the 'porteur', and the girl the 'agile'. It is very interesting to apply this concept in the practice of yoga. We always have to find out which part of the body is the 'porteur', and which part is the 'agile'.

The porteur, the two men holding the bamboo bar, have to be very stable. In this case, the two men that are holding the bar are the two hip joints. By slightly constricting the two hip joints inwards, you create the stability for the buttock bones to elongate downwards, thus creating that rebounding force that then travels back upwards (the agile).

Actually, at the base of your body, there are four points: the two buttock bones, the pubic bone on the front and the coccyx on the back. For a couple of seconds experiment with this: that actually the buttock bones are the real roots, because they are the ones that are on the ground, while the pubic bone and the coccyx are more like air roots of the banyan tree, because they are not really on the floor. What you can experiment with is that those four points should go down equally to the ground. That is not always the case.

There are four possibilities: the possibility that the body goes too much to the left, too much to the right, too much to the front, or too much to the back. To experience this swing the body slightly over the right buttock bone, over the right hip, and feel how that changes your balance. Then come back to the center and then swing the body slowly and carefully over the left buttock bone, and feel how it changes your balance. If you watch the spinal column internally you also see how, when you go over the right buttock bone, the lumbar spine curves to the right, and when you go to the left it curves over the left. Thus you see that the spine always has to compensate on the gravitational line, otherwise the body will fall over. You have to come to a point where you are exactly in balance between the two buttock bones.

Then you can do the same thing with the pubic bone and the coccyx. With some people, especially when the hip joints are not really working properly, the pelvis is rotated backwards; they are sitting more on the coccyx and sacrum area. On the other hand, if you are too enthusiastic, too hard working, you might roll the pelvis too far forward and so you are rolling the pubic bone down to the floor. Just experiment with this and feel the effect is has on the lumbar spine. When you roll the pelvis backwards, bringing the coccyx further down to the floor, you feel how the lumbar spine is pulled backwards, while if you are really trying very hard to roll forwards so that the pubic bone goes down to the floor you can feel how the lumbar spine caves in. Again you have to come to the position where everything is held in an even and easy balance.

Yesterday I isolated the spinal column out of the body, to move everything away from the spinal column. Today I want to talk more about the relationship between the pelvis and the chest. The body has three 'boxes': the head box, the chest box and the pelvis box. For many people the posture is held too high up, either in the chest or in the head.

Yesterday we showed that many people push the head too far forward. In that case you have to bring the head backward, so that the back of the head is floating over the shoulder blades. On the other hand, some people might be too eager to lift the rib cage up, because you are told to do so. Those two boxes are like the top part of a three-deck bus, not a London double-deck bus, but a three-deck bus. You can imagine what happens to the bus if all the weight is held up in the two top stories: the bus is going to be very unstable.

The center of gravity is low in the pelvis. If you shoot an arrow through the two hip joints, and then shoot another arrow from the front of the lower abdomen, halfway between the navel and the pubic bone, and through the second sacral vertebra, where those two arrows cross, in the middle of the body, this is where your center of gravity is, what they call in Japanese hara. This is the center where the body should rest.

It is very easy, when you think of that center in the lower pelvis, to collapse the whole body. You do not want to do that. Keep the head in alignment with the shoulder joints, the ears, and feel that hook on top of the head, with the cord pulling you up towards the sky. The head is being pulled up to the sky, and that helps to elongate the spinal column. Like yesterday, isolate the spinal column out of the chest, and let it elongate upwards towards the head, which is being pulled up.

Then, look at your rib cage, look at your lower ribs, and if you have the habit of pushing those ribs forward and pulling the body up from the ribs, then you can use several images to find your bearings. One image, for instance, for people who have a very big rib cage which always pulls upwards is that the chest is like an umbrella, with the spine as the stick of the umbrella and the ribs like the cloth which is raised high as if it is raining. Some people always walk around as if it is raining, with the umbrella open. So, keeping the head high, gently let the umbrella close, let the cloth fall down onto the pelvis, without losing the height and the respectability of the spinal column, the dignity of the spinal column; let the parachute or the umbrella fall nicely and drop into the lower abdomen, and let the lower abdomen receive that energy and bounce it back up again, without reopening the umbrella.

Another image that I like to use when people hold the body up from the chest and the pelvis and legs are kind of dangling is an image from the aquarium. If you go to an aquarium you can see those beautiful jelly fish: many people are like those jelly fish in the sense that they have this wide and open chest like the body of the jelly fish, and the pelvis, the lumbar spine and the legs are hanging down from this umbrella shaped jelly fish like its tentacles. Bring everything down to the lower abdomen, and then hold the whole structure of the body up from there.

We have three points of reference: first the central point of gravity, which is in the center of the lower abdomen and from which the whole body is held up from, supported by; second, out of that point the lumbar and thoracic spine grow upwards, vertebra per vertebra: third, the fontanel is held high by that small cord attached to the head that is pulling you upwards. These are your three points of reference: the lower abdomen, top of the head and the spinal column.

Then bring your attention to your breathing. Breathing is of course an affair of the lungs, the rib cage, but this is not entirely true, because actually the whole body breathes. First bring your attention to the chest, and watch the lungs inside your chest. Watch the left lung, watch the right one. Find out where you are breathing, are you breathing more on the left, more in the right, more on the front, more on the back. I give you two minutes the time to follow your own breathing internally and find out if your lungs are like a balloon, a round balloon, where the air moves in all directions simultaneously, or whether your lungs are lumpy, and the air goes a little bit here, a little bit there, with empty spaces in the middle. Watch your own breathing.

Then, without paying any special attention to the breathing, we are going to expand this breathing to fill the entire body. This means a little subtlety, and I can give you a bit of help: we are going to play wind chimes. Shift your attention to the outside and listen to the trees, the wind in the trees as it rustles the leaves. Leaves rustling in trees are a very nice tool to use. In a way it is the breathing of the trees, the trees are also inhaling and exhaling, and that makes a rustling sound.

Sound can only move through a vehicle. What you are going to do now in order to continue what we did yesterday, this expansion movement, we are going to do it now from the breathing. You are listening to the rustling of the trees, to the sound of the leaves, and then you are going to breathe into the sound of the leaves.

You can start simply with your chest, your rib cage. When your rib cage expands, you push it outwards as it were; you expand the rib cage out into the sound of the wind in the leaves. You transcend in a way the skin on the rib cage, so your breathing is no longer inside the chest, the rib cage, but you are breathing way beyond the rib cage.

Again, the more you relax the skin, the more you can breathe outward, going into the sound of the wind. Breathe into the sound; on the inhalation you breathe into the sound; on the exhalation, you retreat from the sound.

Then gradually add the rest of the body, so the next wind wave which comes, add your arms and shoulders. Breathe through the arms into the sound, so that you feel that the arms are also participating in this expansion as you breathe. You can actually feel the breathing going through the arms and shoulders outwards. So as the wind comes, go into it. On the inhalation, you go into the sound, on the exhalation, you retreat: a wave action. Go into it, and then retreat.

On the next wind wave you are going to add your pelvis and lumbar, the lumbar region. On the sound, on the wind wave go into it, with the breathing coming out of the pelvis, out of the lumbar spine, out of the lumbar region, out of the kidneys, into the sound of the wind. Go into it as it comes. Out and in, but always way beyond the skin. Breathe from the pelvis, from the lumbar into the sound, into the wind wave, breathe from the lumbar. Like yesterday, the more you relax the muscles, the more you can breathe into the sound.

On the next wind wave, add the legs, the thighs, the feet, the whole body breathing. Go with the legs into the sound on the inhalation, the whole body into the sound, into the sound as it comes at you.

On the next wave you take the last part of your body, which is your head. It is the most difficult and the most fun and the most rewarding. When the sound comes, expand your whole head into the sound, the brain, the face, everything, the muscles of the face, go into the sound with your breathing, so you breathe from the center of your head outward, into the sound. Take a point in the center of your head and already move outwards from there. Go into the wave as it comes. The face, the brain, relaxing from the center outward. Watch your facial muscles, ease into the sound with your relaxation.

You can do this exercise any time you are outside, where you can breathe parallel to the sound of the wind, which is very nice. You can parallel the movement or sound with your inhalation and exhalation, but keep the skin completely non-existent: the body becomes like a huge cloud which expands and retreats according to your own rhythm, but also according to the sound around you.

Then, without opening your eyes, keeping the blindfold on, just change your legs, stretch the knees, stretch the legs, and when you are ready, when the body has come back to normal, you can take your blindfold off.

We have taken ourselves out of nature, out of the world; we do not even remember that we too are a product of nature, that we are an animal, just like all the other animals. Therefore the skin has become very tight, and we are inside the skin. We live inside the skin, and then we try to communicate, but that does not work. The skin prevents us from being in communication with the outside, it prevents us from remembering that we are only an animal, another product of nature, we are only another natural thing, and it prevents us from being a conduit. If we can take the skin away, and really feel that the atoms of the body are like a cloud and expand and expand, so that the energy, the wind, everything goes through, then it means that we are not generating our own energy inside our skin, but we are just taking the energy as it goes through us, and we use it. We are catching it as it goes through us. So there is no barrier.

Tomorrow we can use another image, another way, how to get in touch with our inner body, and how the inner body can use what is around us in order to become bigger and bigger, more in tune with everything. I think it is very important for the health to be completely open for the energy. In one of my books I wrote that if you have water washing over cement, it does not go through, but if you are on the beach and the wave comes, you watch the water and in a couple of seconds it is gone, because it just goes through the sand. If we can be like the sand on the beach and let everything just go through.

The story

There was a young swords man in Japan, who was a champion samurai and very ambitious, he wanted to be number one. He knew that there was an old teacher somewhere whom everybody said was the best. So he challenged him to a fight, but the old man refused. But one day the old man consented, so they set up a meeting. They drew lots, to see who would strike first, and the old man won. So he drew his sword, and hit the young man on the head, but the sword broke, so strong was the young man. Then it was the young man's turn. He took his sword, raised it high, and hit the old man on the head, but to his surprise the sword went straight through the body of the old man without leaving a trace.

Part three: sitting and breathing

Once you are all seated, see if for ten minutes you can not disturb the body, because we do need to go back to the posture and how to sit.

In all the postures we need to find a very fine balance between having certain integrity in the posture, and at the same time not to stress the body. We need to find the place from which to hold the body up, and at the same time a place of rest.

Sitting on the floor in cross legs your base is formed by the pelvis and the crossed legs. This is the image of the cobra, the coiled tail of the snake. We need to find out how to sit straight, with the spinal column growing straight up out of the pelvis, with the pelvis in a vertical position, and at the same time not pulling the body up from wrong body parts, from mistaken body parts.

In this human body the upholding power of the body is in the pelvis, in the lower abdomen. This is a physical point, in the sense that it is in the physical body, but it is also an etheric point, an energy point. Yesterday we were talking about breathing into the sound of the poplar trees, and also that the breathing should come out of the whole body, not just out of the spinal column or out of the rib cage.

If you want to find the center of the body it is good to almost make an x-ray of your own body inside, where the bone structure is visible, while the soft part of the body is like a shadowy outline. Find the x-ray of your body, which is the pelvis and the spinal column, and see if this bone structure is strong, firm. When you pull the body up from the spinal column in the thoracic area, that is bringing it way too high in the body, and therefore it is not efficient. The efficient thing to do is to place all your awareness, all your weight bearing in the pelvis, and then let the spine easily elongate upwards out of there.

In other words, the buttock bones should grow down into the ground underneath you. We were also talking about the air. Air is actually also a substance, so for beginners I might say that you have a hook on top of your head, which pulls you up, or you have a book on top of your head and you have to push up into the book. A nicer and more sophisticated way is to say that the top of the head, the fontanel, is also a root, it can root into the air mass above it. You can almost feel the air mass above the head, and then root the fontanel into the air mass above you.

Then shift your awareness to the energy inside the body. The energy in the body has to do with awareness; you can only detect it by awareness, you cannot detect it normally. Be aware of this energy. Now this energy is not a flimsy entity. It is an actual thing, and it shows for instance in Kirlian photography, where you can see the light coming out of the body. It still has a certain mass, a certain weight. I was always told that when people die, when they weight them after one or two days, the body weighs less than before, because this luminous body, energy body, has gone. This body has weight and bulk. Inside your body, feel where this energy body is sitting.

Usually, because we are so frontal body oriented, this energy body is pressing forward into the frontal body. Feel for instance your chest. That is an easy part to feel. You can feel how this inner weight tends to push forward to the frontal chest. Keeping your spine completely straight, see if you can internally bring the weight of the chest backwards towards the back ribs. If you do so you can feel the back ribs widen.

You can do the same thing with the pelvis. The internal weight on the abdominal area and the pelvis area, which collapses forward into the front wall of the abdomen. That is why people hang in the lumbar. Again, keeping the pelvis vertical and the lumbar spine growing up out of the vertical pelvis, see if you can bring the inner weight of the body back to lodge against the lumbar spine and the sacroiliac joints. Physically you are not shifting the weight; you are shifting the weight psychically. If you do that you can again feel how the lumbar broadens, the sacroiliac joints broaden and ease off.

The most delicate part of course is the head; again because we are such cerebral creatures, we always push the energy forward into the frontal brain. We are also very neurotic creatures, and so we always push the energy forward into the face. This is why people at the age of forty have already deep furrows on the front of the forehead and around the mouth; there are all these creases because the energy is tight in there.

The body has its own mechanism. When you are cold or upset or angry, the body tends to shrink inside. Which means that the energy moves from the skin inwards towards the skeletal structure. That is why people who are shy or upset tend to hunch over with the arms folded in front of the chest. That is a defensive posture.

When you are in a relaxed mood and happy and having a good time, when you are on the beach in the hot sun, the whole body tends to spread-eagle outwards and the energy moves from the skeletal structure outwards towards the skin and out into the air around the skin. This is called relaxation. Tension is from the periphery of the body inward towards the center, and relaxation is from the inner body outward towards the periphery and out through the skin out.

The face is the same thing, only it is more delicate. The face is much more of a barometer for what happens inside. Again the constricting movement inward is a question of tension, while opening is a question of relaxation. We have to understand the front brain and the back brain.

The back brain is the old part. It is the root for seeing, for hearing, for the physical body, which has old knowledge, out of the time of the dinosaurs. That is why the back brain is often called the reptilian brain. It is old and it is cold.

The frontal brain is young, it is the monkey brain; it is only three million years old, and it is a kind of computer. It knows how to calculate. It is also very excited. It is also very presumptuous.

Because it is young, like young things, it thinks that it knows everything. The frontal brain thinks it knows everything. Therefore the frontal brain tends to pull everything along. It pulls all the energy forward into the head. It sucks the energy forward; it sucks the energy into the face. This is why thinking, which is a typical product of the big brain – thinking is the formulation of words, sentence and pictures – belongs to the frontal brain and has the effect on the face in the form of narrowing the face inward, of making the face narrow and pushing forward. The mouth going in and forward, the forehead creasing inward, toward the center, and the eyes following the excitement of the brain.

Thus the eyes bring the focus on the inner corners of the eyes. With the blindfold you can see that you are focusing through the inner corners of the eyes. The effect is tensing the temples inward, making the temples narrow, and making the eyes a little hard and dry. All this has to do with the frontal brain. The frontal brain cannot understand, the frontal brain can only make a lot of excitement. Therefore the face follows the frontal brain, and therefore this whole thinking process, which affects the face, does not take you very far.

We need to come back to the old brain, to the old part of the body. For me personally, this is the meaning of yoga. People are always very presumptuous, saying that yoga is union between man and god, and all that. I do not know if anybody knows what god it. Let us keep closer home, and just say that yoga is the bridge or yoke between the young part of the human being and the old part, and finding a balance, a bridge between the two of them, where both are held in balance. You need to use the young brain, but when you do not need to use it, you put it on hold, and go back to the old one. Most people, however, are stuck and caught and trapped in the frontal brain, in the thinking brain, and it is very difficult for them to turn the internal radio off.

Yoga means that you can turn the internal radio on and off at will, and are not the victim of the frontal brain.

Keep your head exactly where it is, and see if you can bring the energy of the front of the head into the back in the same way as you did with the chest and the pelvis. An easy way to do that is to think of the eyes. The person who looks through the eyes, the 'you' who looks through the eyes, is usually standing right behind the eye balls. That is why you are looking though the inner corners of the eyes and the eyes are sharp and dry. This is concentric vision.

Pull the nerves of the eyes backwards; the roots of the eyes are actually in the back of the brain. Like a thera band stretch the nerves of the eyes backwards, so that you are standing actually in the back of the head, looking out through the whole dark room of your inner head to look out through the eyes. The more you move backwards, the more you notice that you are looking through the outer corners of the eyes. Therefore the eyes become wide and soft and liquid. This is peripheral vision.

The dry and hard qualities belong to the inner corners of the eyes when you are standing right behind the eyes. When you are moving backwards in the head, you move automatically to the outer corners of the eyes, and the eyes lose that hardness and dryness, and become soft and liquid. I think that the old Egyptian paintings with those people with the eyes lined sideways, that is probably what they meant to indicate, that the eyes have to move sideways in order to access the back of the brain.

You can do the same thing with the ears, with the mouth and with the forehead. The more you can go back inside the head using peripheral vision, the more the forehead widens, it loses its creases, the eyes widen and the face widens. As the energy is pulled backwards into the back of the head the face loses its hard quality of the' I know it all 'of the frontal brain. So you bring again a balance between the front and the back; not all in the front, but the whole frontal body yields and brings the energy into the back of the body, so that the spine in the middle, the gravitational line in the middle, divides the energy exactly in two: front and back.

The option or the choice is that if you need to function behind your computer, you can go to the front brain, but when you shut off the computer, the radio, and you want to have a holiday and go into the garden, then you have to move towards the back brain, because the frontal brain is useless in the garden.

At this moment, since we are in the garden, bring the energy on the back, and then go back to the breathing. The other day I was using the sound of the wind in the trees, but if you do not have any sounds around you, you can also visualize that you are sitting in an egg shaped container and that you move outward into the egg shaped container, or just expand the whole body sideways, up, down, forward and back, in all directions.

This is not something you can do; it is something that' happens' when you take the skin all around the body away, when you really make the skin so invisible that at a certain point you do not even know where your body ends and where the space around you begins; the dividing line becomes very fuzzy, invisible.

There is a slight breeze in the trees, and there are some other sounds going on. Just for you to experiment with this, when you are breathing and when you are sitting, listen to the wind sound, listen to the occasional bird sound: you can clearly feel that most of the time your body 'feels' the sound on the front of the body. The sound of the wind is like one of those rain sticks, you can 'feel' it on the front of the chest, on the front of the abdomen.

Now see if you can 'feel' it on the back too, on your shoulder blades, 'feel' the sound with your shoulder blades, hear the sound with the back of your waist, the back of the lumbar. Again you can clearly see that the more you listen to the sounds with the back of the lumbar, the back of the chest, the shoulder blades, the more the tension dissolves and your back gets bigger and broader. Not because you are 'doing' that, but because it happens, because you are listening.

Listen to the bird sounds with your shoulders, the shoulders reaching out to listen to the birds, not reaching out in a motoric, physical sense, but reaching out in an energetic sense, in a psychic sense. And the sound of the traffic, see if you can hear, listen, to the sound of the traffic with the base of the head, with the back, the base of the head meeting the sound halfway. The sound is a wave, so your listening energy waves out to meet the wave of the traffic sounds. Then there are also the little lightning streaks of bird song going through the whole thing, sharp jittery lightning streaks.

This kind of practice is easy to do when you are sitting still and do not have to worry about anything. You can just play this game of seeing if you can bring the front and the back of the body in balance, but in reality this should be applied to all the postures. In all the postures, if you want to take notes, you have to use the front part of the body and the frontal brain, but if you want to actually do the postures from a place of relaxation and elongation, you have to move into the back of the body. So when you are doing back bends, or forward bends, or standing poses, if you can slide the posture out of the back of the body it will have a very different flavor from doing it from the front of the body.

Now slowly take the blindfold off, but keep your eyes closed, because the light will be very sharp, and gradually let your eyelids absorb the light before you open your eyes.

part four
on the artful teacher

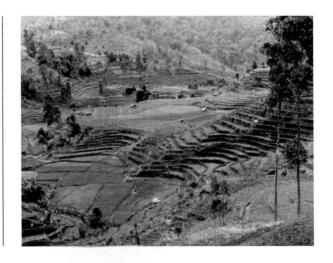

It is an art to be a student, and it is an even greater art to be teacher. Learning is at the base of being a teacher, as it is at the base of being a student, but learning and teaching are arts that have to be learned, and the place where to start is with oneself.

To explain certain concepts we sometimes have to borrow from other disciplines to fill in the gaps not covered by the practice of yoga. In this way we can enrich yoga beyond its boundaries and show new roads to old goals.

I would like to use the following concepts borrowed from the Japanese culture and from classical horse riding.

These are:
> **Being centered in hara**
> **Being pro-active**
> **Being *durchlaessig***
> **To have *schwung***

The first concept is *hara*

Being centered in hara is the one and most important concept to understand for the artful teacher.

The word hara derives from the Japanese culture and stands, on the physical level, for the center of gravity, and on the spiritual level for the seat of the spirit. Where exactly is this center in the body? We find hara in the lower abdomen in the center of the pelvis, between the navel and the pubic bone.

This is the point through which the vertical force of gravity travels and it is therefore the center of gravity or the point around which the human being keeps itself in balance. Any disturbance here will disturb the balance of the body. The disturbance of the body contributes to the disturbance of the mind and the emotions.

Hara is the first area the artful teacher has to be aware of and the first one to be firmly established. This center is an automatic center, and at the same time it is not. Without an intense awareness of its existence and therefore of its use, this center loses 80% of its power as a balancing center of stability.

The asanas in the practice of yoga are nothing else than the reorganizing of the various parts of the body around hara.

In order to make the body light and fluid, all the asanas have to be done in relationship to the center of gravity, like the chairs of the children's merry-go-round which, turning around the central pole, maintain the same distance from that pole.

Thus every asana begins and ends with the center of gravity and the body moves soft and relaxed around this center.

However, the center of gravity or hara does not only have a balancing quality from a physical point of view, but it has also a mental and emotional stabilizing effect.

Whoever is well balanced in hara has little problem being healthy on an intellectual, mental, emotional and physical level.

The second concept I would like to introduce is being *pro-active*, and not re-active

To be pro-active means to make things happen, not wait till they happen by themselves. One could define a pro-active person someone who ties the horse before the cart. Whoever is pro-active is lightly ahead of things – programming the course of action and then following it.

This is the opposite from the person who is re-active: one could say that this is a person that puts the cart before the horse. Someone who allows himself to be swept up by events, often impotent before these.

A pro-active teacher is one who is ahead of the situation, one who has a plan and understands the consequences of this plan. If there is an asana to be done, this teacher has a profound understanding of the asana with its benefits and dangers. She is therefore in a position to prevent possible accidents.

In contrast, a re-active teacher does not have a well-defined program with which to begin, and therefore can only re-act when things go bad, trying to solve the problems that may come up to the best of her ability.

Not only is the pro-active teacher aware of the problems inherent in a certain asana, but she is also aware of the capacity and the limitations of her student. She has the clarity to stop before the physical, mental and emotional problems arise.

The teacher needs to be aware of the limitations and the capacity of the student on all levels: mental, intellectual, emotional and physical, and not push the student beyond the limits within which the student can deal with the demands of the teacher.

The third concept is the German word *durchlaessigkeit* and its opposite: *opposition reflex*

These two forces are inherent in all living beings.

Durchlaessig is a German word that I have borrowed from classical riding. The German word durchlaessig means literally 'to let go through' and is used to describe a horse that is well trained and that accepts the aids of his rider and executes them willingly and precisely without rebelling. It is the quality of being porous, to allow things to go through without resistance, without opposition. It is the state of being receptive, fluid, of not fighting that which is presented to it, but to allow it to go through without leaving any physical, emotional or mental residue.

The concept of durchlaessigkeit is applied on all four levels: intellectual, mental, emotional and physical.

The opposite of durchlaessigkeit is the opposition reflex.

The opposition reflex is what the name says. Body, mind and emotions oppose whatever is presented; it is the reflex of fighting or fleeing which every living being has when confronted with situations which it considers dangerous for the survival of the body or for the usual way of thinking or feeling.

This fight-or-flight reflex belongs to all living beings, be they insects, birds or mammals. It is a powerful survival tool common to everybody, including human beings.

Even though this opposition reflex is useful at times, like when we find ourselves in a moment in which it is legitimate to defend ourselves, at other times it creates problems, like when we want to explore a new territory, for instance learn a new asana, or change our way of thinking or feeling.

Fear is at the root of the opposition reflex. The artful teacher does not only need to be aware of this phenomenon in herself, but also in the student. She needs to be able to guide the student into this new territory, avoiding the fight-or-flight reflex, knowing how far to go, how fast to go and when to stop before provoking the fight-or-flight reflex. She needs to know the art of 'tocca-e-fuga' or 'advance and retreat', presenting lightly a new asana to the student, stay for a short time and then retreat again, without insisting too much, too long and too heavily, so as not to give the student the time to go into the opposition reflex.

The fourth concept is the German word *schwung*

This is again a German word that is difficult to translate. It means literally 'swing' and stands for a forward movement on all levels.

In classical riding, the definition of a horse that has schwung, is that he has an energetic and free walk and a sharp mind to follow the instructions of the rider.

With an attitude of not opposing new situations or new information, but to accept them as a means of moving into a new territory and therefore of growing and expanding, schwung means the enthusiasm and the forward pushing energy with which you do what you do.

Schwung in the development of the teacher herself means the enthusiasm to learn more about the anatomy of the body as an intellectual exercise, and a fearlessness to explore her mental and emotional states and their connection to the body as cause of durchlaessigkeit or opposition reflex.

It is in general that energy that takes you forward with brio.

In her relationship with the student, the artful teacher who possesses schwung is in a position to awaken the enthusiasm in the student, to awaken the internal energy in the student that then will take the student forward.

A dull teacher can only create dull students.

Therefore the three concepts of being pro-active, durchlaessig and to have schwung are intimately connected and find their source of security and stability in the fact of being centered in hara or the center of gravity.

The art of the teacher is to integrate these concepts on four levels, to create health and well-being.

What is intellectual health?

The teacher is intellectually healthy when she understands the necessity to study the human body from the anatomical and physiological point of view, before dealing with it.

The asanas have a profound effect on the body; they deal not only with the muscles and the skeletal structure, but they also interfere with the organism and therefore the teacher should not only have a profound knowledge of anatomy and physiology, but also know in which way each asana influences the body.

The teacher should never have the presumption to know everything, but should always leave ample space for research.

She should realize that learning never finishes, that every moment is a new moment and that that which could be applied in the previous moment, may not be suitable in this present moment, since the body is a mutating being (it is alive, grows and changes).

Thus the meaning of intellectual health is the capacity to continue studying the body from all points of view and to apply this knowledge in the teaching of the asanas.

What is mental health?

At the basis of every movement and of every action is the mind. The mind is the initiator and the mind is the controller.

A mind that is not clear, that does not have a clear intent, can never produce a clear movement. What is intent? Intent is the image in our mind of what we want to do. This image has to be clear, well defined, free from doubts and uncertainties. It is not simply visualization. Intent is the visualization that has the power of self-fulfillment, which is so strong that the movement, the action comes by itself as a result.

This is the meaning of mental health: to have an image that does not vacillate and which allows the body to transform the image in action.

It is a mind that does not get distracted, that does not get confused, but is calm and collected. This mind is capable to see clearly and to decide which action to undertake under the given circumstances.

What is emotional health?

Emotional health is the most difficult to cultivate and on which many teachers shipwreck.

The Greek poet Homer describes the hero as a man who stands like a rock in the boiling waters. One can say the same thing of the artful teacher. The art of the teacher is to not be influenced by the emotional states of the students, not to be re-active. The teacher possesses the art of durchlaessigkeit, allowing the emotions to pass through and go out again without retaining them for re-active use.

It is the most difficult health to acquire because emotions are contagious and create a dependency at the same time. Often they have the tendency to create a landslide effect, impeding any further progress. We all know that if we stand next to a sad person, that sadness is communicated to us and if we allow that to happen, we end up in the same way. This is what it means, that emotions are contagious.

They are also a source of dependency. Some scientists have discovered that emotions are in reality small molecules that have the capacity to group together. If we allow ourselves to be sad about something for a small period of time, this can become a dependency and to change our state of mind needs then a certain 'reset' (reprogramming). Therefore the teacher should never allow the students to communicate their negative moods, and should always maintain emotional distance.

What is physical health?

For the common doctor physical health is the absence of an obvious disease. This is far from real health. A healthy body is a body that, even if there is a disease, carries itself with a certain brio, a certain joy-de-vivre. It is a body that is confident, that has a strong aura and has self-carriage, another concept borrowed from classical riding, where self-carriage is the definition of a horse that shows a proud and collected posture. It is the opposite of the collapsed posture that one often sees and that can only communicate a depressed and collapsed personality.

The teacher is a role model and her first thought is to communicate to her students that brio and that health that she herself possesses.

This is done through example, not through descriptions. Words can never produce that effect. The human body is a photocopy machine: it copies what it sees and therefore the responsibility of the teacher is to present the right image in such a way that the student can copy it.

Thus the art of the teacher is to show health on these four levels with the application of being centered in hara, to be pro-active, to possess durchlaessigkeit and schwung and to be able to communicate these to her students.

epilogue

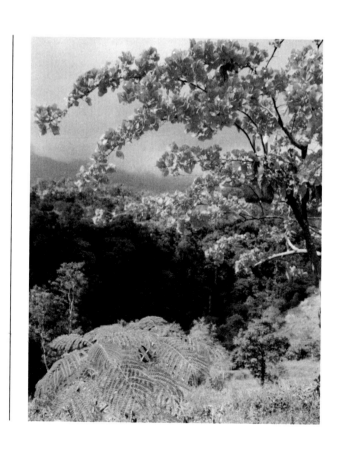

Introduction to Megamendung

The following chapter was written while I was visiting Indonesia in 1996. After the Second World War my family moved back to Indonesia, where my mother had been born and raised, and where she met and married my father. I spent part of my childhood there, and the Indonesian sounds, sights and smells are an integral part of my being.

Due to political turmoil my family was forced to leave the country in 1956. In 1958 I started practicing yoga while living in Holland. When I went back for a visit to Indonesia after forty years, I carried with me thirty-eight years of yoga practice with me.

Patanjali calls the final samadhi the dharma-mega-samadhi, the rain-cloud of samadhi. My uncle's family used to live in a small town in the mountains, called Megamendung, which, in the Indonesian language, means 'big rain cloud'.

The impact of Indonesia after so many years galvanized me into summarizing my personal understanding of yoga. I say personal, because each yoga practitioner has her or his own personal interpretation of yoga, her or his own vision.

Having gone through so many upheavals in my life – world war, civil war, revolution, changing countries, changing cities, I came to realize that philosophies and religions cannot – can never – explain or substitute life, the universe, or us. It is when we are empty of words and concepts that the universe can reveal its ultimate goodness that can fill the human heart with a joy that goes beyond explanations. This joy is not something that we can solicit. It has its own momentum, and can only come to us in that moment when the past and the future are absent, and we face the absolute present, the absolute here-and-now. Words can only stand between us and that goodness that goes beyond the human capacity to comprehend, even the words here-and-now. In that moment of being face to face with the ultimate present is the human heart broken and flooded by the rain cloud of joy, of beauty, of love.

MEGAMENDUNG (Tropical Rain cloud)

Meditations of an old yogini

I came to Indonesia because I had some business to do. Apart from being ecstatically happy to walk the streets of Bandung again after so many years I had to see if I could get rid of some of the old skeletons in my cupboard, doing some house cleaning, as it were. To proceed in life with the new, one has to first get rid of the old, so that one is fresh and unencumbered.

Seems a small task? Well, let's begin at the beginning.

My father. His early death made me idolize him as a child. Classical, would any psychologist tell you.

When my mother died, I suddenly had this sense of a second loss. Where, during my mother's life, my dead father had 'belonged' to me, now suddenly he 'belonged' again to my equally dead mother. They were again together, and I felt left out.

Lesson number one: Nobody belongs to anybody. Everybody belongs only to him or herself. Let go of people and the dependency on them, and learn to see each human being as a luminous, self-contained parcel, floating in an infinite universe, alone in utter aloneness, and yet bumping into and joining with other balls of luminosity for a while, to again continue afterwards on this lonely journey through eternity.

Some interesting perspectives here.

Like compassion. Where does compassion come from? From our own judgments, based on what others tell us or show us. Sad stories and our reaction to the sad stories, which have nothing to do with eternity and the great journey. As such, compassion is a terrible thing, an illusion based on fear and presumptuousness. Fear of the eternal, the unknown, death, and presumptuousness in thinking that we know what is good and what is bad. Between these two they form a sandwich with the human being squashed in the middle, dripping tears.

I am sitting in my hotel room with the door wide open on the patio. It is pouring with rain, and the sound of the drops on the big leafed tropical plants is like music.

This is happiness – listening to the rain, smelling the smells of Indonesia, the sound of the Indonesian language drifting up to my room, thinking, thinking . . .

My Indonesian childhood, and then thrown out of the garden of Eden into the cold and frosty streets of Holland. The sounds, the smells, the faces that were locked in the cells of my blood in a static picture of a skinny girl bicycling along the streets, horse riding among the tea bushes, doing home work on the large, triangular, stone veranda of the house called home.

It is all there, walled-in by many years of living, of gathering new experiences, of learning new lessons.

But they are there, and the minute I peek through a hole in the wall, there she is, the fourteen year old girl, lying in bed on a winter morning in Holland, waiting for the familiar morning sounds, the peanut vendor, the tea vendor, that would not come, not this morning, not tomorrow morning, not ever again. Bicycling to school through snow, looking at white faces, blue eyes, big, slow, awkward moving bodies, big, slow, awkward moving minds. Looking backwards, always looking backwards, to a future which would never come back.

Now the skinny girl is a fifty-year-old woman, and there is work to be done. Picking up bits and pieces of myself off the streets of Bandung, out of the university gardens where my mother taught biology, listening to the echo of the laughter of a young girl between the drops of a tropical rainstorm, searching the faces around me for recognition, looks and gestures mirrored through the amber colored blood of a great grand mother in my body, my face, my gestures. Recognizing which gesture, which expression, which turn of a bone comes directly from this mixture of blood and memory. And always the memories, which are right underneath the surface, of love and regret mingled together . . .

Met this man once, actually a friend brought him to my house. He told me he lived in the Himalayas most of the year, being more interested in spiritual yoga than in hatha yoga.

Blue eyes looking into mine and quick flashes of smile, mainly around the mouth and some around the eyes. Not inside the eyes. The smiles come and go too quickly. A really good smile is slow to start and even slower to end. These smiles were like lightning ripples on the surface of the face, with the underlying muscle remaining cold.

My friend, who had brought him, seemed a little overwhelmed by him. He talked about swamis and yoga and bathing in the cold waters of the Ganges at four o'clock in the morning at an altitude of three thousand meters.

He also said he came to Europe every year for a couple of months. To teach, he said, because people asked him. I thought about the four o'clock in the morning dips in the Ganges and wondered. Hot water showers, down beds and western meals might also have something to do with these visits. Being spiritual in the Himalayas is OK for a certain time, but I guess one needs a holiday from it occasionally.

Hidden messages. The word spiritual, as opposed to hatha yoga, frequently cropped up, with the underlying meaning that I was doing physical yoga, while he was on the spiritual path. In the Himalayas.

'A romantic place to be', commented another friend of mine, who is also on the seekers trail. He had tried it, being of an idealistic frame of mind. But being maybe a little more sober than the other man realized soon that being cold, damp, hungry and lonely at three thousand meters altitude was not much fun, and might result in death without achievement. So he came back to the hot showers and the down beds, defeated by the excessive romantic-ness of the Himalayan yoga trip.

Yoga, like everything else in life, is an attention trap, trapping, or corralling the attention of people within a certain fenced-off space, or mental (spiritual) corral.

The mind is more or less allowed to wander freely within the fenced-in area, but is not encouraged to jump the fence.

If we look at the world like a map, we see hundreds, thousands, of these corrals, where people are fenced in, having bartered their free roaming status for security against predators (i.e. other predators than the one who rules the corral), and three meals a day (psychologically or spiritually speaking).

All these groups of people, yoga practitioners, whether physical or spiritual, or others, that swarm around a central figure, the guru, the swami, the man (or woman) who knows what you don't know, like bees around their queen.

I once had a bee swarm like that on the wall of my house. It was amazing, I watched them day in, day out. They would cluster around the queen so tightly in the evening that you could actually scrape them off the wall like a lump of sugar candy, with little lumps of bee clusters dropping off from the big lump, to immediately dissolve itself in so many bees buzzing to get back onto the main cluster again.

Then, for some reason, the queen died, and fell off the wall onto the ground, but the swarm kept covering her dead body on the ground, desperately clinging to the security of her scent, until the last bee was dead, two weeks later.

This fear of the fluidity of the world is so deep rooted that we will do anything, even kill ourselves psychologically, in order to turn that fluidity into a static mass, the static mass being the doctrine, the credo, the concept, the rule, the 'us' against 'them', the 'my guru is better than your guru'.

And so we invent words like hatha yoga and raja yoga, the first being physical yoga and the second being spiritual yoga. But both yoga's are *doings*, whether it is physically or spiritually, both are *doings*. And it is precisely the *doing* which is the corral, the attention trap, which fences the doer off from the rest of the world. The keyword is *doing*. Anything we do is a trap, whether it is physical or spiritual *doing*.

It is not the thing one does which counts. Anything is only anything and, within the vastness of the universe, is equal to everything else. Neither is the one who does it that counts. What counts is whether the one doing it does it because he enjoys doing it, or whether he does it because he thinks is it important, thus giving it a higher status than everything else in the universe.

It is so simple. Nothing being more important or spiritual or true than anything else in the universe, just get on and *do whatever you like doing best, which your nature dictates you,* without labeling it higher or lower.

But wait a minute. With that I do not mean to say that you can do something that *you* like doing, but which infringes on the freedom and right to peaceful existence of another living creature. All the living creatures in the universe being equal they have equal rights to peaceful existence and freedom.

So, there you are. Do whatever you like doing best, but like bats flying on radar in pitch dark *don't bump into other bats,* physically, psychologically, morally or spiritually speaking, causing them to lose their control and fly into a wall instead of into the open skies.

Something else.

The more, as a yogi (or yogini), we profess to be completely and irretrievably right-brained and un-interested in modern technology, like computers and such 'material things' (as if some God somewhere in the universe is busy putting labels on everything saying 'this is material, this is spiritual'), the more people think that we are spiritual, even mystical, mysticism being a more intimate form of spirituality.

Right brain versus left brain, the good versus the bad, the high and the low, the divine world and the material world.

The prophet of the first one is the mystic gazing at the divine, the prophet of the second the man at the computer gazing at the screen, both vertically absorbed in what they are doing, screened off from the rest of the world, the only thing they have in common being that they get a headache if they do their gazing for too long.

All our lives we have been told that there is a divine world and a material world, separated from each other by an invisible Berlin wall, which raises some very basic questions, like: *'who says so'*.

Scriptures, prophets, saints, they all exist because other people have said that they exist, and so to believe the scriptures, prophets and saints, we have to first believe the other people. We can make this chain as long as we want, without getting anywhere, really, in the end.

Second basic question.

I think everybody would agree that the divine world belongs to the divine, so to whom does the material world belong? If it belongs to some dark entity, we are then left with two equally powerful and creative entities. If the so-called material world, however, also belongs to the divine, that makes it automatically also divine, and worthy of consideration, study and respect.

So, going out from that premise, that the universe is a yin-yang symbol with both worlds contained within one circle, I bought myself a personal computer.

Because, if you are only right brain, or, for that matter, only left brain oriented, then half the circle is missing, and one tips on one's side, being lop-sided.

And so, clicking and double-clicking the mouse all over the screen, I say to myself: 'Hey, I have seen this before'. Double click on your icon and lo and behold, there it is, life size on the screen, just like in the movies of real life. Double click on an item of, say, twenty years ago, or two days ago, and lo, there it is, life size in front of your eyes, in Technicolor, with full sound and A(utomatic) E(motional) R(ecall) to top it off. Much better than any computer, who may have the technicolor and sound recall, but misses the A E R.

In that sense, however, the computer may be better off than we are, because what he recalls is the unembellished truth, while our recollection is usually a rather confused affair, tainted by positive or negative emotions, that make us see things that are not there, or not see things which are there. Love and hate, happiness and sadness, are equally unreliable companions if it comes to seeing the truth.

I am sitting in Dago teahouse, looking out over the hill called Cimbuleuit. On the table in front of me is a black and white photograph of the same teahouse forty-five years ago. A little girl, all curly, sitting on the lap of her mother, also all curly, both of them a ninety-fiftieth look on their faces. Classical, straight out of an old Shirley Temple movie. In the background the same hill of Cimbuleuit, with more trees and less houses.

Once the emotions are stuck to your skin, they are difficult to peel off again. Because that is how deep most emotions run, skin deep. Only a few manage to worm their way in, to lodge themselves in your guts, where they slowly start chewing you, until everything you look at is seen through the colors produced by those emotions.

What we do to our mothers and fathers, turning them into toys for our monstrous egoism and self-centeredness. Blaming them for the fungus in us, as if one eternal soul can ever be blamed for the fungus of another eternal soul.

And so the fifty year old woman is looking at the little six year old girl in the photograph looking back at her with that 1950-ish look on her face which says: 'Wait till I am as old as you are, then we'll talk again'.

Now she is as old as I am, and we look at each other, and then we laugh and hug and say to each other: 'Didn't we have a wonderful childhood, all those adventures, thanks to my impossible mother, who could not sit still in one place for very long, and who made the whole world, material as well as spiritual, look like one huge toy shop to browse in and enjoy. Hurray for all the mothers and fathers and children in this world, and for the pathos of their dance. And hurray for my mother, who never feared of opening new doors, and kept her windows open in a 360-degree arch.

Once we have decided that our parents are more or less a failure and have outgrown the illusion that they are omnipresent, omnipotent and omniscient, we start seriously looking for a surrogate parent who *is* all those things and who will not fail us, in other words, who will obediently conform to the image that we have built of such a mythological super being. And thus the game starts all over again, but this time the stakes are no longer childish thoughts and feelings, but adult ones, and so the situation is more fraught with danger than before.

All this reminds me of that girl scout camping trip we made in the Pengalengan mountains north of Bandung.

There must have been around twenty of us, sleeping in sleeping bags on straw mats on the floor, to be woken up suddenly in the middle of the night by one girl zipping and unzipping her sleeping bag. On being asked what on earth she thought she was doing, she explained that she was practicing unzipping in the event of the arrival of burglars, so that she would be ready to flee in an instant.

Well, come to think of it, that is really what most of us are doing all the time, zipping and unzipping our sleeping bags to be ready for the burglars, if they come, when they come, to stand or flee.

Actually, some of us may keep the bag even permanently unzipped. It is not so much the material things that we are worried about, or rather not only. I think we are actually more worried about burglars breaking into our psychological storeroom, snatching away our beliefs, our convictions, our judgments, our gurus, our gods. Like drowning rats we cling to them for dear life, terrified to lose our raft and be swept away by the current of life, to be stranded on some God knows what kind of other worldly beach. And so every time the raft bumps over a stone, we mend the hole, getting wetter and wetter all the time.

Talking about getting wet.

I remember the day we took this little hike in the woods, in the middle of the night, when finally we realized we had gotten ourselves lost.

At that point the most boisterous of the group jumped in front and cried convincingly: 'Follow me, I know the road'. So, like little lambs of Mary, we trustingly followed her, to be suddenly startled by a loud SPLASH, and there she was, sitting in the middle of the river, which she hadn't seen, and which she didn't know was there. To our fortune we hadn't followed her too closely and therefore could enjoy the scene standing on dry land. Well, so far for this follow-me-I-know-the-road business.

So, if you do want to follow somebody else, do so by all means, but keep your ears open for the SPLASH, which is bound to come, sooner or later.

Why did I come here, to walk the streets of this city for ten whole days? The past is a terrible burden to carry around, and the older you get, the more there is of it.

I am sitting in the ice-cream parlor on Jalan Haji Juanda, formerly called Jalan Dago. On the screen of the street outside they are projecting two films at the same time.

One is of the present, with hundreds, thousands of cars, honking, racing, going somewhere, going nowhere. The other film superimposed on this one is an empty Jalan Dago, a few becaks, a dog car with a tired pony listlessly pulling its burden. A couple of girls running along the street, one of them falling on her face every couple of minutes. Legs don't work too well. Beriberi, a common children's disease out of the Japanese prison-of-war camps.

How do we get rid of the past? I am looking at this double screen outside and think: 'There must be a way of separating those two images, of putting them into two separate boxes, robbing both images of their emotional content'.

Because it is not the images that bother us. It is the emotional content that sticks to those images that bother us and which create that funny dualism. On the one hand we suffer under the impact of the emotions, on the other hand we cling to those emotions with a fierceness that defies any burglar who wants to take them away. And suddenly I am struck by a thought, and I am back at the corral again, with the leaders, the gurus and the systems. They are not meant to *help* us get rid of the past, but to *prevent* us from getting rid of the past, and the present, and the future. They are not meant to *liberate* us, but to imprison us.

There you are. I have done thirty-five years of yoga, following the system, and in the end I do not know how to use the computer, I have twenty-five thumbs when I have to drill a hole in the wall to put up a picture, and I cry all over the black and white photograph of the little girl sitting primly erect on the giant horse, under the fond gaze of her horse riding teacher.

My first guru. I worshipped the ground he stood on. When I was ten, my horse and I fell in a ditch, trying to jump over it. The horse had to be shot, the little girl was sobbing in the stables, and did the teacher show any sympathy? Did he say: 'There, there, little one, cry your little heart out?' No. Instead he had another horse saddled up, an even bigger one, and 'Up you go, raise your leg, back in the saddle again, and off you go'.

Yes, I worshipped the ground he stood on. His face is number one on the list of faces filed away in the memory of the computer that sits in my head.

So, something went wrong somewhere, if I can't even put a nail in the wall without bringing half the wall down, or use the computer, without getting into horrendous quarrels with it.

Reading through the *Bhagavad Gita* one comes across the phrase: 'Yoga karmasu kausalam'. This means: 'Yoga is skill in action'.

I look suspiciously at my Black & Decker drill. Two thousand years ago the yogis didn't have Black & Decker's, but surely they must have had something analogous?

So, if yoga is skill in action, then something is wrong with me. Or maybe not wrong, but incomplete. Half the world consists of drills and computers. The other half consists of the breeze going swooooosh through the bamboo leaves outside my window, and the sound of the tropical rainstorm sweeping over the city, drenching everything and everybody in a matter of seconds.

We are back at the yin-yang symbol.

It is only by entwining the black and the white that we can draw the circle. And it is the circle that is important, but the circle can only be made by joining the two halves, by going beyond them, by making them so *equal* that it does not matter that one is black and the other white.

It is by making everything *equal* that makes the universe and ourselves whole, or holy. As long as things are not *equal*, as long as one thing is more important than the other, more spiritual than the other, we are not whole, not holy, and the universe we live in is only half a universe.

While I am eating my lechee ice cream, the teenage girl next to me turns her head to look at me. Perfect almond eyes, set in a perfect oval face with perfect, smooth, amber colored skin. She smiles shyly at me, and I smile shyly back. I remember that these people already made me feel shy as a child. Next to their tiny, delicate bodies with the quick, nimble movements, I used to feel like a rusty locomotive going puff puff puff with every move.

Rrrrrrrng goes the telephone in the hotel room and 'Would-Miss Dona-want-to-go-to-Saung-Angklung-of-Pak-Ujo-your-driver-is-waiting-for-you-please'.

'Yes, please, miss Dona very much wants to go to Saung Angklung, thank you, just give me two minutes to put on my jeans and I'll be with you in a sec.'

And off we go in the minibus of the hotel to the village of Pak Ujo (Pak means literally father and is used as a title of respect towards any older man) famous for his children's performances of Sundanese dancing and angklung music, bamboo instruments that are shaken to produce a sound similar to that of wind chimes in the breeze.

Little children holding the delicate instruments, the youngest child must be four, and the oldest fifteen. About thirty of them playing the music and twenty dancing, looking for all the world like tiny dragonflies, hardly touching the ground with their bare feet and up they are again in the air. Looking unreal in their bright colored clothes, obsidian eyes sparkling at the group of overfed tourists. A strange symbiosis. Again the yin and the yang.

In between the songs and dances Pak Ujo sits beside me and we talk about dance and yoga.

'I am a business man', he says proudly, sweeping the hall with his hand, and, switching inconsequently to Dutch (those sudden switches between Indonesian, English and Dutch occur rather often and with startling abruptness) continues: 'De beste business is lief geven aan iedereen' (the best business is to give love to everybody). Something went wrong with the Dutch grammar, but otherwise it is an interesting concept. I am imagining everybody in Wall Street: 'Just one moment, please, ladies and gentlemen, could you all stop doing whatever you are doing for a moment and give love to each other?'

Up goes the Dow Jones, and the titles soar to dizzying heights. Quite a thought.

At the end of the performance the children all run into the crowd of tourists, each one grabbing someone to join in the dance, the big, white men and women in their too tight clothes, and the tiny amber dragonflies. Yin and yang.

I have to refrain myself from picking my dragonfly right up and kissing its oval face. Don't be sentimental, Miss Dona.

But the children go to school with the money of the performances, and Pak Ujo goes back to his bamboo hut. His fee for the evening is Rupiah 15.000 (about eight US Dollar).

He is right. The best businessman is he who gives love.

Love.

A big word to tackle. Do I really want to go into this? It might get me into some deep water, and I might end up doing some splashing myself. Well, let's take a deep breath and JUMP.

Shri Maharishi once pointed at a young girl, ravishingly beautiful, who was just passing him and his group of disciples. The disciples all looked at her with delight.

Along came an old woman, long past youth. Said Maharishi: 'If your eyes can look at the young girl and the old woman in the same way, that is equanimity, that is yoga'.

If you love one person, and not the other one, it is not love, but self-interest.

If I love A, but not B and C, it is because A is giving me something that makes me feel good and cheerful, while B and C do not do that to my system. Not to even mention D, who makes me feel outright disgusted, maybe because he is doing something that reminds me too much of something that I am doing and of which I am secretly ashamed.

There we are again, back to the dualities. Love and hate, good and bad. The split universe, the yin and the yang not in symbiosis, but in opposition to each other.

It is not that I love A.

What I love is the feeling that A produces in me, the feeling of warmth and security and safety. The reassuring feeling that everything is fine and that the universe is proceeding on the right course.

And it not B that I hate, but the feeling that he produces in me of un-safety, of insecurity, of doubt. The terrifying feeling that the universe is not all roses, but that between the roses there are as many thorns.

Those feelings are the things that we love and hate. Not other people. How can we hate or love another person? How can we hate or love the unknown?

The greatest illusion in history is the phrase: 'Know yourself'.

There is no way I can ever know myself.

I am a mystery, a total mystery, and all I can do is sit here, looking at the clouds in the tropical skies, and shout at them inside my mind: 'WHAT AM I'.

Note the wording. Not 'WHO'. WHAT am I? What is this thing sitting here looking up at the clouds and being aware of them?

It is not the clouds that are a mystery. It is me being aware of them, which is the mystery. Me being aware of being aware of the clouds.

I am a luminous ball of awareness floating in something that I call universe. To get rid of the terrifying feeling of loneliness that this produces in me I am busy all my life giving names to things, creating thus the illusion that I know those things and that I know what is going on in the universe: Car, house, tree, flower, man, woman, God, all game names to cover up the fact that I am an unknowable ball of awareness traveling through an unknowable space, meeting all the time other unknowable balls of awareness that I call people to cover up the fact that I don't know what they are.

Well, that was a long sentence. And a rather complicated one too.

The clouds have burst open and the tropical rainstorm is turning the holes in the road into so many tiny swimming pools for the ants.

The naming of things that are ultimately unnamable is the *doing* that we do all our lives, and which creates the illusion that we *know*, that we are in control.

To have the courage and the transparency to see and acknowledge that in reality we *do not know*, that we will never know, and to make our peace with that, is *not doing* or *wu-wei*.

In that state everything is equal to everything else, being unknown and unknowable. People, trees, airplanes, nothing being more or less than the other, we then become aware of the substratum in which all this exists, which permeates everything and in which all things float like goldfish in a pond. Philosophers have tried to name even this: God, Love, Reality, Brahman, Tao, whichever you prefer.

Or one can leave it as it is, the Nameless.

Rrrrrrrng goes the telephone and 'Would-Miss-Dona-want-to-go-to-Pabrik-Teh-of-Malabar-your-driver-is-waiting-for-you- please'.

This sounds like one of those repeating dreams or déjà vue, and 'Yes, please, Miss Dona very much wants to go to the Tea Factory of Malabar, thank you, just give me two minutes to put on my jeans and I'll be with you in a sec'.

This is where the repeating dream ends, because this time we are going into the high mountains of the Priangar, to the famous tea plantation of Malabar.

The Priangar, a name that sounds like magic in my head, the time that my mother and I went there for holiday, she to do nothing, I to do horse riding, living in this little bamboo hut in the mountains. It was Christmas, and there was guerrilla war all around while I steered my pony all day long through the teagardens. I remember the shooting, and the smell of tea, everywhere.

The car winds its painful way out of the streets of Bandung, through the impossible traffic, on the impossible pavement. Cars, cars, cars and cars. But above the cars the huge trees in magnificent explosion of bright orange flames: the flaming tree, the Flamboyant.

Nobody, who has never seen this tree, could ever imagine it.

Nobody, who has ever seen this tree, could ever forget it.

They are breathtaking, and it does not matter, all those crawling cars underneath them.

They are there, and their flames are purification in themselves.

I am getting better at this. They are not showing double screen any more, or maybe only in short flashes.

As the car slowly goes uphill, one by one old things drop off and are left behind beside the road. The air gets cooler and it starts to rain, slowly, gently, almost excusing itself for doing so.

They are all there, the way they were forty-five years ago. The neat rice terraces stacked one on top of each other, an occasional water buffalo standing knee-deep in the mud. The miniature homes, some made of woven bamboo, some of lava stone, snugly tucked away among the greenery; the occasional chicken crossing the road right in front of the car. 'Bikin satay ayam' (I'll make chicken satay), grins the driver, swerving however at the last second to avoid the confused creature.

And then, suddenly, we are in the middle of the tea plantation. Tea bushes everywhere, as far as the eye can see, women in bright colored shirts and straw hats picking the leaves and there, in the background, the mountains, covered in clouds.

Yes, it is all there. But something is missing. And I realize that there is no more double screen. There is only one scenery: the one in front of my eyes.

The view is breathtaking, and I get out of the car, staring, staring.

And then, out of nowhere, comes this feeling as if I am about to be exploded into a million tiny bits of Miss Dona as a tsunami-size wave of joy rolls over me, and over those bushes, and those gorgeous mountains.

Joy is not man made.

Happiness is man made, as is sadness, and anger, and contentment.

These are all man made, and under our control, if we put ourselves a little to it.

But joy is not man made, and is not under our control, will never be under our control.

IT comes and goes as IT wills, leaving its victim gasping for air, like a fish on the beach.

IT decides when to come, to whom to come, and when to leave.

The only thing IT needs is space, a lot of space, all the space available. When there is all the space available, when there is nothing inside, neither of the past, nor of the present, nor of the future, when there is no dogma, no credo, no guru and no god, then, if IT so wills, IT will take you.

The Flamboyants are burning against the stormy skies as the tropical rainstorm sweeps over the land.

index of poses

ALSO FROM
YogaWords

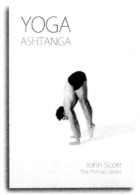

Ashtanga Yoga

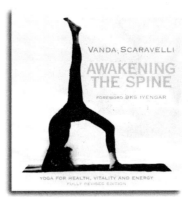

Awakening the Spine*

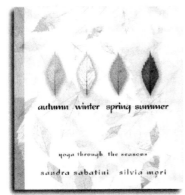

Autumn, Winter, Spring Summer*

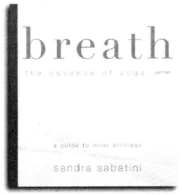

Breath: The Essence of Yoga*

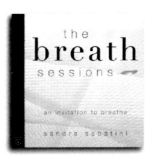

The Breath Sessions (CD)*

*in association with Pinter & Martin Ltd

YOGAWORDS

visit **www.yogawords.com** for further information and special offers